Transformative Healthcare Practice through Patient Engagement

Guendalina Graffigna
Catholic University of the Sacred Heart, Italy

A volume in the Advances in Medical Diagnosis, Treatment, and Care (AMDTC) Book Series

Medical Information Science
REFERENCE
An Imprint of IGI Global

Published in the United States of America by
Medical Information Science Reference (an imprint of IGI Global)
701 E. Chocolate Avenue
Hershey PA 17033
Tel: 717-533-8845
Fax: 717-533-8661
E-mail: cust@igi-global.com
Web site: http://www.igi-global.com

Library of Congress Cataloging-in-Publication Data

Names: Graffigna, Guendalina, 1979- , editor.
Title: Transformative healthcare practice through patient engagement / Guendalina Graffigna, editor.
Description: Hershey PA : Medical Information Science Reference, [2017] | Includes bibliographical references and index.
Identifiers: LCCN 2016014418| ISBN 9781522506638 (hardcover) | ISBN 9781522506645 (ebook)
Subjects: | MESH: Patient Participation | Delivery of Health Care | Biomedical Technology
Classification: LCC R727.42 | NLM W 85 | DDC 610.69/6--dc23 LC record available at http://lccn.loc.gov/2016014418

This book is published in the IGI Global book series Advances in Medical Diagnosis, Treatment, and Care (AMDTC) (ISSN: Pending; eISSN: Pending)

British Cataloguing in Publication Data
A Cataloguing in Publication record for this book is available from the British Library.

Advances in Medical Diagnosis, Treatment, and Care (AMDTC) Book Series

ISSN: Pending
EISSN: Pending

Mission

Advancements in medicine have prolonged the life expectancy of individuals all over the world. Once life-threatening conditions have become significantly easier to treat and even cure in many cases. Continued research in the medical field will further improve the quality of life, longevity, and wellbeing of individuals.

The **Advances in Medical Diagnosis, Treatment, and Care (AMDTC)** book series seeks to highlight publications on innovative treatment methodologies, diagnosis tools and techniques, and best practices for patient care. Comprised of comprehensive resources aimed to assist professionals in the medical field apply the latest innovations in the identification and management of medical conditions as well as patient care and interaction, the books within the AMDTC series are relevant to the research and practical needs of medical practitioners, researchers, students, and hospital administrators.

Coverage

- Chronic Conditions
- Emergency Medicine
- Disease Management
- Disease Prevention
- Patient Interaction
- Critical Care
- Alternative Medicine
- Diagnostic Medicine
- Cancer Treatment
- Medical Procedures

IGI Global is currently accepting manuscripts for publication within this series. To submit a proposal for a volume in this series, please contact our Acquisition Editors at Acquisitions@igi-global.com or visit: http://www.igi-global.com/publish/.

Titles in this Series

For a list of additional titles in this series, please visit: www.igi-global.com

Promoting Patient Engagement and Participation for Effective Healthcare Reform
Guendalina Graffigna (Catholic University of the Sacred Heart of Milan, Italy)
Medical Information Science Reference • copyright 2016 • 357pp • H/C (ISBN: 9781466699922) • US $220.00 (our price)

Effective Methods for Modern Healthcare Service Quality and Evaluation
Panagiotis Manolitzas (Technical University of Crete, Greece) Evangelos Grigoroudis (Technical University of Crete, Greece) Nikolaos Matsatsinis (Technical University of Crete, Greece) and Denis Yannacopoulos (Piraeus University of Applied Sciences, Greece)
Medical Information Science Reference • copyright 2016 • 315pp • H/C (ISBN: 9781466699618) • US $190.00 (our price)

Handbook of Research on Trends in the Diagnosis and Treatment of Chronic Conditions
Dimitrios I. Fotiadis (University of Ioannina, Greece)
Medical Information Science Reference • copyright 2016 • 659pp • H/C (ISBN: 9781466688285) • US $385.00 (our price)

IGI GLOBAL
DISSEMINATOR OF KNOWLEDGE
www.igi-global.com

701 E. Chocolate Ave., Hershey, PA 17033
Order online at www.igi-global.com or call 717-533-8845 x100
To place a standing order for titles released in this series,
contact: cust@igi-global.com
Mon-Fri 8:00 am - 5:00 pm (est) or fax 24 hours a day 717-533-8661

Table of Contents

Detailed Table of Contents

The World Health Organization has estimated that chronic obstructive pulmonary disease (COPD) is the fourth most common cause of death worldwide. Due to the economic and social extent of the problem, patient engagement must be comprised as a new resource for the achievement of higher health outcomes and lower costs. As many key processes involved in the COPD patient engagement consist of communication and education processes, modelling those processes in a whole framework, including actors and content needs, is a requirement. The main scope of this chapter is contributing to design such a framework within the Italian Health System. Final recommendations suggest to create a synergy among patient engagement and a set of legal tools, namely informed consent, integrated care and advance care planning. The synergy is based on the fact that both patient engagement and those legal tools have a common deep root in the universal principle of patient autonomy.

The concept of patient engagement is attracting growing attention from scholars working on doctor-patient interactions. It refers to the condition in which patients are fully aware of their medical condition and willing to be active both in the relationship with their caregivers and towards the health care institutions. However, the operative steps necessary to achieve patient engagement have not yet been fully described. This chapter focuses on the communicative dimension of engagement. Communication is shown to be a pivotal means to improve patient self-efficacy and commitment, both fundamental components of engagement. In particular, the authors take a closer look at the process of decision making in chronic care settings, and propose a normative model to analyze and evaluate the quality of decision making in consultations. It is argued that the model can also be used as a blueprint to create training materials for clinicians.

This chapter uses a patient-centered communication framework to examine observational studies of patient and family engagement in communication about end-of-life care. It analyzes how the literature has connected communication with health outcomes in end-of-life care. Within this analysis, it brings together three main ideas. First, family plays an important and overlooked role in communication about end-of-life care. Second, the literature describes communication that serves multiple functions, and it describes the special challenges presented by end-of-life care communication. Finally, it links these communicative functions with health outcomes and outlines directions for future research.

Societies need solutions to achieve the "triple aim" of improved health outcomes, better patient care, and lower costs; and engaging patients in their care by using technological solutions is claimed as a possible strategy to achieve this vital goal. On this basis, the chapter focuses on reviewing, categorizing and synthesizing technological tools currently available in the market today designed to engage patients in their own care process. In particular, the goals of medication adherence, reduced hospital readmission, behavior modification, and health literacy - with related technologies - are assessed, since they are considered todays most expensive health care burdens. The advantages, shortcomings, and potential economic impact of such tools are finally discussed.

In this chapter the author describes the challenges of engaging and communicating with patients and how technology can improve communication, elicit honest patient disclosure, and create more productive conversation and help patients engage and

Diabesity could be defined as a new global epidemic of obesity and being overweight with many complications and chronic conditions. The financial direct and indirect burden of diabesity is a real challenge in many Western health-care systems. Even if multidisciplinary protocols have been implemented, significant limitations in the chronic care management of obesity with type 2 diabetes concern costs and long-term adherence and efficacy. mHealth approach could overcome limitations linked with the traditional, restricted and highly expensive in-patient treatment of diabesity. The mHealth approach could help clinicians by motivating patients in remote settings to develop healthier lifestyles and could be implemented in the Chronic Care Model. A practical stepped-care model for diabesity, including mhealth approach and psychological treatments with different intensity, is discussed.

In the last decade, rehabilitation process has shifted from medical management to issues that enhance quality of life, community participation, treatment and cost effectiveness. In this context physiotherapists design and implement new and/or tailored interventions that enhance physical and functional abilities, restore, maintain, and promote optimal physical function, wellness, fitness and quality of life. The aim of this review was to assess the extent, content, and outcomes of in-home physiotherapy interventions. A search was conducted in Medline, PEDro, and Cochrane Library and IEEE Xplore. RE-AIM and GRADE guidelines were used to report this review. The findings suggest that in-home physiotherapy tailored specifically to the people needs, functioning and disability has positive results, including patients' engagement in their healthcare. Integration of information and communication technology in-home physiotherapy has great potential to increase accessibility, quality and effectiveness of various interventions provided by physiotherapists.

Recent literature shows that new technologies can be used to promote patient engagement. The present contribution focuses on Virtual Worlds (VWs), namely virtual environments that multiple users can experience together thanks to the use

Preface

In recent years, the engagement of patients in health management has become an increasingly crucial challenge for healthcare organizations. At a time when demands to improve quality compete with savage demands for cuts in healthcare spending, the 'patient resource' promises to play a key role in resolving a seemingly insoluble dilemma.

Indeed, the importance of the topic has stimulated growing scientific interest, both theoretical and applied. Another recently published book by G. Graffigna, *Promoting Patient Engagement and Participation*, has taken stock of theoretical developments of the paradigm; this book instead explores practical and applicative ones.

How can the patient's effective engagement in health management be developed? How can healthcare practitioners (doctors, nurses, etc.) work to promote patient engagement? How can the peers and social context (caregivers, networks, communities, etc.) support the patient's active and participative role in health management? What role can be played by the new technologies (virtual worlds, positive technology, e-health, etc.)? These are the main questions addressed by the book.

Exploration of the various studies collected in the book yields a composite – though provisional – picture of the 'state of the art'. Whilst leaving to the reader the task of constructing a personal view on the subject, I think it useful to direct his or her attention to some key suggestions made by the book on how best to steer developments in patient engagement.

- **Processual Approach:** Developing effective patient engagement requires abandoning a 'state-based approach' and adopting a 'process-based one'. Engagement of the patient, in fact, is not an 'on-off' status, but rather a dynamic process; a process diversified in its quantitative aspects (e.g. levels of engagement) and qualitative ones (e.g. crucial contents of engagement), and in any case characterized by non-linear developments (i.e. both progressive and regressive). Taking a "process-based vision" is essential for non-trivial and non-trivializing applications of the paradigm.

- **Systemic Approach:** The book focuses on patient engagement. But this does not mean adopting an individualistic view on the subject. Patient engagement is the outcome of systemic action in which the patient interacts with other expert actors (doctors, nurses, etc.), with social networks (caregivers, networks, communities, etc.), and within differently organized contexts (hospital, local services, etc.). These various components combine to configure an action system which may foster or impede patient engagement. The patient, therefore, is the final outcome of complex action which ranges far beyond the individual.
- **Communicative and Relational Dimension:** Interventions to promote patient engagement refer to a communicative-relational dimension as their specific area of action. Simple mechanical behavioural replication does not seem sufficient to generate the activation-participation that engagement requires. It is therefore necessary to specify the functionings activated in an engagement development process, and the skills required for the formative action to be performed appropriately. Put otherwise, engagement seems to require a conception of the patient as co-author of the process, not as the mere final executor of a process guided by others.
- **Good Practices:** Development of the paradigm requires the devising and applying of good practices: without good practices, there is a risk that the patient engagement operative evolution will be rather superficial. Two conditions seem necessary: a) intervention on patient engagement should be allocated adequate space, at least equal to that given to construction of the theory; b) the intervention should be provided with methodological foundations of a level similar to those given to development of basic research on the paradigm.

Overall, the methodological foundation of action in favour of patient engagement is a new frontier, to the exploration of which this book makes a significant and involving contribution.

A. Claudio Bosio
Catholic University of the Sacred Heart, Milan, Italy

Introduction

PROMOTING PATIENT ENGAGEMENT: FROM THEORY INTO PRACTICE

The key word patient engagement is worldwide becoming a "must do" for academics, industries and policy makers in the healthcare arena. The academic and managerial "buzz" on patient engagement is growing at a dizzying pace. In 2015, 665,300 new web indices were found on Google.com with the key words "patient engagement," including 1,230 news pages and 6,200 dedicated blogs. During this same period, over 3,500 new academic papers focused on patient engagement (see Figure 1)

The idea of patient engagement moves from the assumption that making patients co-producer of their health can enhance their satisfaction towards the healthcare system, as well as their responsibility in care, cure and prevention. A previous Book entitled *Promoting Patient Engagement and Participation for Effective Healthcare Reform* (Graffigna, 2016) has been dedicated to discuss the clinical and pragmatic value of favoring the active role of patients along their care journey. The different chapters of that Book well testified the different elements and ingredients which may play a role in promoting patient engagement. However, despite this growing

Figure 1. Trend of Google Scholar sources indexed with patient engagement from 1954 to 2014

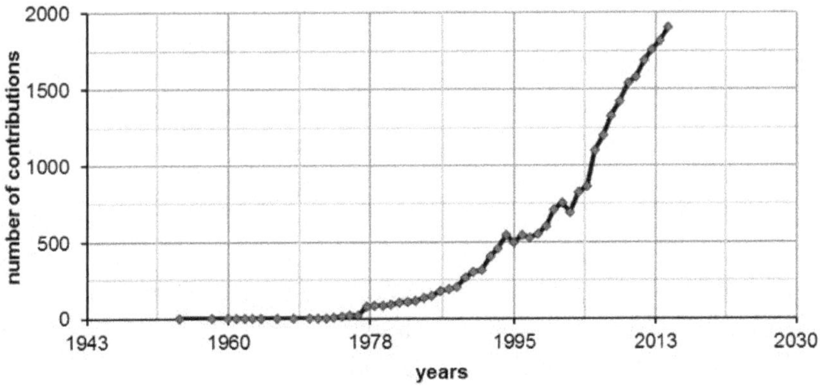

interest and the shared research efforts to come to a unique theoretical definition of what patient engagement is and how it may be promoted, concrete guidelines for practices are still awaited. A question spontaneously arises: *Is patient engagement a fashionable claim or a real guidance for practice?*

PROMOTING PATIENT ENGAGEMENT: MAIN AREAS OF INTERVENTION

Initiatives aimed at promoting patient engagement are growing across the world, also thank to the input posed by policy makers on this issue. In the majority of the western countries, patient engagement in healthcare is well established with the government's commitment in fostering interventions, research and innovative methodologies aimed at prioritizing the "patient's voice" and the "patient's active roles in their own healthcare" (Health Affairs, Feb 2013), but scarce have been the efforts putted into the analysis of effectiveness of such initiatives. Furthermore, still rare are the occasions to put into dialogue the different experiences mastered in this area in order jointly work at a shared set of rules and best practices for the promotion of patient engagement. Not to say, the level of scientific and clinical evidences reached in this areas are still scarce, often because the early stage of the initiatives promoted: as discussed elsewhere (Graffigna, 2016) patient engagement and participation are new phenomena, which are advocating for an important shift of paradigm in medical practices. This justifies the fact that new initiatives finalized to innovate healthcare organizations are still ongoing and needing further evidences.

Moving from these premises, in this Book we shall offer a contribution in this direction by hosting the description of best practices aimed at enhancing the active role of patients in their care management. The areas covered by the best practices reported in this Book are related to the initiatives that in the literature appear more suitable to promote change in patients' attitudes and behaviour towards their enhanced self-management. Those are in particular:

- The area of *patient's education* interventions: here we may conceptually gather all the initiatives aimed at improving patients' level of health literacy and at forming patients' skills and behaviour related to medication adherence and self-management.
- The area of *medical communication* initiatives: this is a broad area of initiatives mainly finalized: 1) on the one hand to support the communication and relational skills of healthcare professionals and their ability to sustain the engagement of the patients in health management; 2) on the other hand to sustain the patients' question-asking ability and their attitude to legitimize

themselves as agents in the medical encounter, able to play a more negotiating role in the shared decision making about their treatments.

- The area of *self-monitoring* supports: in this area are gathered initiatives and tools dedicated to the patients and finalized to support them cognitively and pragmatically in the daily managements of therapies and of medical requirements.

PROMOTING PATIENT ENGAGEMENT: THE ROLE OF NEW TECHNOLOGIES

In this regards, it is important to acknowledge the growing body of literature dedicated to attest the potentiality of new technologies in improving patient's engagement and participations. There is consensus that health technologies are crucial in supporting patient engagement in their own care, in terms of enhanced self-management and responsibility. As stated above, the concept of patient engagement advocate for a shift from the classical "doctor-centred model" of healthcare to new healthcare management models that improve communication and more democratic interaction between patients and healthcare professionals, particularly in an integrated approach to care and in the aim of a better linkage between hospital and territory. Some scholars suggested that E-health may be a useful framework in this direction (Barello et al., 2016) by allowing the connection between the different systems and actors involved in the health management process (Eysenbach, 2001; Phalen & Eaton, 2008). Scholars define e-health as: "electronic communication-based technologies to aid or provide healthcare in some form" (Keogh, Rosser & Eccleston 2010; p. 18), considering everything to be connected to both health and technology (Oh, *et al.* 2005*)* as "designed to improve health surveillance, health-system management, health education and clinical decision-making, and to support behavioral changes related to public-health priorities and disease management". However, in line with other scholars (Ricciardi, Mostashari, Murphy, 2013), we emphasize the infancy of the literature debate on this topic and the lack of shared guidelines for orienting e-health interventions that are really able to enhance patient engagement. Some of the initiatives reported in this book may offer an advancement in this direction.

THE AIMS AND STRUCTURE OF THIS BOOK

On the basis of these premises, this book is conceived as the virtual extension of the discussion started in the previous book entitled "Promoting Patient Engagement and Participation for effective Healthcare Reform" (Graffigna, 2016) and collects some exemplary initiatives promoted across the world and in different pathological areas to improve patient engagement. The selection of best practices here commented didn't follow the criterion of systematicity, rather it was inspired by a qualitative logic of maximum variety of cases reported.

In order to improve the readability of the Book, its chapters have been organized in the following two thematic sections.

Section one ("Best practices in promoting patient's participation and engagement: strategies for patient education and medical communication") is dedicated to review theoretical insights and empirical best practices in the area of patients' education and medical communication in order to proactively contribute to the practical promotion of patient participation and engagement in healthcare. The chapters hosted in this section addressed different but crucial patient populations, by highlighting the specific needs of engagement in each one of them.

Chapter 1, "Best Practices to Promote Patient and Donor Engagement to Care in Living Donor Transplant" by Emanuela Saita, Susanna Zanini, Enrico Minetti and Chiara Acquati, reviews the literature about patient engagement in the context of chronic kidney disease and discusses the importance of understanding the patients' emotional and affective dynamics and the relational implications that may influence the elaboration of the information given by healthcare providers. These assumptions are at the basis of the innovative educational protocol developed to promote potential donors and recipients' participation and adherence to care at the Niguarda Ca' Granda Hospital in Milan (Italy), which the chapter describes into details.

Chapter 2, "Communication and Education processes involved in COPD patient Engagement within the Italian Health System" by Virginia Recchia, Antonio Dodaro, Rosita B. Maglie and Carlo G. Leo, focuses on chronic obstructive pulmonary disease (COPD) and on the specific requirements of engagement of this target population. On the basis of this analysis, authors propose an innovative framework, experienced within the Italian Health System, finalized to create synergy among a set of legal tools, namely informed consent, integrated care and advance care planning, in order to innovate the healthcare system and to improve patient's engagement and participation in the process.

Chapter 3, "The Power of Words: Deliberation Dialogue as a Model to Favor Patient Engagement in Chronic Care" by Sarah Bigi and Giulia Lamiani, focuses on the communicative dimension of engagement, conceived as the pivotal means to improve patient self-efficacy and commitment. In particular, the authors take a closer look at the process of decision making in chronic care settings, and propose a normative model to analyze and evaluate the quality of decision making in consultations.

Chapter 4, "Patient and Family Engagement in THE Conversation: Pathways from Communication to Care Outcomes" by Jennifer Freytag and Richard L. Street,

Jr., focuses on communication strategies to engage families in end-of-life care. The authors discuss the major advancements of the literature about communication of health outcomes in end-of-life care by discussing their implication for engagement of families in this delicate care moment. The authors conclude by outlining future research lines in the field.

The second section of this book ("The potentiality of new technologies to promote patient's participation and engagement in health management") is dedicated to a selection of technological tools and interventions able to sustain patients' participation and engagement in healthcare.

Chapter 5, "Engaging Patients and Lowering Costs: Technology to the Rescue" by Tony Zordich and Julia Menichetti Delor, review the technological tools today available to sustain patient participation and engagement. New technologies are regarded as the best strategy to improve clinical outcomes today, to sustain patients' satisfaction for healthcare management and to reduce cost of service delivery. Furthermore, the new communication solutions offered by these tools improve the relations between patients and their healthcare providers and make possible the continuous and remote monitoring of patient's behaviors. The overview provided by this chapter is a useful premise to the technological interventions reported in the following chapters.

Chapter 6, "Meeting Patients Where They Are: Using Multimedia and Interactive Voice Technology to Humanize Communication and Engage Patients" by Geri Lynn Baumblatt, deeply discusses the relational, emotional and psychological advantages of new technologies for patient engagement. The author describes the specific function of different technological devices and argument on the value of adopting multimedia technologies to inform and motivate patients along their care journey.

Chapter 7, "Using the Communication AssessmenT Checklist in Health to assess the communication quality of web based resources for prostate cancer" by Juliana Genova, Curtis A. Olson and Jackie Bender, focuses on the specific population of prostate cancer patients. The chapter introduces the new Communication AssessmenT Checklist in Health (CATCH) specifically developed to assess the quality of information reported on websites dedicated to this target population and highlight interesting gaps and problems in these resources that open interesting new direction for future practices.

Chapter 8, "A stepped care mHealth-based approach for promoting patient engagement in chronic care management of obesity with type 2 diabetes" by Gianluca Castelnuovo, Giada Pietrabissa, Gian Mauro Manzoni, Stefania Corti, Margherita Novelli, Maria Borrello, Emanuele Maria Giusti, Francesco Borgia, Enrico Molinari, Nicole Ann Middleton, Roberto Cattivelli and Susan Simpson, targets diabetes patient population and their specific problem to engage in healthcare management.

In particular, the authors present a practical stepped-care model of intervention for patients suffering from obesity and diabetes, based on the mhealth approach and psychological treatments modulated with different intensity along the care journey.

Chapter 9, "Why, What and When in-Home Physiotherapy?" by Gabriela Postolache, Raul Oliveira, Isabel Moreira, Octavian Postolache, focuses on rehabilitation programs and, on the bases of a systematic review of scientific evidences, systematize the effectiveness of different kind of tools and interventions to promote patients participation and engagement in in-home physiotherapy. The authors conclude by describing a road map for future interventions and research in the field.

Chapter 10, "Healthy Avatars, Healthy People: Care Engagement Through the Shared Experience of Virtual Worlds" by Stefano Triberti and Alice Chirico, focuses on the ability of virtual worlds to foster patient's participation and engagement in their care. The authors, by discussing evidences from recent scientific research, argue that virtual environments allow multiple users to learn in an engaging and transformative way healthier conducts and better effective healthcare management behaviours. The chapter illuminates new emerging opportunities for clinical and cost effective patient engagement interventions.

Chapter 11, "Waiting for Health Care Services" by Stefan Janzek-Hawlat and Hilda Tellioğlu, discusses the impact of waiting times for healthcare services on the patients' perceived quality of services, on the healthcare professional performance and on the effectiveness of the healthcare system in the whole. The authors base their examination both on the analysis of the recent literature in the field and on the result of an empirical research focused on these aspects. The chapter concludes with advices to reduce the waiting time in healthcare systems.

Guendalina Graffigna
Catholic University of the Sacred Heart, Italy

REFERENCES

Eysenbach, G. (2001). What is e-health? *Journal of Medical Internet Research*, (3): e20.

Keogh, E., Rosser, B. A., & Eccleston, C. (2010). e-Health and chronic pain management: Current status and developments. *Pain*, (151): 18–21.

Oh, H., Rizo, C., & Enkin, M. et al.. (2005). What Is e-health (3): A systematic review of published definitions. *Journal of Medical Internet Research*, (7): e1.

Phalen, J. M., & Eaton, C. B. (2008). *The role of e-health in patient engagement and quality improvement. e-health solutions for healthcare disparities*. New York: Springer.

Ricciardi, L., Mostashari, F., & Murphy, J. et al.. (2013). A national action plan to support consumer engagement via e-health. *Health Affairs (Project Hope)*, (32): 376–384.

Section 1
Best Practices in Promoting Patient's Participation and Engagement:
Strategies for Patient Education and Medical Communication

Chapter 1
Best Practices to Promote Patient and Donor Engagement to Care in Living Donor Transplant

Emanuela Saita
Catholic University of the Sacred Heart, Italy

Susanna Zanini
Niguarda Ca' Granda Hospital, Italy

Enrico Minetti
Careggi University Hospital, Italy

Chiara Acquati
University of Houston, USA

ABSTRACT

Increasing evidence has demonstrated that patients' involvement promotes better health care outcomes and cost-effectiveness of services. However, limited literature is available about the experience of living donor kidney transplantation and best practices to promote patients and donors' engagement. Aim of the present chapter is to review the literature about patient engagement in the context of chronic kidney disease, and to introduce an innovative protocol developed to promote potential donors and recipients' participation and adherence to care at the Niguarda Ca' Granda Hospital in Milan (Italy). Results are critical to reflect on the identification of best practices for patients' engagement in the context of chronic kidney disease. Through a better understanding of the emotional and affective dynamics and the relational implications that may influence the elaboration of the information given by health care providers, it will be possible to develop evidence-informed interventions.

DOI: 10.4018/978-1-5225-0663-8.ch001

INTRODUCTION

Increasing evidence has demonstrated that patients' involvement in decision making about their treatment and care promotes better health care outcomes, higher satisfaction with care and cost-effectiveness of services (Majani & Cavallini, 2010; Stockie, 2012; Berwick, 2010; Ocloo & Fulop, 2012; Hibbard & Greene, 2013; Provenzi, Borgatti, Menozzi, & Montirosso, 2015). With increasing demand for a more active role of patients in the management of their health (Crawford et al., 2002; Davis, Schoenbaum, & Audet, 2005; Bellardita et al., 2012; Barello, Graffigna, Savarese, & Bosio, 2014a; Barello, Graffigna, Vegni, & Bosio, 2014b; Menichetti, Libreri, Lozza, & Graffigna, 2014; Graffigna, Barello, & Riva, 2013; Barello & Graffigna, 2015), patient engagement (PE) is more and more considered as a key factor in the improvement of health behaviors and outcomes in the context of chronic diseases (Graffigna, Barello, Libreri, & Bosio, 2014). However, limited literature is available about the experience of living donor kidney transplantation and best practices to promote patients and donors' activation and engagement (Boulware et al., 2013).

Until sixty years ago kidney insufficiency was a lethal disease. Nowadays the scenario has changed, although this illness is still a life-threatening disease in some underdeveloped areas where dialysis is not provided by the healthcare system. Despite its severity, symptoms of the progressive loss of renal function are often absent and the patient does not perceive to be "ill" or the individual is simply not aware of the seriousness of the condition. It has been noticed that the body of the patient suffering from renal insufficiency often adjusts to the disease and its evolution over time, with the consequence that indications from the medical team about changes in diet or medications are difficult to be negotiated (Polaschek, 2003). It therefore follows that a discrepancy exists between the recommendations of the medical team and the subjective experience of the patient, who often becomes non-compliant if the changes in care and treatments are not well-communicated (Kugler, Vlaminck, Haverich, & Maes 2005; Schell, Green, Tulsky, & Arnold, 2013). It follows that behavioral changes and best adherence to therapies are achieved only if patients internalize the need for self-change (McCarley, 2009).

The provision of information to the patient is critical since the moment of diagnosis for two main reasons. First, an effective communication with the patient is essential to address concerns and questions about the medical treatment (in particular, the surgery). Second, as the individual will need to take several medications and undergo numerous medical examinations, it is important that the process is clearly explained and understood in its complexity. Hence, information is key to engage patients evaluated as clinically and psychologically eligible for a transplant (Saita, Zanini, & Fenaroli, 2012).

The practice of living-donor kidney transplantation has significantly increased in the recent past and it represents an effective way to address the growing demand for organs (Fehrman-Ekholm, Duner, Brink, Tyden, & Elinder, 2001). Furthermore, it ensures a shorter waiting period and fewer complications. Within the context of chronic kidney disease, living-donation has registered a growing interest among individuals with this illness, their relatives and friends. As family members and close ones have started to consider themselves potential donors, greater demand for information has occurred and an increased number of health care professionals are now involved in explaining practices and evaluating potential kidney donors and recipients (LaPointe Rudow et al., 2015).

In the midst of this complexity, the present chapter has two objectives: (1) to review the literature about patient engagement in the context of chronic kidney disease and (2) to present an innovative protocol developed at the Niguarda Ca' Granda Hospital in Milan (Italy) to promote patients and relatives' participation and adherence to care.

BACKGROUND

Chronic kidney disease has been defined as a "reduced glomerular filtration rate, increased urinary albumin excretion, or both" (Jha et al., 2013; p. 260) and represents an increasingly concerning public health issues. Data from the Global Burden Disease study (2010) indicate that in an interval of 20 years, from 1990 to 2010, chronic kidney disease became the 18th cause of deaths worldwide, with an increment second only to HIV and AIDS (Lozano et al., 2013). Most recent data indicate that more than 70 million people worldwide are affected by the disease (Braun, Sood, Hogue, Lieberman, & Copley-Merriman, 2012; Levey et al., 2009), and this number is expected to grow in the near future (Diamantidis & Becker, 2014). End-stage kidney disease (ESKD) requires life-saving dialysis or kidney transplantation. Worldwide, the number of patients receiving renal replacement therapy (RRT) is estimated to be more than 1.4 million with an increase in incidence of 8% annually (Schieppati & Remuzzi, 2005).

Complications from chronic kidney disease include cardiovascular mortality, increased mortality at all stages, kidney disease progression, acute kidney injury, cognitive decline, anemia and bone disorders. (Jha et al., 2013; Go, Chertow, Fan, McCulloch, & Hsu, 2004). Several strategies to reduce these complications and to assist patients' management of the disease are available. However, adherence to the recommended treatments, diet and lifestyle changes is challenging, as it is expected that the patient and his support network are able to understand, implement and maintain over time kidney-related self-care strategies (Tout, Davis, Velasquez,

Banerjee, & Powe, 2013; Dageforde & Cavanaugh, 2013; Bear & Stokie, 2014). This limited adherence to self-management behaviors like managing medications, dietary recommendations and co-morbid conditions next to renal replacement therapies is confirmed extensively by the literature, as non-adherence among patients on dialysis ranges from 25% to 86%. (Kluger et al., 2005; Denhaerynck et al., 2007; Gerbino et al., 2011).

The patient suffering from kidney disease is therefore expected not only to make significant changes in his lifestyle, but also to develop communication skills necessary to improve the quality of the interaction with the health care system (Dageforde & Cavanaugh, 2013; Berkman, Sheridan, Donahue, Halpern, & Crotty, 2011). The Institute of Medicine defines health literacy as "the degree to which individuals can obtain, process, understand and communicate about health-related information needed to make informed health decisions" (cited in Berkman, Davis, & McCormack, 2010; Institute of Medicine, 2012). It has been identified as a critical competence to master, as low health literacy is associated with limited prevention, more hospital stays and higher mortality (Berkman et al., 2011). Studies consistently indicate that limited health literacy among kidney disease patients is associated with greater risk of mortality, higher blood pressure, more missed dialysis treatments and more frequent ER visits (Boulware, Carson, Troll, Powe, & Cooper, 2009; Wright, Wallston, Elasy, Ikizler, & Cavanaugh, 2011; Kleinpeter, 2003; Pollock & Jaffrey, 2007; Cavanaugh et al., 2010; Foster et al., 2011; Grubbs, Gregorich, Perez-Stable, & Hsu, 2009; Green et al., 2011; Adeseun, Bonney, & Rosas, 2012; Osborn, Cavanaugh, Wallston, White, & Rothman, 2009; Green et al., 2013).

Berkman and colleagues report that in the last decade more than forty health literacy interventions have been published (Berkman et al., 2011) with the objective to improve the effectiveness of information delivered and increase opportunities for shared decision-making. Despite the availability of educational materials (Bear & Stockie, 2014; Dageforde & Cavanaugh, 2013), approximately one-third of patients with advanced chronic kidney disease and end-stage renal disease still report low health literacy about their illness (Fraser et al., 2013; Fadem et al., 2011; Young, 2013; Finkelstein et al., 2008; Pierratos, 2013; Schell, 2012; Green et al., 2011) and education tools are not routinely implemented as part of clinical protocols (Bear & Stockie, 2014).

However, findings from a recent report confirms that patients are interested in research that targets improved communication with their providers, the selection of dialysis modality, next to the management of emotional and physical symptoms (Manns et al., 2014).

Among the available treatments, kidney transplantation is an option for patients with advanced chronic kidney disease and end-stage renal disease when a patient is considered medically and psychologically eligible. The evaluation process that precedes the approval requires an intense level of patient engagement. Despite this, the literature about kidney transplant is limited (Devraj & Gordon, 2009). Furthermore, it is now well accepted that support from significant others plays a critical role to a successful kidney transplant, as caregivers are expected to facilitate self-care and promote effective health decisions. Difficulties with the administration of medicine, errors in the dosage of medications and poor health outcomes are some of the problems associated with limited literacy of caregivers (Yin, Dreyer, Foltin, van Schaick, & Mendelsohn, 2007; Lau et al., 2010).

Therefore, the attention of the multidisciplinary healthcare team should be placed on the development of programs and educational materials aimed at increasing patients and caregivers' engagement and adherence to treatment protocols. In the case of kidney transplant from living donor, this is extremely challenging given the relationship between donors and recipients, as well as the impact on their respective quality of life. Despite this, a review of the literature conducted by the authors has revealed a gap about protocols to promote patients and donors' engagement. Although a few centers have started to develop some experiences (see this link https://www.youtube.com/watch?v=fvdL8_WNxLA for the protocol used by the Azienda ospedaliero-universitaria in Novara), protocols from both the Italian and the international context and -more importantly- evidence of their efficacy/effectiveness have not been published yet. Hence, the present contribution aims to fill this gap by introducing the Informative Groups on Kidney Transplantation from Living Donor.

MAIN FOCUS OF THE CHAPTER

Issues, Controversies, Problems

Since 1979, one hundred eighty-six kidney transplants have been successfully completed at the Nephrology Unit of the Ca' Granda Niguarda Hospital. The first transplant from a blood-related donor took place in 1979, while the first transplant from a living donor not blood related was completed in 1987. Within the Unit, in 2002 the Clinical Psychology Service has received the mandate to conduct psychological assessments of living donor transplant candidates. This process is aimed at identifying possible psychological risks for the donor and the recipient, and to report about the psychological well-being of candidates as requested by the Italian public administration. The first assessment is conducted through meetings with potential donors and recipients, as mandated by the guidelines of Italian Society of Nephrology, the National Centre for Transplants, and the law number 458 of June 26th, 1967. However, this strategy soon appeared to be insufficient and incomplete because of the limited information and feedback provided by participants.

An initial reflection on the experience led the investigators to identify key topics to assess. In particular, motivation and self-determination of the possible donor next to psychosocial characteristics of the recipient were rated as crucial, since personality traits like psychoticism, limited adherence to treatment and ability to deal with stress have been associated to higher chance of rejection (Calia, Ferrarese, Zecchini, & Orlandelli, 2006; Lovera et al., 2000; Fisher, 2003; Rupolo & Poznanzki, 1999). The difficulty to follow indication from the healthcare team, both at the present time and earlier, represents another core aspect to investigate. Predictors of non-adherence among kidney recipients have been identified in four categories: socio-economic and cultural variables (occupation and dimension of social network), psychological and psychiatric characteristics (thought process, anxiety disorders, mood disorders, substance abuse), pre-transplant non adherence (for the renal disease or other associated illnesses), and the health literacy of the patient (information about illness, treatments, risks factors, etc). This last category is of particular interest for psychologists, as it gives the professional the opportunity to guide the patient in a process of knowledge and management of the illness that prevents complications and promote quality of life. To reduce non-adherence to the transplantation protocol, the first step was then to develop a program to increase patients' engagement.

Despite it is generally accepted that engagement reduces drop-outs and complications, to date procedures that involve the team as a whole do not exists. This is the reason to offer the readers a description of the protocol implemented in the last years at the Ca' Granda Niguarda Hospital, where this program precedes the medical evaluation. In particular, this protocol is truly multidisciplinary, as doctors, nurses and psychologists contribute to the selection of contents and to its implementation. Finally, the program has been inspired by a first standardization of the psychological assessment of patients and donors candidates and it represents an active strategy of engagement.

DESCRIPTION OF THE PROTOCOLS

Step One: The Development of the SICADR (Fact Sheet for the Potential Kidney Donor)

A central component of the new protocol is the SICADR - Scheda Informativa per il Candidato Alla Donazione di Rene/*Fact Sheet for the Potential Kidney Donor* (Minetti, Zanini, & Saita. 2011) which summarizes the essential information in simple sentences with the best balance of scientific precision and comprehensibility. This informative sheet, initially implemented in 2004 (Lennerling & Nyberg, 2004;

Minetti, Zanini, & Civati, 2004), has multiple purposes. First, it was introduced to standardize the information given by different health care professionals. Second, it contributed to limit the amount of missing information in the patient-doctor meeting. Similarly, it assisted balancing pros and cons to promote awareness and self-determination in the decision-making process about care and treatment. Finally, it promoted a mutual feedback between the individual and the health care professional to improve the quality of the informative exchange.

This form is designed to meet the informational needs of the donor, with the goal to involve the individual from the beginning of the transplant experience. It has been reported in the literature that potential donors sometimes show a tendency to not listen and remember only part of the information given during the consultation with the medical team; especially details about potential risks associated with the removal of a kidney (Saita & Zanini, 2011). This behavior seems to reflect defensive tendencies from the anxiety associated with the surgery and the following impact on the quality of life of the potential donor. Hence, it is crucial to provide the donor with multiple opportunities to review significant information during the decision process, as highlighted by all the guidelines for living donor transplants.

The SICADR has been introduced as a routine step of the evaluation: it is provided during a meeting with the psychologist after the potential donor has already met with the physician. Copies are also made available to the primary care physician of the potential donor, to the Third Party Committee and the judge. The SICADR has been consistently reviewed over time and a final version (available in English – see Appendix 1) has been prepared in 2009 using the data from follow-up calls with donors. Its efficacy has also been evaluated in following studies and results have been presented at the Technical-Scientific Meeting of the Nord Italian Transplant network and at the 2010 ELPAT International Congress (Minetti et al., 2004; Minetti, Zanini, & Saita, 2011).

However, the clinical experience has highlighted that informational support, although necessary, it is not sufficient to promote donors and recipients' engagement because of the role intra-psychical and relational factors have in this process. Given the limited literature available about this topic, the research team has then decided to engage in a qualitative study to better understand the emotional and affective dynamics that may contribute to a different processing of the information provided by the healthcare team. The project was aimed at exploring representations and meanings associated with the living donor transplant experience. Two were the objectives of the study: first, to examine how organ donation and transplant were experienced by potential donors and recipients, trying to identify which aspects contribute to the difficulties of making the decision. Second, authors wanted to explore the effects organ donation has on the family dynamics, with the long term goal to confirm the hypothesis that the organ donation can only take place in families where giving and receiving are characterized by authenticity and positive exchange. This qualitative research was conducted through the methodology of the focus group, which involves that a group of people are asked questions about perceptions, beliefs and attitudes about a certain topic. It is a method extremely used in social sciences, especially when the investigator is trying to collect preliminary knowledge (Krueger, 1994).

Focus groups were conducted by two researchers with extensive knowledge of renal disease and the meetings were aimed at examining three different areas: the individuals' representations of what organ donation is and the meanings associated with the word; the motivations for organ donation; and the information needed to make the decision (both for donors and recipients). Each focus group meeting was audiotaped and transcribed by the researchers. Participants, 12 potential donors and recipients, completed informed consent form before the beginning of the study. Transcripts of the meetings were then analyzed with T-LAB (Lancia, 2004; Lancia 2012), a statistical software aimed at analyzing, comparing and graphically representing contents. Results indicate that the kidney transplant from a living donor can be placed within a relational dynamic: the motivation to give and to receive are both influenced by the relationship between the donor and the recipient. The level of intimacy and closeness between donor and recipient emerges as the most relevant factor in the decision making process: the higher the bond between them, the higher the desire to donate (Saita et al., 2012).

Step Two: GITREV Groups (Informative Groups on Kidney Transplantation from Living Donor)

From these initial results, the authors have developed informative groups about kidney transplant from living donor dedicated to potential recipients and donors treated at the Ca' Granda Niguarda Hospital. Called GITREV (Gruppi Informativi sul Trapianto di Rene da Vivente/ *Informative Groups on Kidney Transplantation from Living Donor*), they represent a multidisciplinary strategy to increase the level of participants' engagement.

While it is known from the literature that the first level of patient engagement is direct patient care (Carman et al., 2013), in which subjects get information about a condition and answer questions about treatment preferences, this is not enough in living-donor kidney transplantation. In the selection of living donors, guiding ethical principles are important (the absence of coercion or monetary reward, autonomy, beneficence, and no maleficence) and a psychological assessment is required. Furthermore, deciding for living-kidney transplantation requires an ongoing discussion with the patient and the family because of the numerous psychological implications which affect both the kidney donor and the recipient. As a consequence, past donors and recipients were invited to be part of the meeting along with the multidisciplinary team. The GITREV groups represent an essential step of the educational journey of patients and potential donors, as they are not limited to the provision of information but they recognize the ability of the individual to make informed decisions about health issues (Rossi Ferrario et al., 2009).

The GITREV meetings are organized in two moments. At first a nephrologist, a surgeon, a nurse, and a psychologist present information about kidney transplantation (the same information included in SICADR) according to the criteria of gradual disclosure, choosing non-technical language, and using images to support the description of the procedures involved. Some time for questions is included to address issues and needs of participants. In the second part of the meeting, a small group approach is used. Under the guidance of two facilitators trained in group work and with expertise in kidney transplantation's psychosocial issues, potential donors and recipients discuss about the information received. The goal is to promote free expression of emotions, worries and concerns from the participants, without fear of negative evaluation by the health care providers. The use of a peer to peer approach, for both donors and recipients, helps to provide understanding of the transplantation procedure and to improve their health and well-being. In addition to surgical information, the candidate to transplantation may learn something about a real experience and receive informal knowledge from other donors or recipients. Furthermore, a group setting is useful to facilitate discussion and to collect information about the adequacy of candidates (possible coercion, expectations, aspirations, hopes, and the quality of the relationships) and to explore the real motivation (Saita & Zanini, 2011; Saita et al., 2012).

THE EVALUATION OF GITREV

The Efficacy of GITREV Groups: Preliminary Findings

A comprehensive evaluation of the efficacy of the GITREV groups is currently underway, and preliminary findings are presented here. To date, data have been collected and analyzed about the first three GITREV groups. Two perspectives have been considered: the experiences of the members of the healthcare team leading these groups and those of potential donors and recipients. Between 4 to 6 team members have been involved in the evaluation of each group, for a total of 14 professionals. Semi-structured interviews were conducted by psychologists about topics like: satisfaction of the healthcare team members, satisfaction of the participants and feedback about the experience. The interviews were audiotaped, transcribed and analyzed with the textual analysis software ATLAS.ti (Chiarolanza & De Gregorio, 2007).

For every area investigated codes have been created, with a procedure similar to the one used by the Grounded Theory methodology (Glaser & Strauss, 1967). The goal was to identify theoretical models underlying the data by examining the relationship between codes. From codes, categories have been created and narrative themes have been investigated in the texts. The analysis of the participation of potential donors and recipients has been conducted focusing on the questions subjects asked to members of the team and group leaders during the informative and discussion session. Questions from 25 participants (12 potential recipients: 9 men and 3 women, and 13 potential donors: 11 women and 2 men) have been analyzed with the T-LAB software (Lancia, 2004). This software allows researchers to conduct a number of statistical analysis to gain a more detailed understanding of the text compared to the paper-pencil strategy. Using this software, a text (in this case the transcripts from the three GITREV group sessions) is prepared for analysis through a series of steps, which include text segmentation, automatic lemmatization and key-term selection. Subsequently, researchers are given the choice to conduct three main types of analysis: co-occurrence analysis, thematic analysis, and comparative analysis. In the present work, a Thematic Analysis of Elementary Contexts has been conducted, with the goal to extract thematic clusters from the transcripts of the meetings. Separate analyses have been conducted on the two moments of the GITREV groups: during and after the informative session, and during the group discussion.

Participants' and Team Members' Experience of the GITREV Groups

Seven codes (major themes) have been identified from the researchers, using the same words used by the participants as suggested by the literature (Tarozzi, 2008). Connections between codes have been established through similarities and juxtaposition, to create two categories.

The first category, called "*exhaustive contents*" refers to the comprehensiveness of the information provided and the possibility to deepen and to examine more in detail questions or concerns of potential donors and recipients. Both members of the healthcare team and participants highlighted this as the key characteristic of the group experience. The second category, called "*participation*" refers to the satisfaction reported from health care professionals and participants about the way the GITREV groups have been conducted. They all positively commented on the fact that communication was not univocal (from the "expert" to the audience) but bi-directional. Furthermore, participants particularly enjoyed the closeness experienced with the other members of the group, the opportunity to get to know better other potential donors and recipients, and to share the emotional aspects associated with the disease. It is very interesting to comment about reported concerns and positive consequences of the transplant, which were similar among potential donors and recipients. Donors were concerned about the change in the quality of life of the patient moving from dialysis to transplant and the following treatment regime, while recipients reported worries about the risks of nephrectomy for donors. Both, however, anticipate reciprocal positive changes for their relationship. For example, among married couple's partners expected a positive change due to the end of dialysis and to an increased physical well-being of the patient. Among dyads composed by a parent and a son or a daughter, the identified improvement was the higher quality of life of the patient, while among siblings the act of organ donation represented a way to strengthen their affective bond.

Throughout a series of following analysis the core category has emerged. Using the words of a members of the healthcare team, it has been named "*As Virgil for Dante*" to illustrate how the informative groups were perceived as a guide and support in a challenging moment of their lives. Like Virgil in the Divine Comedy has walked with Dante in the afterlife, guiding him through Hell, Purgatory and Paradise, so the groups have assisted potential donors and recipients walking through the different challenges of the transplant experience. This core category has been placed in relation with the others, in order to describe how members of the healthcare team have perceived and experienced from an intra-psychic point of view the participation in the GITREV groups (see Figure 1).

Figure 1. Professionals: Core category and its relations with the other categories

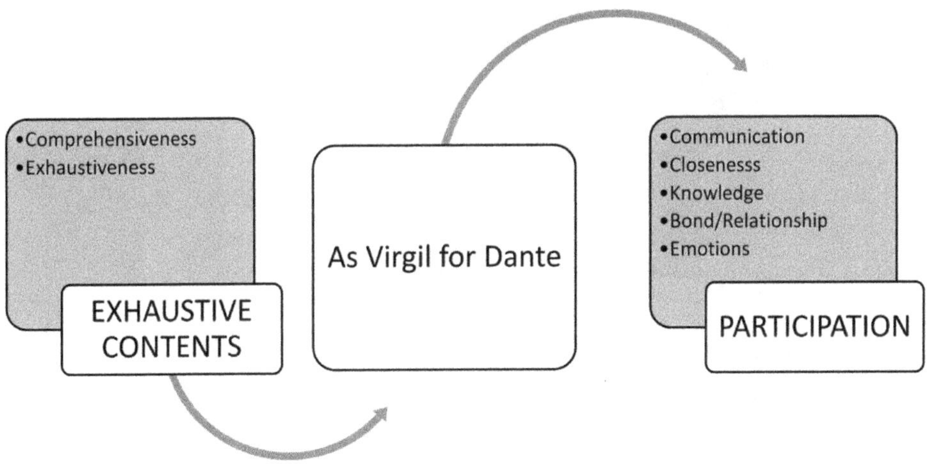

Potential Donors and Recipients' Experience on the GITREV

It is, however, the analysis of the questions asked by potential donors and recipients that is essential to describe the aspect of participation. Among the questions asked at the end of the first part of the GITREV, which account for 15% of the total (see Figure 2), four thematic clusters emerge (see Figure 3). The first one refers to *medical aspects* like pain management, or the efficacy of anti-rejection therapy and accounts for 24.23% of the variance. The second cluster, accounting for 28.39% of the variance, is organized around information that pertains to *nursing*. In the third cluster (29.06% of variance), lemmas refer to *psychological issues* like the risks for depressive disorders associated to a failed transplant. Finally, the fourth cluster, which accounts for 18.32% of the variance, is organized around *legal implications* of organ donation like healthcare coverage for the donor (see Figure 3).

Figure 2. Potential donors and recipients: percentages of questions in first part (1) and in the second part (2) of the GITREV

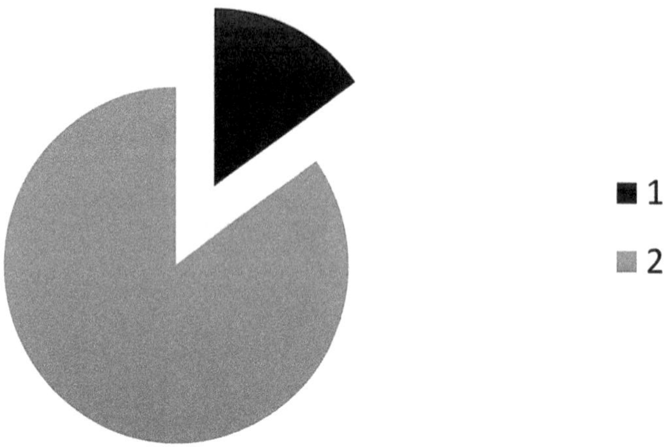

Figure 3. Thematic cluster in the first part of the GITREV

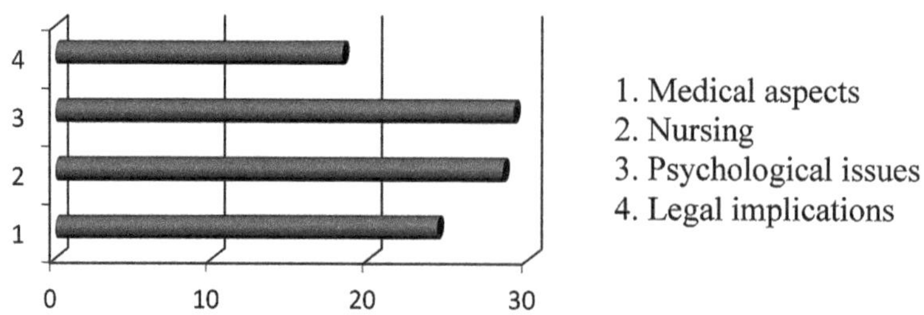

Questions asked during the group discussion, in the second half of the GITREV meeting, represent 85% of the questions asked during the whole session. Five are the thematic clusters identified through the analysis, which can be summarized in two macro areas: *information* and *emotions*. Among the macro area of information, one cluster pertains to confirm the information given by the healthcare team in the first part (20.23% of variance). A second cluster, which explains 19.07% of the variance, refers only to the need of information and clarification about post-operative pain and its management (for example, about the intensity of post-operative pain, and the dosage of anti-pain medication)

Focusing on the macro area of emotions, one cluster (accounting for 26.25% of variance) refers to the expressions of fear that both donors and recipients communicated to the team about aspects that couldn't be controlled like the survival of the donor during the surgical procedure. Hope and joy were part of another cluster explaining 24.27% of variance, while the relationship between donor and recipient is addressed in the third one (which accounts for 10.18%). From the way the questions are organized in the two moments of the group meeting, it is possible to affirm that the opportunity to meet and exchange perspectives and questions with peers promotes the active engagement of potential donors and recipients. In a similar way, participation and discussion contribute to higher satisfaction also among members of the healthcare team (see Figure 4).

SOLUTIONS AND RECOMMENDATIONS

The study has strong implications for clinical practice and patient engagement. First of all, the experience presented in this chapter is unique within the field of patient engagement in the context of chronic kidney disease. While previous studies have been limited to motivational interviewing in nursing and patient navigation programs

Figure 4. Thematic cluster in the second part of the GITREV

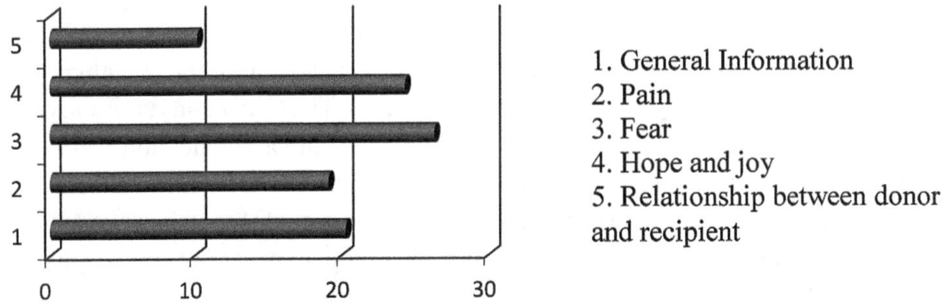

(McCarley, 2009; Jolly et al., 2015), the GITREV contributes to foster patient engagement as a "process-like and multidimensional experience" (Graffigna et al., 2014, p. 1). Similarly, our findings are in line with previous studies identifying a positive relationship between engagement and quality of life (Barello & Graffigna, 2014).

From this initial analysis it is possible to appreciate how the GITREV group experience represents a setting where a tapestry of communication occurs: the medical description of the transplant process provided by the medical team is intertwined with questions and concerns of potential donors and recipients. Similarly, cognitive aspects intersect with the emotional dimensions of fear and hope. These last themes have been addressed only in a limited way by the literature. However, they tend to strongly emerge in the moment there is the opportunity for an open confrontation and a bi-directional communication between the healthcare team and potential organ donors and recipients. As health professionals explain the protocol and its side-effects to patients and their caregivers, so they are also in a position to ask questions and -more importantly- to voice their concerns and emotions.

In particular, this type of analysis has allowed the researchers to investigate the psychological implications of the introduction of a model of patient engagement as well as to evaluate attitudes towards transplantation. Results of the present work are therefore critical to reflect on the identification of best practices for patients' engagement and adherence to care in the context of chronic kidney disease. Through a better understanding of the emotional and affective dynamics and the relational implications that may influence the elaboration of the information given by health care providers, it will be possible to develop evidence-informed intervention with this population. Specifically, from our experience, donors are interested in knowing what could be the benefits for the recipients, while recipients' focus of attention is to understand risks for donors. It is therefore possible to affirm that both donors and recipients expect mutual and dyadic benefits.

We have mentioned earlier that this work was inspired by the desire to address barriers to effective communication between the team and potential organ donors and recipients as they occur in the clinical practice. One of the most delicate moment of the renal disease is the passage from conservative treatments to the dialysis or transplant. This passage is discussed with the patient by considering pros and cons of the different treatment options, giving priority to the patient's and his/her family's quality of life. In the case a living donor is available, a transplant can be completed before the dialysis (preemptive transplant). The transplant represents the best therapy for chronic renal insufficiency for the right candidate, and it is considered as life-extending because of its ability to improve the individual's quality of life and postpone death. A study has in fact demonstrated that Italian patients in dialysis show lower quality of life than transplanted patients (Mazzoni, Laghi, & Cicognani, 2013).

It is however well-known the limited availability of organs and, when an organ from a dead donor is not available, family members often offer themselves as potential donors. In case of blood-relatives, they are encouraged because of higher immunological compatibility and the lower risk of organ rejection, while for non-blood related potential donors it is often the desire to improve the health of their loved ones. Living organ donation is a topic that is creating increasing attention among patients and their relatives with the subsequent need for more information (Minetti et al, 2004). This information should be not only exhaustive, but also easy to understand for the patient in order to not compromise the success of the transplant.

FUTURE RESEARCH DIRECTIONS

The present contribution presents some limitations and it cannot be considered exemplificative of all the informative protocols about kidney transplant. On the contrary, it has been the absence of shared procedures both in the International and in the Italian context that has supported the description of the protocol implemented at the Ca' Granda Niguarda Hospital and its preliminary evaluation. Subjects, methodologies and statistical analyses have been inspired by an ethical dimension, aimed at listening to the needs of the individual with chronic kidney disease and the desire to help potential donors. In the future, this humanistic perspective should be supported by a stronger scientific rigor, in line with the directions of evidence-based medicine. However, the process leading to kidney transplant from living donor -because of its intrinsic complexity- requires analyses and strategies of study flexible and adjustable for the clinical practice. An integrative approach is necessary to assess situations and personal characteristics that poorly fit with the transplant but also to activate resources from the family and social context of the patient.

This type of transplant offers the opportunity to give without the certainty of a restitution: the aim of organ donation is then placed within the relationship between individuals and family members (Cigoli, 2006). Donation is characterized by positive connotations, and it is perceived as an idealistic and altruistic act because it requires to overcome a natural and genetically strong instinct to self-conservation, which is manifested through the care for one's integrity and safety (Saita, 2012). Given these considerations, chronic kidney disease can be considered a *we-disease* (Bodenmann, 2005; Kayser, Watson, & Andrade, 2007), an illness that affects both members of the dyad and their relationship. By assuming this perspective, it is within the relationship that it is possible to find a cure characterized by taking care of the patient, the close one and their relationship (Saita et al., 2012).

CONCLUSION

In this chapter we wanted to offer an initial reflection about some clinical practices influenced by the problems experienced by healthcare professionals working with patients with chronic kidney disease. These practices have promoted new spaces of communication among disciplines. The hope is that this first experience will contribute to increased confrontation between Medicine and Psychology with the long term goal to a more effective work with the patient, as suggested by some recent contributions (Saba, Saita & Novelli, 2011).

Summarizing, this chapter has originated from a serious clinical problem: patients and caregivers' engagement and adherence to transplant's protocol procedures and requirements, next to the efficacy of these protocols. These issues are at the core of the transplantation practice, because the success of the surgery is influenced by the adherence of the patient to the treatment and by the engagement of both potential donors and recipients. It is necessary to move from the idea that donors and recipients simply have to obey to prescribed guidelines, and to introduce the idea of a true partnership between them and the healthcare team.

Starting from issues and problems experienced by the members of the healthcare team, the protocol presented in the chapter has been developed. In its current form, the GITREV represents a multidisciplinary educational intervention that involves medical, nursing and psychological information. Informative aspects about the illness and its treatment are mixed with more expressive contents, like the possibility to share in a group setting emotional aspects and to take an active role. In this sense the GITREV promotes that ability of the members of the healthcare team to manage the diversity of situations that arise when health consumers are engaged in clinical decision making described by Barello and Graffigna (2015). This practice is coherent with the literature (Majani & Cavallini, 2010), which highlights how adherence in kidney transplant from a living donor requires higher active engagement from the patient, the donor and the family members who are expected to become involved in the preparation for the transplant.

As described before, in order to create the current protocol numerous steps have been taken and several instruments have been used. However, over time their limitations in the ability to address issues and concerns raised by patients and their relatives have emerged. Through an ongoing reflection, it has been possible to review and make adjustments to a previous clinical practice unable to address the complexity of the living donor transplant. As a consequence, a new dialogue between disciplines has started, and new strategies have emerged.

Chronic kidney disease therefore requires a constant exchange between Medicine, Psychology and Social Sciences. They all contribute to the promotion of care for patients and their relatives, as Medicine is focused on the promotion of prevention and care, Psychology assists understanding emotions and meanings associated to health and illness, and Social Sciences take in consideration the context and the multiple systems people are part of. Finally, the methodology adopted to improve patient engagement involves patient, family and health care providers in an active partnership aimed at ensuring the best quality of care. For this reason the protocol presented can be easily adapted into routine practice.

REFERENCES

Adeseun, G. A., Bonney, C. C., & Rosas, S. E. (2012). Health literacy associated with blood pressure but not other cardiovascular disease risk factors among dialysis patients. *American Journal of Hypertension*, *25*(3), 348–353. doi:10.1038/ajh.2011.252 PMID:22237154

Barello, S., & Graffigna, G. (2014). Engaging patients to recover life projectuality: An Italian cross-disease framework.[Epubaheadofprint]. *Quality of Life Research: An International Journal of Quality of Life Aspects of Treatment, Care and Rehabilitation*. doi:10.1007/s11136-014- 0846-x PMID:25373927

Barello, S., & Graffigna, G. (2015). Engagement-sensitive decision making: training doctors to sustain patient engagement in medical consultations. In G. Graffigna, S. Barello, & S. Triberti (Eds.), *Patient Engagement: A Consumer-Centered Model to Innovate Healthcare* (pp. 78–93). Berlin: De Gruyter Open. doi:10.1515/9783110452440-008

Barello, S., Graffigna, G., Savarese, M., & Bosio, A. C. (2014a). Engaging patients in health management: Towards a preliminary theoretical conceptualization. *Psicologia Della Salute*, *3*(3), 11–33. doi:10.3280/PDS2014-003002

Barello, S., Graffigna, G., Vegni, E., & Bosio, A. C. (2014b). The challenges of conceptualizing patient engagement in health care: A lexicographic literature review. *Journal of Participatory Medicine*, *6*, e9.

Bear, R. A., & Stockie, S. (2014). Patient engagement and patient-centred care in the management of advanced chronic kidney disease and chronic kidney failure. *Canadian Journal of Kidney Health and Disease*, *1*(1), 24. Published online21October2014. doi:10.1186/s40697-014-0024-7 PMID:25780613

Bellardita, L., Graffigna, G., Donegani, S., Villani, D., Villa, S., Tresoldi, V., & Valdagni, R. (2012). Patient's choice of observational strategy for early-stage prostate cancer. *Neuropsycholological Trends*, *12*, 107–116. doi:10.7358/neur-2012-012-bell

Berkman, N. D., Davis, T. C., & McCormack, L. (2010). Health literacy: What is it? *Journal of Health Communication*, *15*(sup2Suppl. 2), 9–19. doi:10.1080/10810730.2010.499985 PMID:20845189

Berkman, N. D., Sheridan, S. L., Donahue, K. E., Halpern, D. J., & Crotty, K. (2011). Low health literacy and health outcomes: An updated systematic review. *Annals of Internal Medicine*, *155*(2), 97–107. doi:10.7326/0003-4819-155-2-201107190-00005 PMID:21768583

Berwick, D. M. (2010). *What patient-centered care should mean*. Retrieved from http://patientprivacyrights.org/wp-content/uploads/2010/02/What-Patient-Centered-Should-Mean.pdf

Bodenmann, G. (2005). Dyadic coping and its significance for marital functioning. In T. A. Revenson, K. Kayser, & G. Bodenmann (Eds.), *Couples coping with stress: Emerging perspectives on dyadic coping* (pp. 35–50). Washington, DC: American Psychological Association. doi:10.1037/11031-002

Boulware, L. E., Carson, K. A., Troll, M. U., Powe, N. R., & Cooper, L. A. (2009). Perceived susceptibility to chronic kidney disease among high-risk patients seen in primary care practices. *Journal of General Internal Medicine*, *24*(10), 1123–1129. doi:10.1007/s11606-009-1086-6 PMID:19711135

Boulware, L. E., Hill-Briggs, F., Kraus, E. S., Melancon, J. K., Falcone, B., Ephraim, P. L., & Powe, N. R. et al. (2013). Effectiveness of educational and social worker interventions to activate patients' discussion and pursuit of preemptive living donor kidney transplantation: A randomized controlled trial. *American Journal of Kidney Diseases*, *61*(3), 476–486. doi:10.1053/j.ajkd.2012.08.039 PMID:23089512

Braun, L., Sood, V., Hogue, S., Lieberman, B., & Copley-Merriman, C. (2012). High burden and unmet patient needs in chronic kidney disease. *International Journal of Nephrology and Renovascular Disease*, *5*, 151–163. doi:10.2147/IJNRD.S37766 PMID:23293534

Calia, R., Ferrarese, D., Zecchini, J., & Orlandelli, E. (2006). *Vissuti Psicosociali nel Trapianto di rene: Pazienti in lista di attesa, nel post-trapianto e nel ri-trapianto* [Psychosocial Experiences in Kidney Transplant: Patients waiting for transplant, post-transplant and re-transplant]. Roma: Accademia Lancisiana.

Carman, K. L., Dardess, P., Maurer, M., Sofaer, S., Adams, K., Bechtel, C., & Sweeney, J. (2013). Patient And Family Engagement: A Framework For Understanding The Elements And Developing Interventions And Policies. *Health Affairs*, *32*(2), 223–231. doi:10.1377/hlthaff.2012.1133 PMID:23381514

Cavanaugh, K. L., Wingard, R. M., Hakim, R. M., Eden, S., Shintani, A., Wallston, K. A., & Ikizier, T. A. et al. (2010). Low health literacy associates with increased mortality in ESRD. *Journal of the American Society of Nephrology*, *21*(11), 1979–1985. doi:10.1681/ASN.2009111163 PMID:20671215

Chiarolanza, C., & De Gregorio, E. (2007). *Lavorare con ATLAS.ti. Come analizzare i processi psicosociali* [*Working with ATLAS.ti. How to Analyze Psychosocial Processes*]. Roma: Carocci.

Cigoli, V. (2006). *L'albero della discendenza. Clinica dei corpi familiari* [*The Descendents' Tree. A Clinical Approach to Family Bodies*]. Milano: Franco Angeli.

Crawford, M. J., Rutter, D., Manley, C., Weaver, T., & Bhui, K. (2002). Systematic review of involving patients in the planning and development of healthcare. *BMJ (Clinical Research Ed.)*, *325*(7375), 1263. doi:10.1136/bmj.325.7375.1263 PMID:12458240

Dageforde, L. A., & Cavanaugh, K. L. (2013). Health Literacy: Emerging Evidence and Applications in Kidney Disease Care. *Advances in Chronic Kidney Disease*, *20*(4), 311–319. doi:10.1053/j.ackd.2013.04.005 PMID:23809283

Davis, K., Schoenbaum, S. C., & Audet, A. M. (2005). A 2020 vision of patient-centered primary care. *Journal of General Internal Medicine*, *20*(10), 953–957. doi:10.1111/j.1525-1497.2005.0178.x PMID:16191145

Denhaerynck, K., Manhaeve, D., Dobbels, F., Garzoni, D., Nolte, C., & De Geest, S. (2007). Prevalence and consequences of nonadherence to hemodialysis regimens. *American Journal of Critical Care*, *16*(3), 222–235. PMID:17460313

Devraj, R., & Gordon, E. J. (2009). Health literacy and kidney disease: Toward a new line of research. *American Journal of Kidney Diseases*, *53*(5), 884–889. doi:10.1053/j.ajkd.2008.12.028 PMID:19324481

Diamantidis, C. J., & Becker, S. (2014). Health information technology (IT) to improve the care of patients with chronic kidney disease (CKD). *BMC Nephrology*, *15*(7). Available at http://www.biomedcentral.com/1471-2369/15/7. doi:10.1186/1471-2369-15-7 PMID:24405907

Fadem, S. Z., Walker, D. R., Abbott, G., Friedman, A. L., Goldman, R., Sexton, S., & Peters, T. G. et al. (2011). Satisfaction with renal replacement therapy and education: The American Association of Kidney Patients Survey. *Clinical Journal of the American Society of Nephrology; CJASN, 6*(3), 605–612. doi:10.2215/CJN.06970810 PMID:21330485

Fehrman-Ekholm, I., Dunér, F., Brink, B., Tydén, G., & Elinder, C. G. (2001). No Evidence of Accelerated Loss of Kidney Function in Living Kidney Donors: Results from a cross-cultural follow-up. *Transplantation, 72*(3), 444–449. doi:10.1097/00007890-200108150-00015 PMID:11502974

Finkelstein, F. O., Story, K., Firanek, C., Barre, P., Takano, T., Soroka, S., & Mendelssohn, D. et al. (2008). Perceived knowledge among patients cared for by Nephrologists about chronic kidney disease and ESRD therapies. *Kidney International, 74*(9), 1178–1184. doi:10.1038/ki.2008.376 PMID:18668024

Fisher, M. S. Sr. (2003). Psychosocial evaluation interview protocol for living related and living unrelated kidney donors. *Social Work in Health Care, 38*(1), 39–61. doi:10.1300/J010v38n01_03 PMID:14984248

Foster, M., Brice, J. H., Shofer, F., Principe, S., DeWalt, D., Falk, R., & Ferris, M. (2011). Personal disaster preparedness of dialysis patients in North Carolina. *Clinical Journal of the American Society of Nephrology; CJASN, 6*(10), 2478–2484. doi:10.2215/CJN.03590411 PMID:21852660

Fraser, S. D., Roderick, P. J., Casey, M., Taal, M. W., Yuen, H. M., & Nutbeam, D. (2013). Prevalence and associations of limited health literacy in chronic kidney disease: A systematic review. *Nephrology, Dialysis, Transplantation, 28*(1), 129–137. doi:10.1093/ndt/gfs371 PMID:23222414

Gerbino, G., Dimonte, V., Albasi, C., Lasorsa, C., Vitale, C., & Marangella, M. (2011). Adesione Alla Terapia Del Paziente In Emodialisi[Adherence to Care for the Patient in Dyalisis]. *Giornale Italiano di Nefrologia, 28*(4), 416–424. PMID:21809311

Glaser, B., & Strauss, A. (1967). *The Discovery of Grounded Theory: Strategies for Qualitative Research*. New York: Aldine.

Go, A. S., Chertow, G. M., Fan, D., McCulloch, C. E., & Hsu, C. Y. (2004). Chronic kidney disease and the risks of death, cardiovascular events, and hospitalization. *The New England Journal of Medicine, 351*(13), 1296–1305. doi:10.1056/NEJMoa041031 PMID:15385656

Graffigna, G., Barello, S., Libreri, C., & Bosio, C. A. (2014). How to engage type-2 diabetic patients in their own health management: Implications for clinical practice. *BMC Public Health, 14*(1), 648. doi:10.1186/1471-2458-14-648 PMID:24966036

Graffigna, G., Barello, S., & Riva, G. (2013). Technologies for patient engagement. *Health Affairs, 32*(6), 1172–1172. doi:10.1377/hlthaff.2013.0279 PMID:23733998

Green, J. A., Mor, M. K., Schields, A. M., Sevick, M. A., Palevsky, P. M., Fine, M. J., & Weisbord, S. D. et al. (2011). Prevalence and demographic and clinical associations of health literacy in patients on maintenance hemodialysis. *Clinical Journal of the American Society of Nephrology; CJASN, 6*(6), 1354–1360. doi:10.2215/CJN.09761110 PMID:21551025

Green, J. A., Mor, M. K., Shields, A. M., Sevick, M. A., Arnold, R. M., Palevsky, P. M., & Weisbord, S. D. et al. (2013). Associations of health literacy with dialysis adherence and health resource utilization in patients receiving maintenance hemodialysis. *American Journal of Kidney Diseases, 62*(1), 73–80. doi:10.1053/j.ajkd.2012.12.014 PMID:23352380

Grubbs, V., Gregorich, S. E., Perez-Stable, E. J., & Hsu, C. Y. (2009). Health literacy and access to kidney transplantation. *Clinical Journal of the American Society of Nephrology; CJASN, 4*(1), 195–200. doi:10.2215/CJN.03290708 PMID:19056617

Hibbard, J., & Greene, J. (2013). What the evidence shows about patient activation: Better health outcomes and care experiences; fewer data on costs. *Health Affairs, 32*(2), 207–214. doi:10.1377/hlthaff.2012.1061 PMID:23381511

Institute of Medicine. (2012). *How Can Health Care Organizations Become More Health Literate? Workshop Summary*. Washington, DC: National Academies Press.

Jha, V., Garcia-Garcia, G., Iseki, K., Li, Z., Naicker, S., Plattner, B., & Yang, C. W. et al. (2013). Chronic kidney disease: Global dimension and perspectives. *Lancet, 382*(9888), 260–272. http://www.ncbi.nlm.nih.gov/pubmed/23727169. doi:10.1016/S0140-6736(13)60687-X PMID:23727169

Jolly, S. E., Navaneethan, S. D., Schold, J. D., Arrigain, S., Koning, V., Burrucker, Y. K., & Nally, J. V. et al. (2015). Development of a chronic kidney disease patient navigator program. *BMC Nephrology, 16*(1), 69. doi:10.1186/s12882-015-0060-2 PMID:26024966

Kayser, K., Watson, E., & Andrade, J. T. (2007). Cancer as a we-disease: Examining the process of coping from a relational perspective. *Families, Systems & Health, 25*(4), 404–418. doi:10.1037/1091-7527.25.4.404

Kleinpeter, M. A. (2003). Health literacy affects peritoneal dialysis performance and outcomes. *Advances in Peritoneal Dialysis. Conference on Peritoneal Dialysis, 19*, 115–119. PMID:14763046

Krueger, R. A. (1994). *Focus groups. A practical Guide for Applied Research*. Thousand Oaks, CA: Sage Publications.

Kugler, C., Vlaminck, H., Haverich, A., & Maes, B. (2005). Nonadherence with diet and fluid restrictions among adults having hemodialysis. *Journal of Nursing Scholarship, 37*(1), 25–29. doi:10.1111/j.1547-5069.2005.00009.x PMID:15813583

Lancia, F. (2004). *Strumenti per l'analisi dei testi. Introduzione all'uso di T-LAB* [*Instruments for Textual Analysis. An Introduction to the Use of T-LAB*]. Milano: Franco Angeli.

Lancia, F. (2012). T-LAB 8.0 – User's Manual. Available at http://tlab.it/it/bibliography.php

LaPointe Rudow, D., Hays, R., Baliga, P., Cohen, DJ, Cooper, M., & Danovitch, G, M., ... & Rodrigue, J. R. (2015). Consensus conference on best practices in live kidney donation: Recommendations to optimize education, access, and care. *American Journal ofTransplantation, 15*(4), 914–922. doi:10.1111/ajt.13173 PMID:25648884

Lau, D. T., Berman, R., Halpern, L., Pickard, A. S., Schrauf, R., & Witt, W. (2010). Exploring factors that influence informal caregiving in medication management for home hospice patients. *Journal of Palliative Medicine, 13*(9), 1085–1090. doi:10.1089/jpm.2010.0082 PMID:20836633

Lennerling, A., & Nyberg, G. (2004). Written information for potential living kidney donors. *Transplant International, 17*(8), 449–452. doi:10.1111/j.1432-2277.2004.tb00468.x PMID:15322746

Levey, A. S., Schoolwerth, A. C., Burrows, N. R., Williams, D. E., Stith, K. R., & McClellan, W. (2009). Comprehensive public health strategies for preventing the development, progression, and complications of CKD: Report of an expert panel convened by the Centers for Disease Control and Prevention. *American Journal of Kidney Diseases, 53*(3), 522–535. doi:10.1053/j.ajkd.2008.11.019 PMID:19231739

Lovera, G., Basile, A., Bertolotti, M., Comazzi, A. M., Clerici, C. A., Gandione, M., & Ponton, P. et al. (2000). L'assistenza psicologica nei trapianti d'organo.[Psychological Care in Organ Transplants]. *Annali dell'Istituto Superiore di Sanita, 36*(2), 225–246. PMID:11213654

Lozano, R., Naghavi, M., Foreman, K., Lim, S., Shibuya, K., Aboyans, V., & AlMazroa, M. A. et al. (2013). Global and regional mortality from 235 causes of death for 20 age groups in 1990 and 2010: A systematic analysis for the Global Burden of Disease Study. *Lancet, 380*(9859), 2095–2128. doi:10.1016/S0140-6736(12)61728-0 PMID:23245604

Majani, G., & Cavallini, L. (2010). Il ruolo del paziente nella gestione di una terapia a lungo termine. Dalla compliance all'adherence.[Patient's role in the management of a long term treatment. From compliance to adherence]. *Giornale Italiano di Nefrologia, 27*(3), 316–318. PMID:20540027

Manns, B., Hemmelgarn, B., Lillie, E., Crowe, S., Cyr, A., Gladish, M., & Laupacis, A. et al. (2014). Setting research priorities for patients on or nearing dialysis. *Clinical Journal of the American Society of Nephrology; CJASN, 9*(10), 1813–1821. doi:10.2215/CJN.01610214 PMID:24832095

Mazzoni, D., Laghi, M., & Cicognani, E. (2013). Qualità della vita e fattori psicosociali nei pazienti con insufficienza renale[Quality of life and psychosocial factors in patients with Renal Insufficiency]. *Psicologia della Salute, 3*, 5–27. doi:10.3280/PDS2013-003001

McCarley, P. (2009). Patient empowerment and motivational interviewing: Engaging patients to self-manage their own care. *Nephrology Nursing Journal, 36*(4), 409–413. PMID:19715108

Menichetti, J., Libreri, C., Lozza, E., & Graffigna, G. (2014). Giving patients a starring role in their own care: A bibliometric analysis of the on-going literature debate.[Epubaheadof print]. *Health Expectations*, n/a. doi:10.1111/hex.12299 PMID:25369557

Minetti, E., Zanini, S., & Civati, G. (2004). *Scheda informativa per il potenziale donatore vivente di rene* [[*Fact Sheet for the Potential Kidney Donor]*]. Ancona: Riunione Scientifica Nord Italia Transplant Program.

Minetti, E., Zanini, S., & Saita, E. (2011). Evaluation of Effectiveness of Information for the Candidate to Kidney Donation. In W. Weimar, M. Bos, & J. van Buschbach (Eds.), Organ Transplantation: Ethical, Legal and Psychological Aspects (pp. 322-328), Vol II, Pabst Science Publisher.

Ocloo, J. E., & Fulop, N. J. (2012). Developing a 'Critical' approach to patient and public involvement in patient safety in the NHS: Learning lessons from other parts of the public sector? *Health Expectations*, *15*(4), 424–432. doi:10.1111/j.1369-7625.2011.00695.x PMID:21711471

Osborn, C. Y., Cavanaugh, K., Wallston, K. A., White, R. O., & Rothman, R. L. (2009). Diabetes numeracy: An overlooked factor in understanding racial disparities in glycemic control. *Diabetes Care*, *32*(9), 1614–1619. doi:10.2337/dc09-0425 PMID:19401443

Pierratos, A. (2013). Patient Education in Chronic Kidney Disease and Dialysis. *Seminars in Dialysis*, *26*(2), 135–137. doi:10.1111/sdi.12081 PMID:23520986

Polaschek, N. (2003). Negotiated care: A model for nursing work in the renal setting. *Journal of Advanced Nursing*, *42*(4), 355–363. doi:10.1046/j.1365-2648.2003.02627.x PMID:12752880

Pollock, J. B., & Jaffery, J. B. (2007). Knowledge of phosphorus compared with other nutrients in maintenance dialysis patients. *Journal of Renal Nutrition*, *17*(5), 323–328. doi:10.1053/j.jrn.2007.05.009 PMID:17720101

Provenzi, L., Borgatti, R., Menozzi, G., & Montirosso, R. (2015). A dynamic system analysis of dyadic flexibility and stability across the Face-to-Face Still-Face procedure: Application of the State Space Grid. *Infant Behavior and Development*, *38*, 1–10. doi:10.1016/j.infbeh.2014.10.001 PMID:25463152

Rossi Ferrario, S., Zotti, A. M., Pasetti, C., Comazzi, F., Giorgi, I., Negri, M., & Omarini, P. et al. (2009). Communicating medical information: A little lesson from italian patients. *Giornale Italiano di Medicina del Lavoro Ed Ergonomia*, *31*(3Suppl B), b12–b16. PMID:20518222

Rupolo, G., & Poznanzki, C. (1999). *Psicologia e psichiatria del trapianto d'organi* [*Psychology and Psychiatry on Organ Tranplants*]. Milano: Masson.

Saba, G. W., Saita, E., & Novelli, M. (2011). Pearls Toolbox: l'equipaggiamento psicologico per il medico [Pearls Toolbox: Psychological tools for the medical doctor]. In E. Saita (a cura di) Pensare alla salute e alla malattia [Thinking of Health and Illness] (pp. 53-67). Milano: EDUcatt.

Saita, E. (2012). Il corpo condiviso. La motivazione a donare parti di sé.[The Shared Body. The motivation to donate a part of him/herSelf]. *Ricerche di Psicologia*, *4*, 639–641.

Saita, E., & Zanini, S. (2011). Donare un rene: le determinanti di una scelta. (Donating a Kidney: determinants of the choice). In G. Castelnuovo, R. Menici, & M. Fedi (Eds.), *La donazione in Italia. Situazione e prospettive della donazione di sangue, organi, tessuti, cellule e midollo osseo* [Donation in Italy. Current Status and Prospectives in Blood, Organs, Tissues, Cells and Bone-Marrow]. (pp. 195–205). Milano: Springer-Verlag.

Saita, E., Zanini, S., & Fenaroli, V. (2012). Il trapianto di rene da vivente: Le motivazioni a donare e a ricevere un rene.[Kidney Transplant from Living Donor: Motivations to Give and Receive a Kidney]. *Ricerche di Psicologia*, *4*, 693–711. doi:10.3280/RIP2012-004008

Schell, J. O., Green, J. A., Tulsky, J. A., & Arnold, R. M. (2013). Communication Skills Training for Dialysis Decision-Making and End-of-Life Care in Nephrology. *Clinical Journal of American Society of Nephrology*, *8*(4), 675–680. doi:10.2215/CJN.05220512 PMID:23143502

Schell, J. O., Patel, U. D., Steinhauser, K. E., Ammarell, N., & Tulsky, J. A. (2012). Discussion of kidney disease trajectory by elderly patients and Nephrologists: A qualitative study. *American Journal of Kidney Diseases*, *59*(4), 495–503. doi:10.1053/j.ajkd.2011.11.023 PMID:22221483

Schieppati, A., & Remuzzi, G. (2005). Chronic renal disease as a public health problem: Epidemiology, social, and economic implications. *Kidney International*, *68*(Suppl. 98), S7–S10. doi:10.1111/j.1523-1755.2005.09801.x PMID:16108976

Stockie, S. (2012). *Making patient-centred care a reality for Ontario Hospitals* [Unpublished MBA Thesis]. York University, Toronto.

Tarozzi, M. (2008). *Che cos'è la grounded theory* [*What Grounded Theory is*]. Roma: Carocci.

Tout, D. S., Davis, E., Velasquez, A., Banerjee, T., & Powe, N. R. (2013). Assessment of Printed Patient-Educational Materials for Chronic Kidney Disease. *American Journal of Nephrology*, *38*(3), 184–194. doi:10.1159/000354314 PMID:23970127

Wright, J. A., Wallston, K. A., Elasy, T. A., Ikizler, T. A., & Cavanaugh, K. L. (2011). Development and results of a kidney disease knowledge survey given to patients with CKD. *American Journal of Kidney Diseases*, *57*(3), 387–395. doi:10.1053/j.ajkd.2010.09.018 PMID:21168943

Yin, H. S., Dreyer, B. P., Foltin, G., van Schaick, L., & Mendelsohn, A. L. (2007). Association of low caregiver health literacy with reported use of non-standardized dosing instruments and lack of knowledge of weight-based dosing. *Ambulatory Pediatrics*, *7*(4), 292–298. doi:10.1016/j.ambp.2007.04.004 PMID:17660100

Young, B. A. (2013). Health Literacy in Nephrology: Why is it Important? *American Journal of Kidney Diseases*, *62*(1), 3–6. doi:10.1053/j.ajkd.2013.04.003 PMID:23773837

KEY TERMS AND DEFINITIONS

SICADR: Scheda Informativa per i Candidati alla Donazione di Rene.
GITREV: Gruppo Informativo Trapianto di Rene tra Viventi.

APPENDIX

SICADR: Fact Sheet for the Potential Kidney Donor

Information for Potential Kidney Donors

During the presentation of the process of evaluating your suitability to donate a kidney, the nephrologist and clinical psychologist described many aspects in order to help you make a free and informed decision concerning the donation.

We here summarise the key points and ask you to indicate whether you have clearly understood the information received.

1. Living donor kidney transplant represents an alternative to cadaveric donor kidney transplant and to dialysis.
   I understand [ ] *yes* [ ] *no*
2. The evaluation of the suitability of a donor is intended to minimise the following risks:
   - The risk of an unwilling donation.
   - The risk of the operation.
   - The risk of diseases affecting the remaining kidney.
   - The risk of the failure of the kidney transplantation.
   - The risk of transmitting a disease to the recipient.

   Minimising these risks does not mean excluding them with absolute certainty.
   I understand [ ] *yes* [ ] *no*
3. The evaluation process provides an opportunity of discovering any diseases and initiating possible treatments.
   I understand [ ] *yes* [ ] *no*
4. The decision as to which surgical technique is used to harvest the kidney (traditional or video-laparascopic) is made by the surgeon on the basis of the specific characteristics of the donor. The average duration of hospitalisation is seven days.
   I understand [ ] *yes* [ ] *no*
5. The complications depend on the surgical procedure; they tend to be higher with the video laparascopic technique. It is essential that, before the operation, donors give their consent to receive transfusions in the case of intra- or postoperative haemorrhaging.
   I understand [ ] *yes* [ ] *no*

6. A transplanted kidney has an average life of about 15 years. A kidney transplant does not constitute a complete recovery since the recipient will need pharmacologic therapy to prevent rejection for all the kidney life.
   I understand [ ] *yes* [ ] *no*
7. The results of kidney transplantation from a living donor (a relative or otherwise) are better than those of transplantation from a cadaveric donor.
   I understand [ ] *yes* [ ] *no*
8. While convalescing, donors cannot undertake any strenuous physical activities for a period of about two months. Subsequently, all physical activities can be resumed without any limitation. Check-up examinations at our Centre are foreseen one, three, six and twelve months after the operation, and are subsequently recommended every year.
   I understand [ ] *yes* [ ] *no*
9. The evaluation of the suitability of a donor involves many resources, and can therefore only be started if the donor is convinced that he/she really intends to make the donation.
   I understand [ ] *yes* [ ] *no*
10. Donors can freely interrupt the process at any time before the operation.
   I understand [ ] *yes* [ ] *no*
11. Years after having made a donation, donors describe the experience positively regardless of its outcome.
   I understand [ ] *yes* [ ] *no*
12. The donation of a kidney must be totally voluntary and so no form of payment is allowed; donors must feel free of any responsibility towards the recipient if the process of donation is interrupted for any reason.
   I understand [ ] *yes* [ ] *no*

   Date................................ Signature....................................

   This information sheet was jointly drawn up by:

   Struttura Complessa di Nefrologia, Struttura Semplice Dipartimentale Dialisi e Terapia del Trapianto Renale Servizio di Psicologia Clinica

   Responsabile: Dott. Enrico Minetti Referente per la SC di Nefrologia: Dr.ssa Susanna Zanini, Ambulatorio Trapianti Tel. 02.6444.2670 Ambulatorio Tel. 02.6444.2306

   Version 2.0 6/2009.

   Azienda Ospedaliera

   Ospedale Niguarda Ca' Granda

   Piazza Ospedale Maggiore, 3 - 20162 Milano

   Tel. 02/6444.2521 – Fax: 02/6444.2909

Chapter 2
Communication and Education Processes Involved in COPD Patient Engagement within the Italian Health System

Virginia Recchia
CNR Institute of Clinical Physiology, Italy

Antonio Dodaro
Independent Researcher, Italy

Rosita B. Maglie
University of Bari, Italy

Carlo G. Leo
CNR Institute of Clinical Physiology, Italy

ABSTRACT

The World Health Organization has estimated that chronic obstructive pulmonary disease (COPD) is the fourth most common cause of death worldwide. Due to the economic and social extent of the problem, patient engagement must be comprised as a new resource for the achievement of higher health outcomes and lower costs. As many key processes involved in the COPD patient engagement consist of communication and education processes, modelling those processes in a whole framework, including actors and content needs, is a requirement. The main scope of this chapter is contributing to design such a framework within the Italian Health System. Final recommendations suggest to create a synergy among patient engagement and a set of legal tools, namely informed consent, integrated care and advance care planning. The synergy is based on the fact that both patient engagement and those legal tools have a common deep root in the universal principle of patient autonomy.

DOI: 10.4018/978-1-5225-0663-8.ch002

INTRODUCTION

Noncommunicable diseases (NCDs) - that is medical conditions or illnesses that are non-infectious or non-transmissible - constitute the primary causes of death worldwide (World Health Organization, 2008a). In 2008, 57 million deaths occurred in the world; 36 million (63%) were due to NCDs, mainly cardiovascular diseases, diabetes, cancer and chronic respiratory diseases (Alwan et al., 2010). NCD deaths are estimated to rise by 15% between 2010 and 2020 (to 44 million deaths) (WHO, 2008b). The foremost causes of NCD deaths in 2008 were: cardiovascular diseases (48% of NCD deaths); cancers (21% of NCD deaths); and respiratory diseases, comprising asthma and chronic obstructive pulmonary disease (COPD) (11% of NCD deaths). In the EU, the estimated costs for COPD varied from 133.7 million in the Netherlands to 1.1 billion USD in Sweden (Van Boven, Vegter, Van Der Molen, & Postma, 2013). This trend consequently results in an enormous, steadily increasing economic and social burden (Lopez & Murray, 2006). In the last years, Italy carefully pondered the epidemiological and social impact of respiratory diseases. As a consequence, chronic respiratory diseases were comprised in the priority areas of intervention in the National Prevention Plan (Ministero della Salute, 2010–2012).

Being COPD a chronic and not completely reversible disease, its treatment needs to develop new health care models targeted on chronic conditions. This is necessary, in order to overcome the traditional approaches based on a concept of illnesses with abrupt onset and restricted duration - which can be typically cured by health professionals - towards new models of patient activation, participation and self-management. Patients with COPD often develop multiple disease-related symptoms as breathlessness, pain, fatigue, loss of appetite, dyspnoea, cough, phlegm, chest tightness, exercise intolerance, sleep disorders as well as loneliness and restriction of social activities (Shipman, White, Gysels, & White, 2009). COPD patients must also cope with the side-effects of treatment, such as anxiety and depression, which can significantly upsurge physical disability, morbidity, co-morbidity, and health-care services utilization, affecting compliance with medical treatment (Maurer et al., 2008). All these aspects make COPD a disease with an extensive impact on the quality of life for both patients and their families (Grant, Cavanagh, & Yorke, 2012).

Due to the economic and social extent of the problem, patient engagement must be comprised as a new resource for the achievement of higher health outcomes and lower costs. Many key processes involved in the COPD patient engagement consist of communication and education processes. Nevertheless, many studies suggest that communication among COPD patients, health professionals and caregivers is a noteworthy problem which requires several improvements (Giacomini, DeJean, Simeonov, & Smith, 2012). Although modelling those processes in a whole framework, including actors and topics (or content needs), is clearly a requirement, this conceptualization had never been conceived. The main scope of this chapter is contributing to design such a framework within the Italian Health Service. A descending objective is that of providing legal and ethical recommendations to create a synergy among patient engagement and a set of legal tools, namely informed consent, integrated care and advance care planning.

BACKGROUND

Nowadays, health care providers and health plans design swiftly changing expectations about patient participation. Currently, patients will not benefit from their health care unless they make use of considerable knowledge, skills and motivation to actively participate in the available care (Gruman et al., 2010). The notion of patient engagement consists of the assumption that patients are co-producers of their health and this should augment their satisfaction about the healthcare system, as well as their accountability, by improving positive clinical outcomes and reducing health delivery costs (Graffigna, Barello, & Triberti, 2015). This is particularly important for COPD patients, since a study demonstrated that an increased activation is related to an advance of a multiplicity of self-management behaviors (Hibbard, Mahoney, Stock, & Tusler, 2007). Engagement regards not only the patient's knowledge related to his/her health literacy level, but also the emotional aspects related to his/her motivation, behavioral changes and personal acceptance of the health condition (Graffigna et al., 2015). Thus, understanding the strategic levers that sustain patient engagement is a key priority to innovate healthcare systems and to improve their sustainability (Graffigna et al., 2015).

Based on the results shown by Gruman et al. (2010), it is essential to affirm that the first strategic lever and prerequisite of COPD patient engagement is communication and education as qualified interchange among patients/caregivers, physicians and health operators. Although we are aware that the terms communication and education refer to different notions, we will use them in a nearly interchangeable way. In fact, many authors (Spruit et al., 2013; Stoilkova, Janssen, & Wouters, 2013; Giacomini et al., 2012; Gruman et al., 2010) agree that - in the healthcare context - education and communication are distinct yet similar interaction modes that focus on equivalent contents (e.g. self-management, end-of-life care) and on the same goals (e.g. enhancing satisfaction, knowledge, skills, adherence, and outcomes).

A recent research suggests that only one third of the oxygen-dependent COPD patients discuss with their physicians the type of care they would desire if they were too sick to speak for themselves (Knauft, Nielsen, Engelberg, Patrick, & Curtis, 2005). When these discussions do occur, although patient satisfaction with physician communication may be relatively high (Curtis, Engelberg, Nielsen, Au, & Patrick, 2004), patient understanding of advance-care planning is poor, physician understanding of patient preferences is poor, even nurses rarely plan the consultations on an individual basis and rarely use motivational dialogue in self-management education, and there are significant shortcomings in the quality of this communication (Osterlund Efraimsson, Klang, Larsson, Ehrenberg, & Fossum, 2009; Curtis, 2008; Knauft et al., 2005; The SUPPORT Principal Investigators, 1995). Furthermore, in a recent survey, results indicate that a worthy patient-physician relationship represents one of the most important aspects of a successful management in respiratory disease population (Santus et al., 2012). All these outcomes suggest that communication and education is one of the main issues in improving quality of life and COPD management. This consideration is especially important in the perspective of healthcare continuity of patients suffering from chronic pathologies, where de-hospitalization and in-home patient care should be balanced by an optimal interaction among patients, caregivers, general practitioners, case managers, nurses, pulmonologists, other specialists, physiotherapists.

Following other authors (Graffigna et al., 2015; Spruit et al., 2013; Dodaro & Recchia, 2011), the paragraph about recommendations and solutions finally describe how to practically use a second strategic lever to promote COPD patient engagement. The key for advances is raising awareness about the main current ethico-legal tools that protect patients' rights in COPD management, such as: informed consent, integrated care, advance care planning. Actually, the possible synergy is attributable to the fact that both patient engagement and those ethico-legal tools have a common deep root in the universal principle of patient autonomy. Nevertheless, patient engagement - as a scientific subject - is commonly treated separately from subjects regarding patients' rights and ethical matters. Being those legal tools widely recognized in many national systems, they represent as a whole a powerful and concrete lever for enhancing patient engagement.

MAIN FOCUS OF THE CHAPTER

Communication and Education in Copd Management: Actors, Their Roles and Their Perspectives

The main actors involved in communication and education processes in COPD management are various: the patient, the caregiver, the general practitioner, the case manager, the respiratory nurse, the pulmonologist, the social worker, the psychiatrist and/or psychologist, the dietician, the physiotherapist, the community physician the pharmacist, the palliative physician, the manager of the medical implants company. In this analysis, the role of caregivers inhabits a peculiar place similar to a bridge, since it embodies both an active part in COPD management and a series of communication and education needs associated with relationship dynamics with health professionals as well as with patients themselves. Moreover, all the health professionals should communicate with patients, caregivers and other health professionals by means of being involved in specific communication and education topics which will be deepened in the following paragraphs.

Patient

In the management of chronic diseases, the patient often takes a central role (Wagner, 2000). The measures described in the literature to improve the results in the treatment of chronic conditions are based on the theories of human behavior (Glasgow et al., 1989). These theories are based on the idea that: 1) the ability to manage the disease can be learned by the patient; 2) motivation and participation are important determinants for the care effectiveness; 3) the social, family, work and health context can facilitate or hinder the active role of the patient; 4) monitoring and immediate response to changes improve disease management (Sabato, Leo, & Sabina, 2009).

In this perspective, even in the Italian context, doctor and patient have complementary roles (GOLD, 2015, Italian version). The doctor is focused on defining the problem in terms of diagnosis, poor adherence to treatment and definition of risk behaviors (e.g., smoking); the patient, however, is able to better define the problem in terms of suffering, symptoms, difficult to make changes in lifestyle, and to express the improvement in quality of life (Sabato et al., 2009). Moreover, the patient – as well as the caregiver – is always involved in communication and education processes.

Caregiver

The caregiver is the person who provides the patient with the most part of assistance and thus must be involved in all the communication and education programs often associated with COPD management. This role, in Italy as well as in many countries, is usually held by family members, although friends or paid caregivers are also a possibility. Severe and progressive dyspnoea are the most hurtful and frequent whiniest of COPD patients (Ahleit, 1995), terrifying also caregivers. Moreover, COPD can cause physical disability, altered cognition, memory disorders, touchiness, and behavioral changes that may further amplify the burden of caregivers (Cain & Wicks, 2006). A partner caregiver can experience a mixture of anger, powerlessness, guiltiness and isolation, together with the satisfaction from lessening his/her spouse suffering and helping him/her to stay at home as long as possible. Moreover, caregivers of COPD patients often play additional roles, as decision-maker and finance manager (Sexton & Munro, 1985). In fact, they are often called upon to decide about treatment on behalf of patients without detecting their preferences (Winzelberg, Hanson, & Tulsky, 2005). Many caregivers express a desire for communication, but feel restricted because of the patient's short breath and because they worry about causing further respiratory distress (Grant et al., 2012; Bergs, 2002). In spite of this burden, there has been a lack of consideration of their important roles. As described in the following paragraphs, these concerns have generated a new conceptualization of advance care planning as a communication process among patients and caregivers that goes beyond the specific treatment interventions.

COPD patients' partners reported some ways of coping with their role: finding personal gratification, successfully managing patients' behavior, finding meaning in the situation, managing their own distress, and finding support when to communicate their feelings (Buffum & Brod, 1998). Some authors argue that the caregivers' need for social support and for communication on their high burden indicates that inadequate social support (Payne, Smith, & Dean, 1999), social isolation (Bergs, 2002), lack of communication with physicians, and concerns about the patients' future (Aldred, Gott, & Gariballa, 2005) are important aspects of caregiver psychological wellbeing (Garlo, O'Leary, Van Ness, & Fried, 2010).

General Practitioner

The General Practitioner (GP) is the patient's main reference person and hence he/she must be informed about everything concerning the patient (Sabato, Sabina, & Leo, 2014). First of all, in Italy, the GP should be responsible for the early detection of COPD, focusing on smokers and ex-smokers over 35 years old with at least one lung symptom, before requiring a referral to a pulmonologist (Gulati, 2011). Another role of the GP is that of designing individualized treatment plans for pulmonary rehabilitation, in collaboration with specialists, nurses and patients (Kruis & Chavannes, 2010). After discharge from hospital, connecting acute care to continuous care in the community may be supported by the development of a discharge care plan, for instance by involving the patient's GP in a case conference (Walters, 2010; Casas et al., 2006). Moreover, the role of telephone follow up is remarkable, in order to steadily thicken support to patients and increase their coping strategies at home (Walters, 2010; Casas et al., 2006). Although the GPs role may vary, depending on the whole integrated care system, they are encouraged to play the role of "gatekeepers".

In a study (Shipman et al. 2009), patients described three categories of need to contact their GPs: routine, urgent and emergency. Routine contacts were reported to be necessary for getting prescriptions, for regular appointments to monitor progress or undertake tests, as well as for drug treatment or referral to other services. Urgent contacts were described to be essential to help with the onset of worsening symptoms when the patient had developed a chest infection or a cold, due either to COPD or to other conditions. Emergency contacts were generally needed for acute exacerbations of COPD or for acute onset of other conditions. Moreover, in another study (Seamark et al., 2012) some patients approved the chance to share decisions about end-of-life care and advance care planning, and they felt that their GP would have been the person best placed to do this.

Case Manager

A case manager usually is the health professional - an experienced nurse or a respiratory therapist, with a specific training - who coordinates the services required by the patient at different stages along the continuing care (Bourbeau, 2004). Moreover, an assigned case manager facilitates communication with the other health professionals belonging to the team, warranting steady progress and problem solving, setting common goal, building motivation and confidence, facilitating access to resources (Bourbeau, 2010). Even in Italy, the case managers play a coordination role: work to satisfy the patients' needs; intervene in the relationship with caregivers, institutions and medical staff; remove obstacles; plan, monitor and evaluate the programs to be implemented; ensure appropriate use of resources; plan training events (Sabato et al., 2014). Nevertheless, the case manager may play his/her role, depending on the complementary involvement of the GP (Casas et al., 2006). In a study, for instance, one joint visit of the case manager and the primary care team was completed at the patient's home within 72 hours from discharge (Casas et al, 2006). Following another study, self-management training for behavioral change in conjunction with case manager assistance are the most crucial strategies for the accomplishment of action plans (Walters, Turnock, Walters, & Wood-Baker, 2010). Another successful strategy is that of encouraging patients to call the case manager during regular working hours if they take action plan medications or if they have questions relating to their medical care. The models conceived by Evercare and Keiser Permanente for case management, which have been adapted in the UK (Hudson, 2005) employ experienced primary care nurses to identify and monitor individuals with long term conditions, intensively manage their care, integrate and coordinate services, support self care and implement specific disease management strategies to progress outcomes.

Respiratory Nurse

The health professionals involved in new service models and even in Italy are often nurses, mostly those with respiratory specialist roles (Stoilkova et al., 2013; Sabato et al., 2009; Candy et al., 2007). In this perspective, there is a multiplicity of roles that a nurse can play in the management of COPD at the hospital and/or territory levels. In some real settings, for instance, practice nurses can support physiotherapists in the delivery - at the level of the general practice - of education pulmonary rehabilitation programs (Murphy et al., 2011). In other healthcare environments, nurses can improve the structure of the visit by means of planning the consultations on an individual basis and use motivational dialogue for self-management education, smoking cessation, and patient communication (Osterlund Efraimsson et al., 2009). Despite all those differences, nurses act as the primary main practitioners and/or as service coordinators, aiming to promoting the service integration and to enabling the satisfaction of individualized care needs (Candy et al., 2007).

Pulmonologist

In Italy, pulmonologists are usually involved by GPs for a more accurate diagnostic assessment of COPD or other pulmonary diseases (Gulati, 2011). After prescribing and/or performing extensive laboratory testing and other diagnostic exams, they typically prescribe the most appropriate therapy (Gulati, 2011). Pulmonologists involved in the Pulmonologist Hospital Unit should also contribute to guarantee the integration activities between hospital and territory services, as well as to provide training for patients and caregivers (Sabato et al., 2014). In the perspective of a more efficient use of healthcare facilities - there is an increasing need of referral guidelines for pulmonologists and GPs, in order to establish their complementary roles. Adequate referral from the GP to pulmonologist and back-referral to the GP delineates a vital part of this challenge. Moreover, pulmonologists should provide clear advice about the treatment when they refer patients back to the GP. Finally, pulmonologists have a key role in the early follow-up after acute hospitalization. Some authors, in fact, found that COPD patients who have an early follow-up with their GP or pulmonologist after acute hospitalization have a lower probability of a 30-day Emergency Department visit or hospital readmission if compared with patients who do not receive such follow-up (Sharma, Kuo, Freeman, Zhang, & Goodwin, 2010).

Although the role of a pulmonologist in communicating with patients is peculiar and important, patients can experience more difficulties in communicating with pulmonologist than with other health professionals. In an interesting study (Visse, Teunissen, Peters, Widdershoven, & Abma, 2010), whereas a pulmonologist declared that his patients did not have difficulties in taking medicine, one of his/her COPD patients noted that the way he/she explained the use of medication could be improved. This patient evaluated the physiotherapists as more clear in this regard. The patient also noted that the conversation with the pulmonologist was a "one way" conversation. Unlike his/her relationship with the physiotherapists, he/she felt less understood by the pulmonologist. Hence, the pulmonologist needs to be trained to show a genuine involvement and an empathy with the patient (Visse et al., 2010). This implies a non-hierarchical relationship among health professionals and a perspective of shared responsibilities which is chiefly necessary in COPD self-management and disease management. The medical specialist needs to develop a new role, that of a teacher, educating the patient to identify his limits and to find new ways of dealing with the disease (Visse et al., 2010). Similarly, patients have to become more active in both defining their problems and in determining the appropriate treatment even when communication barriers occurr.

Social Worker

Rather few experiential data exist, related to the utility of social workers' involvement in patient care teams and in communication/education processes (Stoilkova et al., 2013). However, social workers are considered essential members of evaluation and management teams of elderly people, where the acquisition of community resources and the integration of patients back into the community are fundamental characteristics of the management plan (Wagner, 2000). In Italy, social workers are involved in hospital discharge planning, counseling and crisis intervention, patient and family education, information and referral to hospital and community resources and services. They also facilitate communication, end-of-life care, practical assistance, patient and caregiver support groups (Thomas, 2014; Bettoncelli et al., 2014). Some authors provide more details about the role of social worker in chronic care. If patients have weighty interpersonal or family conflicts, referral to a clinical social worker, psychologist, or other counselor for family/relationship counseling is recommended. Patients with COPD can be seen by a hospital social worker also before discharge from hospital in order to assess whether the patient required apparatus for the home (Gore, Brophy, & Greenstone, 2000). Finally, the involvement of a social worker might address the patients' need for education about welfare and benefits systems (Stoilkova et al., 2013).

Psychiatrist and/or Psychologist

As social workers, also psychiatrists and/or psychologists are healthcare professionals rarely involved in the education of patients. An active role of psychiatrists and/or psychologists in the process of education, may be an important determinant for facilitating and sustaining successful patient's behavior change, which in turn, is the goal of a self-management education. Nonetheless, to date, skills of healthcare professionals needed to provide effective patient education, are - even in the Italian context - rather vague and generally covered in the guidelines and position statements (Stoilkova et al., 2013).

Dietician

Low body weight or recent weight loss and in particular depleted lean body mass in patients with COPD have been proven to be independent predictors of mortality, outcomes after acute exacerbations, hospital admission rates, and the need for mechanical ventilation. The factors contributing to nutritional depletion in these patients include elevated sleeping and activity-related energy consumption, reduced dietary intake relative to sleeping energy expenditure, accelerated negative nitrogen balance, particularly during acute exacerbations of COPD, medication effects, and most importantly an elevated systemic inflammatory response (Mallampalli, 2004). Evidence shows that nutritional support encourages a substantial gain in weight and fat-free mass among malnourished COPD patients, especially when provided as part of an integrated rehabilitation program, including a structured exercise component as an anabolic stimulus (GOLD, 2015, English version). These recommendations are proposed in the Italian context (GOLD, 2015, Italian version).

Physiotherapist

Within the Italian healthcare system, the professionalism of physiotherapists is highly involved when pulmonary rehabilitation programs - that include exercise training - are necessary for COPD patients (Sabato et al., 2009). Rehabilitation is essential to alleviate dyspnea and fatigue, as well as to improve patients' sense of control over their condition (Lacasse et al., 2002). These improvements, which are moderately large and clinically significant, constitute an important part of COPD management (Lacasse et al., 2002). In their hospital-based outpatient pulmonary rehabilitation program, some authors (Cockram, Cecins, & Jenkins, 2006) established that patients and their caregivers should be persuaded to attend group education sessions carried out by a multidisciplinary team including a physiotherapist, a respiratory physician, a dietician and a pharmacist. The physiotherapist lessons can concentrate, for instance, on breathing patterns, coughing, management of attacks and how to exercise. In the same program, when considered necessary, patients should be individually referred to appropriate specialists (Cockram et al., 2006). Following the pulmonary rehabilitation program, those patients who are considered eligible on the basis of their oxygen saturation during exercise are encouraged to attend a community physiotherapy service class (Cockram et al., 2006). Moreover, treatment protocols need to be developed, allowing at the same time sufficient flexibility to preserve the necessity of providing treatment, according to individual need. These data were confirmed by Stoilkova et al. (2013), through the fact that physiotherapists are - in addition to nurses and physicians - the healthcare professionals most frequently involved in communication/education programs regarding COPD patients and caregivers.

Community Physician

Outpatient Pulmonary Rehabilitation, proper management of oxygen, nutritional counseling, compliance with medications, smoking cessation, should be coordinated in communication and education activities with the community physician for each patient (Bao et al., 2015). It is demonstrated that preventing admission in people with COPD exacerbations must be carefully and cautiously managed working closely with the patients own general practitioners and the community physicians. In Italy, they also manage quality improvement system through the analysis of the training needs of professionals and the implementation of training processes (Bettoncelli et al., 2014). Moreover, they collaborate in the construction of service networks and partnerships for the integrated management of COPD (Bettoncelli et al., 2014). They should finally help patients using available resources in the community, and modify work and role functions (Stoilkova et al., 2013), but this role is not enclosed in the Italian context.

Pharmacist

According to Stoilkova et al. (2013), pharmacists – along with psychologists, and social workers - are less likely to be involved in communication and education programs. This situation is experienced even in Italy and is in contrast with the fact that some authors underline the specific role of this professional operator (Wagner, 2000; Fromer, 2011). Adherence and perseverance with medications are crucial to therapeutic efficacy. Pharmacist team members may especially contribute to the care of chronic illness by optimizing drug regimens to reduce adverse effects and increase efficacy (Wagner, 2000). Visits involving medication management or patient education may be led by a nurse or by a clinical pharmacist using protocols or standing orders written by physicians (Fromer, 2011). Each chronic care visit should have a specific agenda (e.g., pharmacotherapy initiation, inhaler training, pharmacotherapy and support, long term oxygen therapy), so that all aspects of COPD management are consciously targeted (Fromer, 2011). For instance, by following the “brown bag” technique, a patient carries all his/her medications to a primary care meeting and describes how the medications are taken, allowing the clinical pharmacist to monitor adherence and settle potential interactions or errors at every visit (Fromer, 2011).

Palliative Physician

Although palliative care improves symptom management, health-related quality of life, cost savings, and mortality, the majority of COPD patients die without palliative care (Vermylen, Szmuilowicz, & Kalhan, 2015). In Italy, there are many barriers to providing palliative care to COPD patients, including the difficulty in prognosticating the illness trajectory, which cause referrals to occur late in the patient's disease (Vitacca & Comini, 2012; Carlucci, Guerrieri, & Nava, 2012). Additionally, physicians elude dialogues about advance care planning, due to communication barriers specifically occurring in patients with COPD (Vitacca & Comini, 2012; Carlucci et al., 2012). Although many health systems are not set up to provide trained palliative care physicians to COPD patients, this is not the case of Italy. Only in 1999 palliative care has been officially recognized and included in the Italian National Health System. Nevertheless, since then, it has had an exponential development and now there are more than 250 centers scattered throughout the country, which offer both residential and home care services (Casale & Calvieri, 2014). However, as described in the following paragraphs, the diffusion of those centers in Italy does not automatically implies that advance care planning is correspondingly a common practice.

Manager of the Implants Company

In Italy, as well as in many countries, the managers of the implants companies accomplish important communication/education activities which regard: the compatibility of the patient's home with the oxygen equipment; the effective use of respiratory devices, the correct use of inhalation therapy, the long term oxygen therapy (Sabato et al., 2014; Lavorini, Levy, Corrigan, Crompton, & ADMIT Working Group, 2010; Sabato et al., 2009).

Communication and Education Topics

Good communication which embraces listening, mutual understanding and collaboration is highly valuable in patient education and counselling and generates a positive influence on emotional health, symptom management, functional status and pain control (Stewart, 1995). Both the patient and the caregiver have needs about specific contents that should be addressed through effective communication and education processes led by the health professionals. These contents have been considered in a series of studies that will be reviewed in this section, in order to provide a clear synthesis of the main concepts that should be shared with patients and caregivers in COPD management. The strength and content of communication and education messages should vary depending on the knowledge areas of disease management, considering also the severity of the patient's disease. The most crucial communication and education topics mainly belong to four knowledge areas related to COPD management: 1) primary prevention and diagnosis; 2) symptom management and self-management; 3) drug consumption and administration; 4) end-of-life care. Each knowledge area includes a series of specific communication and education topics; and each specific topic involves a group of actors.

Table 1a describes the comprehensive framework by means of a matrix including knowledge areas, specific communication and education topics, and all the actors described (see Table 1b) who are considered at international level as well as in the Italian context. The specific communication and education topics have been listed by means of fitting and integrating the topics systematically reviewed by Stoilkova et al. (2013) and by Zwerink et al. (2014).

Findings displayed in Table 2 show that many communication and education topics are recommended in the international as well as in the Italian context. Nevertheless, there are some topics which are recommended in the international context and are lacking in the Italian system: in Table 1 and in Table 2, they are bolded (for instance, "Communicating with healthcare providers"). The actors involved in the bolded background topics (which are marginalised in the Italian guidelines) are logically suggested only by the international guidelines. The actors to be involved are similarly mentioned in the international as well as in the Italian guidelines and best practices. Nevertheless, their concrete involvement in each topic depends on the specific organizational context, which differently integrates some complementary roles. In the following paragraphs, we describe the four main knowledge areas about COPD management and all the related specific communication and education topics enclosed in Table 1a.

Primary Prevention and Diagnosis

Despite COPD is a major health problem, it still leads to a suboptimal diagnosis and an ineffective treatment (NHLBI/WHO, 2001). As above mentioned, the role of GPs is essential in the COPD prevention and early diagnosis, in order to identify and treat people before they reach end-stage lung disease. It is also widely acknowledged as a key step in decreasing management costs and improving quality of life (Lusuardi et al., 2006). Office spirometry by GPs is a good and feasible technique to reduce the underdiagnosis or misdiagnosis of chronic respiratory disorders (Lusuardi et al., 2006). In order to reinforce the usefulness of this technique, GPs should also communicate with patients about a series of prevention contents. For instance, the use of detailed anamnestic questionnaires probably help to address the clinical suppositions on the way to a more reliable diagnosis (Lusuardi et al., 2006; Voelkel, 2000). Moreover, earlier diagnosis has focused awareness on the multiple non-pulmonary

Table 1a. Visual representation of knowledge areas, communication/education topics, and actors involved in COPD management.

Knowledge Areas in COPD Management	Communication and Education Topics	Involved Actors													
		1 PAT	2 CAR	3 GP	4 CM	5 RN	6 PULM	7 SW	8 PSY	9 DIET	10 PHYS	11 CP	12 PHAR	13 PP	14 MIC
Primary prevention and diagnosis	1. Normal pulmonary anatomy and physiology	x	x	x			x								
	2. Interpretation of medical testing	x	x	x		x	x								
	3. Multiple non-pulmonary morbidities	x	x	x			x					x			
	4. Pathophysiology of chronic respiratory disease	x	x	x			x								
Symptom management, self-management	5. Early recognition and treatment of exacerbations	x	x	x	x	x	x					x			
	6. Breathing techniques	x	x			x					x				
	7. Effective use of respiratory devices	x	x		x	x					x				x
	8. Secretion clearance and coughing techniques	x	x		x	x					x				
	9. Action plan for self-treatment of exacerbations	x	x		x	x	x				x				
	10. Controlling acute episodes and emergencies	x	x		x	x					x	x			
	11. Healthy food intake	x	x	x	x	x				x					
	12. Benefits of exercise and physical activities	x	x	x	x	x				x	x				
	13. Energy conservation during activities of daily living	x	x			x					x				
	14. Communicating with healthcare providers	x	x		x	x			x						
	15. Irritant avoidance, including smoking cessation	x	x	x	x	x	x		x						
	16. Asking for information and help; using available resources in the community	x	x	x	x	x		x	x			x			
	17. Modifying work and role functions	x	x	x	x		x		x			x			
	18. Communicating with significant people	x	x		x				x						
	19. Anxiety and panic control, relaxation techniques	x	x			x			x						
	20. Leisure activities and traveling	x	x		x		x		x		x				

continued on following page

Table 1. Continued

Knowledge Areas in COPD Management	Communication and Education Topics	Involved Actors													
		1 PAT	2 CAR	3 GP	4 CM	5 RN	6 PULM	7 SW	8 PSY	9 DIET	10 PHYS	11 CP	12 PHAR	13 PP	14 MIC
Drugs consumption and administration	21. Role and rationale for medications	x	x	x	x		x						x		
	22. Drugs used during the therapy of stable COPD	x	x	x	x		x						x		
	23. Drugs used during exacerbations	x	x	x	x		x						x		
	24. Correct use of inhalation therapy	x	x	x	x	x	x						x		x
	25. Managing long-term oxygen therapy	x	x	x	x	x	x	x			x		x		x
End-of-life care	**26. Role of the treatments in improving quality and duration of life**	x	x		x	x	x							x	
	27. Advance Care Planning	x	x		x	x	x	x	x					x	
	28. End-of-life decision making	x	x		x	x	x	x	x					x	
	29. Prognosis for survival and for quality of life	x	x	x	x		x	x	x					x	
	30. Understanding what dying might be like	x	x	x	x		x	x	x					x	

Table 1b. Explanatory legend for Table 1a

Actor	Acronym
Patient	PAT
Caregiver	CAR
General Practitioner	GP
Case Manager	CM
Respiratory Nurse	RN
Pulmonologist	PULM
Social Worker	SW
Psychiatrist and/or Psychologist	PSY
Dietician	DIET
Physiotherapist	PHYS
Community Physician	CP
Pharmacist	PHAR
Palliative Physician	PP
Manager – Medical Implants Company	MIC

morbidities that often accompany COPD (Yawn & Kaplan, 2008). GPs are often called upon to investigate these multiple problems and to try to integrate the therapy suggested by several specialists into a total care (Yawn & Kaplan, 2008). This is another key concept that in Italy is shared with patients by GPs, case managers, respiratory nurses and community physicians in primary prevention. The common irritant - tobacco smoke - and the common response - inflammation - may underlie many of the multiple morbidities seen in people with COPD (Yawn & Kaplan, 2008).-

The interpretation of medical testing is an additional specific topic that GPs, pulmonologists and respiratory nurses should share with patients and caregivers, and that is recommended in Italian best practices (Casas et al., 2006; GOLD, 2015, Italian version). Other topics that should be addressed by GPs and pulmonologists in communication about primary prevention in Italy are: the normal pulmonary anatomy and physiology; the pathophysiology of chronic respiratory disease (Stilkova et al., 2013; Carone et al., 2002).

Symptom Management and Self-Management

As day-to-day care responsibilities fall most heavily on patients and their families, caregivers expressed a necessity for support to better cope with some patient's symptoms, such as breathlessness (Grant et al., 2012). Actually, access to and use

Table 2. Communication/education topics and sources documenting the relative actors' involvement in the international and Italian context

Communication and Education Topics	Source International Context	Source Italian Context
1. Normal pulmonary anatomy and physiology	Stoilkova et al., 2013	Carone et al., 2002
2. Interpretation of medical testing	Casas et al., 2006	GOLD, 2015 (Italian version)
3. Multiple non-pulmonary morbidities	Yawn & Kaplan, 2008	Bettoncelli et al., 2014 Doos et al., 2014
4. Pathophysiology of chronic respiratory disease	Stoilkova et al., 2013	Carone et al., 2002
5. Early recognition and treatment of exacerbations	Stoilkova et al., 2013	Bettoncelli et al., 2014 Sabato et al., 2009 Lusuardi et al., 2006
6. Breathing techniques	Bourbeau et al., 2003	Carone et al., 2002
7. Effective use of respiratory devices	Stoilkova et al., 2013	Sabato et al., 2009
8. Secretion clearance and coughing techniques	Stoilkova et al., 2013	Sabato et al., 2009
9. Action plan for self-treatment of exacerbations	Bourbeau et al., 2003	Sabato et al., 2009
10. Controlling acute episodes and emergencies	Stoilkova et al., 2013	Sabato et al., 2009 Sabato et al., 2014
11. Healthy food intake	Chavannes et al., 2009 Casas et al., 2006	Sabato et al., 2009
12. Benefits of exercise and physical activities	Bourbeau et al., 2003	Neri et al., 2006
13. Energy conservation during activities of daily living	Bourbeau et al., 2003	Pasqua et al., 2009 Carone et al., 2002
14. Communicating with healthcare providers	Stoilkova et al., 2013	-
15. Irritant avoidance, including smoking cessation	Casas et al., 2006 Chavannes et al., 2009	GOLD, 2015 (Italian version) Bettoncelli et al., 2014 Carone et al., 2002
16. Asking for information and help; using available resources in the community	Stoilkova et al., 2013	-
17. Modifying work and role functions	Stoilkova et al., 2013	-
18. Communicating with significant people	Stoilkova et al., 2013	-
19. Anxiety and panic control, relaxation techniques	Casas et al., 2006	Bettoncelli et al., 2014
20. Leisure activities and traveling	Bourbeau et al., 2003 Stoilkova et al., 2013	-
21. Role and rationale for medications	Stoilkova et al., 2013	Sabato et al., 2009
22. Drugs used during the therapy of stable COPD	Casas et al., 2006 Chavannes et al., 2009	Bettoncelli et al., 2014 Carone et al., 2002
23. Drugs used during exacerbations	Bourbeau et al., 2003	Sabato et al., 2009 Maglie (in press) Carone et al., 2002

continued on following page

Table 2. Continued

Communication and Education Topics	Source International Context	Source Italian Context
24. Correct use of inhalation therapy	Bourbeau et al., 2003 Monninkhof et al., 2003	Lavorini et al., 2010 Carone et al., 2002
25. Managing long-term oxygen therapy	Bourbeau et al., 2003	Sabato et al., 2014 Dal Negro & Goldberg, 2005
26. Role of the treatments in improving quality and duration of life	Stoilkova et al., 2013 Curtis, 2008	-
27. Advance Care Planning	Stoilkova et al., 2013 Patel et al., 2012	GOLD, 2015 (Italian version) Carlucci et al., 2012 Vitacca & Comini, 2012
28. End-of-life decision making	Casas et al., 2006	Bettoncelli et al., 2014 Carlucci et al., 2012 Vitacca & Comini, 2012
29. Prognosis for survival and for quality of life	Stoilkova et al., 2013 Curtis, 2008	Bettoncelli et al., 2014
30. Understanding what dying might be like	Stoilkova et al., 2013 Curtis, 2008	GOLD, 2015 (Italian version) Carlucci et al., 2012

of support mechanisms can be tricky, with many caregivers stating that they lack knowledge about professional services (Spence et al., 2008; Bergs, 2002). Furthermore, there is a tendency for caregivers to energetically pursue professional support only during acute exacerbations (Spence et al., 2008). This represents a reasonable source of aggravation for caregivers, with some of them trying to cope by means of what is available to them and frantic to avoid placing their loved ones in a nursing home (Spence et al., 2008). Being the determination to help the patient at a great emotional cost to the caregiver, the provision of support services is imperative.

According to Grant et al. (2012), nurses have the ideal role to offer communication, education and management strategies to help caregivers cope with hard symptom management. Programs to increase outcomes of chronic disease and/or reduce hospital readmissions have been mostly developed on the basis of self-management principles (Rich et al., 1995). Self-management refer to any formal patient education program meant to develop skills needed to carry out medical interventions specific to the disease, health behavior change, and emotional support for patients to control their disease and functional lives. The continuum among self-management education and support services can go from self-help methods to more demanding case management, through a case manager. The case management approach promotes continuity, communication, and cooperation among the patient, the family, and various health professionals. As reported by Bourbeau et al. (2003), this continuum provided by trained health professionals can significantly reduce the use of health care services and improve health outcomes.

Communication and education topics related to those activities are recommended even in the Italian context. They consist of: early recognition and treatment of exacerbations (Bettoncelli et al., 2014; Sabato et al., 2009; Lusuardi et al., 2006); breathing techniques (Carone et al., 2002); effective use of respiratory devices (Sabato et al., 2009); secretion clearance and coughing techniques (Sabato et al., 2009); action plan for self-treatment of exacerbations (Sabato et al., 2009); controlling acute episodes and emergencies (Sabato et al., 2014; Sabato et al., 2009); energy conservation during activities of daily living (Pasqua et al., 2009; Carone et al., 2002).

In Italy, recommendations indicate that COPD patients must be also educated to assimilate healthy lifestyle choices, in order to slow disease progression and minimize disease impact. Those healthy lifestyle choices are: correct diet (Sabato et al., 2009), systematic physical workout activities; smoking cessation, (GOLD, 2015, Italian version; Bettoncelli et al., 2014; Carone et al., 2002). Currently, no tests can foresee which smoker will develop COPD, but all smokers are encouraged to smoking cessation (Yawn & Kaplan, 2008). Smoking cessation strategies, including combinations of nicotine replacement significantly augment success and should be suggested to patients. The nurse can be optimally supportive in smoking cessation programs and lifestyle issues (Tunsäter et al., 2007). Nevertheless, a study demonstrates that the self-management education and support to stop smoking is provided by nurses through information, commonly without motivational dialogue and open-ended questions which ponder patients' abilities to self-manage their condition (Osterlund et al., 2009). This is a good reason why also psychiatrists and/or psychologists should be involved. They hold effective methods to educate patients to smoking cessation, as well as to other important topics, such as: how to communicate with healthcare providers (Stoilkova et al., 2013); asking for information and help, using available resources in the community (Stoilkova et al., 2013); modifying work and role functions (Stoilkova et al., 2013); communicating with significant people (Stoilkova et al., 2013); leisure activities and traveling (Bourbeau et al., 2003; Stoilkova et al., 2013); anxiety and panic control, relaxation techniques (Casas et al., 2006; Bettoncelli et al., 2014). Only the last one is recommended as an important communication and education topic even in the Italian context, while all the others are unfortunately eluded.

Drugs Consumption and Administration

In this knowledge area of COPD management, communication and education programs enhance interaction between healthcare professionals, patients and caregivers, emphasizing the role and the rationale for use medication and the correct use of related equipment (Sabato et al., 2014). Given the difficulty and variety of the actions required to use these devices correctly, training programs focusing on them should be delivered. For example, as noted by Tiep and Carter (2008), due to its bulk, oxygen kit can become a critical issue for patients and can reduce participation in rehabilitation programs. Essential communication and education topics which are recommended at the international level as well as in the Italian best practices are: role and rationale for medications (Sabato et al., 2009); drugs used during the therapy of stable COPD (Bettoncelli et al., 2014; Carone et al., 2002); drugs used during exacerbations (Sabato et al., 2009; Maglie, in press; Carone et al., 2002); correct use of inhalation therapy (Lavorini et al., 2010; Carone et al., 2002); managing long-term oxygen therapy (Sabato et al., 2014; Dal Negro & Goldberg, 2005). There is one last important topic that is recommended only at international level and ignored in the Italian context: the role of the treatments in improving quality and duration of life (Stoilkova et al., 2013).

Finally, it is important to underline that COPD patients and caregivers further retrieves information on drug consumption and administration by means of: reading Patient Information Leaflets (PILs) (i.e. leaflets enclosed in the medicines she/he regularly takes), watching TV commercials (only in countries where all drug categories can be advertised), and surfing the Internet. Relying on the literature we can state that, on the one hand, the user-friendliness of PILs has been questioned many times (Pander Maat & Lentz, 2010; Raynor, 2007; Gal & Prigat, 2005). On the other, the promotion of drugs directed to consumers through television and the internet is 'still a largely unexplored field, both in terms of the wider potential impact on health consumers, and on medical communication' (Plastina, in press). Focusing on COPD patients, Maglie (in press) addressed Spiriva and Spiriva Respimat drugs, whose PILs were considered best-practice examples of user-friendliness by the Commission on Human Medicines Expert Advisory Group on Patient Information on November 5, 2010. Moreover, Maglie has been investigating Spiriva and Spiriva Respimat product promotion in the pharmaceutical industry, both through narratives on the internet (i.e. patient-volunteered and/or institutional information on how to take the medicine) and through advertising campaigns (i.e. TV commercials) with the aim of researching on how new media both produce medical knowledge, and reinvent the definition of the physician-patient relationship as something more intense and emotive than detached and informative. With regard to Spiriva and Spiriva Respimat PILs, they prove to be real paragons of readability and user-friendliness as far as information design is concerned (i.e. typography and plain language) (Maglie, in press). Notwithstanding these two positive examples, PILs have a long way to go in ameliorating their user-friendliness. A remedial action that should be taken may be to act in compliance with article 59(3) of Council Directive 2001/83/

EC and use questionnaires or other forms of patient consultation to test the leaflet for understanding and usefulness; where problems arise, changes and translations can be further considered.

End-of-Life Care

Communication and education about end-of-life care and advance care planning gives patients the chance to share decisions about the type of care they want and guarantee that their family, physicians and health operators understand their values, goals, and perspectives (Curtis, 2008). Important communication and education topics which regard end-of-life care are recommended at the international level as well as in the Italian best practices: advance care planning (GOLD, 2015, Italian version; Stoilkova et al., 2013; Patel, Janssen, & Curtis, 2012; Carlucci et al., 2012; Vitacca & Comini, 2012); end-of-life decision making (Bettoncelli et al., 2014; Carlucci et al., 2012; Vitacca & Comini, 2012; Casas et al., 2006); prognosis for survival and for quality of life (Bettoncelli et al., 2014; Stoilkova et al., 2013; Curtis, 2008). Advance care planning consists of the process by which patients designate the type of treatment they want to receive in the future if they were no longer able to join in the decision-making process (Fried & O'Leary, 2008). This process has concentrated on the examination of specific treatment interventions and the completion of forms, for instance the living will or other instructional documents (Gillick, 2004). Many doubts have been upraised about this conceptualization, including patient's incapacity to predict their preferences for future treatments (Fagerlin & Schneider, 2004), the complexity in foreseeing all the states a patient may encounter (Gillick, 2004), and the failure to embrace other aspects of end-of-life care that are important to patients, such as lessening the burden on nearest and dearest (Winzelberg et al., 2005). These considerations have led to an innovative concept of advance care planning as a communication process between patients, health professionals and caregivers that goes beyond the reflection on specific treatment interventions. This new concept includes a broader set of problems than treatment decision-making, recognizing the dynamic nature of preferences, and concentrating on barriers to patient-caregiver communication (Fried and O'Leary, 2008).

Patients and their caregivers personify physical, psycho-social and spiritual needs that can meaningfully differ in relation to the disease trajectory they are following (Murray, Kendall, Boyd, & Sheikh, 2005; Seamark et al., 2007). As above mentioned, it consists of a slow deterioration in quality of life interposed by acute exacerbations that patients can only partially recover, until a final crisis occurs that cannot be treated (Murray et al., 2005). Even the best models of survival in COPD patients have a limited capability to predict death for individuals and unexpected deaths occur frequently. This is the main reason why early patient-physician communication about prognosis, preferences for life-sustaining treatments and end of life care is compulsory (Janssen, Engelberg, Wouters, & Curtis, 2012; Curtis, 2008). In this respect, a study addressed the adequacy of professional support perceived by caregivers in their role (Grant et al., 2012). Some caregivers expressed frustration because they had never been told what to expect with the disease trajectory (Spence et al., 2008). Patients and their closest relatives may differ in their preferences to receive information, and family often appreciates the chance to dialogue directly with physicians. Moreover, Curtis (2008) shows that physicians and nurses place more value on quality of life and less value on protracting life than patients or family members. Nevertheless, the patients give higher rates to physicians for listening and answering questions, while they give lower rates for the discussion about prognosis, dying, and spirituality or religion (Curtis et al., 2004).

In Italy, there is one additional problem, since the topic of "understanding what dying might be like" could help decision making, but is regrettably disused even in the best practices or in the guidelines (GOLD, 2015, Italian version; Carlucci et al., 2012). Physicians correspondingly testify that they often fail to discuss end-of-life care with their patients with advanced COPD (Gott et al., 2009). What is more, despite the fact that physicians admit that the suitable timing for these consultations is when patients are well enough to contribute to decision making, these consultations are often originated when patients are too ill to be able to make decisions (Gott et al., 2009). Therefore, all these topics represent specific objectives for interventions to advance communication about end-of-life care (Curtis et al., 2004).

ETHICO-LEGAL SOLUTIONS AND RECOMMENDATIONS TOWARDS COPD PATIENT ENGAGEMENT

In a rapidly changing world of access to health information and exploitation of patients' rights, there is a limited conceptualization available to understand how people can be protected towards their engagement in chronic disease diagnosis and treatment (Johnson, 2011). This happens despite it is increasingly clear that, in order to better encounter patients' rights and needs, patient engagement is necessary to the forefront of medical practice of chronic disease management. In this viewpoint, a deeper attention on COPD patients' rights could help healthcare providers better encounter patients' needs and improve health outcomes by means of their engagement. Following this ethico-legal perspective, key aspects which should be enforced to enhance patient engagement are: the process-based informed consent, the integrated care, and the advance care planning.

As described in the previous paragraphs, an organized communication and education are necessary to give substance to a tangible improvement in the quality of life of the chronic patient, in his/her compliance as well as in the timely and appropriate intervention on the numerous symptoms and side-effects of COPD. In this perspective, informed consent in COPD management represents a key warranty to affirm the obligation of a good communication and relationship that must always accompany the patient clinical pathway. At the present time, in the Italian Health System, legal actions against physicians are 15,000 per year, and a huge increase of costs to refund people injured by therapeutic and diagnostic errors is expected (Messano et al., 2013). One way to limit the damage from potential risks of certain treatments or medical interventions is to activate an effective informed consent process with patients and caregivers. If there is not a good and valid informed consent, even a successful intervention is a source of responsibility, and it is not accidental that also this kind of legal claims is successful and quickly increasing in Italy. Based on the results shown in Table 1a, it is easy to understand how under a legal view, in COPD management there are diverse compensatory hypotheses of responsibility and also of arbitrary medical acts, namely acts which are not accompanied by valid informed consent procedures (Recchia, Dodaro, & Braga, 2013; Terranova et al., 2012; Dodaro & Recchia, 2011). Under the burden of malpractice lawsuits and narrow time to spend per patient, healthcare professionals may find themselves preferring the passive, acquiescent patient over the informed, engaged one (Johnson, 2011). Quite the opposite, there is ample evidence that the patients who are not receiving adequate communication are less serene, less capable of compliance and self-management, and more inclined to raise disputes (Lafata et al., 2013; Moore, Adler, & Robertson, 2000; Levinson, Roter, Mullooly, Dull, & Frankel, 1997). This is mainly because they feel unduly excluded from decisions that affect them closely, and that regard choices based on risk/benefit evaluations, which are finally guided by subjective values and preferences.

Healthcare professionals who are responsible for managing COPD should, within the limits of their powers, first diagnosis and then plan and monitor continuously, together with the patient and his/her caregiver, the organized and shared progress of the disease. Following an integrated care approach, such a sharing, being the result of a constant communication and interpersonal relationship on clinical activities and provided assistance, should always be coordinated among the contexts of the hospital, the territory and the patient's home. In Italy, although the Health System promotes strategies of integrated care for handling COPD, the care pathway should take into account the entire care network, in which a lack of harmonization among different structures at different levels often persists (Calabro, 2014). Informed consent in general, and especially in this chronic-degenerative disease, must therefore be understood as a "wide" legal basis to develop a comprehensive view of organizational communication processes. This is in contrast with the malpractice of simply signing the written consent form, which is regrettably common in Italy and in many countries (Recchia et al., 2013; Terranova et al., 2012; Dodaro & Recchia, 2011). Under this requirement, the health professionals must communicate with the patient before, during and after the execution of any invasive and/or risky act for any disease, being it acute or chronic as COPD. In terms of strict law, in fact, the will of the chronic patient and his/her caregiver cannot be debased merely in the execution of certain medical or nursing treatment without any communicative act. There are circumstances in which patients pursue outcomes such as quality of life and these outcomes do overthrow the defeat of death and disease as the main goals of medical interventions. In these cases, patients' lives rather than patients' bodies should be the focus of medical interventions. This means that - especially in chronic diseases - patients' values should shape the goals as well as the means of medical care. Neither society, nor physicians can assume where pathophysiology fits into the lives of patients (Johnson, 2011; Sullivan, 2003).

On the other hand, in shifting from a paternalistic to a collaborative role, health professionals would have the satisfaction of contributing to the health of more grateful and responsive patients who share decisions, and that indeed would represent a significant progress in health care (Badcott, 2005). This does not mean leaving the patient alone with his/her decisions. On the contrary, this means providing the patient with all the needed information to improve knowledge about risks and benefits, to adjust unrealistic expectations, to elicit values about desired benefits and the degree of individual acceptable risks, in order to autonomously decide. The living wills and advance care planning (which is an ethico-legal approach in addition to a communication/education topic) are affirming, in Italy as well as in other healthcare systems, the right to autonomously decide even though the patient is no longer able to make decisions because of illness or incapacity.

Many communication and education topics and procedures illustrated in the previous paragraphs would enforce patient engagement, but are often neglected or undervalued in the real clinical practice. Those topics and procedures cannot be eluded as far as informed consent, integrated care and advance care planning are fully applied as undeniable patients' rights. Those rights are - as well as patient engagement - all grounded on the universal principle of patient autonomy. This is the common root which should enforce healthcare systems towards improving patient engagement to achieve the best available health outcomes.

FUTURE RESEARCH DIRECTIONS

The main findings from this review provide a conceptual framework to suggest which communication and education topics and actors should be comprehensively implemented to engage patients and caregivers in managing COPD. Many of these communication and education topics should be enclosed in patient and caregiver shared understanding, shared decision-making and responsibility, action taking, motivational dialogues (Osterlund Efraimsson et al., 2009). Although these communication and education topics as well as the involvement of related actors would steadily improve patient engagement and are recommended by international and Italian guidelines about COPD, some of them are ignored in the Italian guidelines, and some of them - although recommended - are neglected or suboptimally implemented in the real clinical practice. These findings open the way to further research opportunities to identify, contextualise and remove barriers which impede the application of those recommendations in each healthcare system and organizational context. Other eventual research opportunities regard the modelling of those topics and actors into specific communication and education processes and their integration into the COPD clinical pathways.

Moreover, it is clear that, within the Italian Health System, each Local Health Unit can involve the recommended actors in different ways and at different levels, on the basis of the specific organizational needs. Modelling each specific communication and education process is not envisaged in the objectives of our article. Nevertheless, we believe that the whole framework illustrated in Table 1a can be used as a good foundation to achieve - in future research efforts - the goals of modelling those processes and integrating them into the COPD clinical pathways.

Finally, the solutions and recommendations descending from the present review highlight the importance of a set of ethico-legal tools - namely informed consent, integrated care, advance care planning - which are suggested to be applied as levers to improve patient engagement, especially wherever the topics enclosed in Table 1a are undervalued in the routine clinical practice. Since patient engagement - as a scientific subject - is commonly treated separately from subjects regarding patients' rights and ethical matters, creating a synergy among those issues in the future research is highly suggested.

CONCLUSION

Results from this review show all the communication and education needs belonging to COPD patients and caregivers, underlining that some of them still remain uncovered in the Italian Health System. Moreover, key actors who should be involved for each specific topic are identified in the whole framework. These findings allow future research to model a communication and education process for each topic as well as to integrate all those processes into the existing COPD clinical pathways. A further support to COPD patients and their caregivers should be provided, aimed at helping the patients better manage their disease and the caregivers cope with their role to reduce their burden and improve their outcomes. All those outcomes should be pursued to achieve a real patient engagement, by way of communication and education programs which should mainly enhance empathy for family emotions as well as the patients' and caregivers' motivation and ability to adapt to COPD.

Moreover, it is highly recommended that already existing legal tools, such as informed consent, integrated care and advance care planning should be better implemented in the healthcare contexts where patient engagement is regarded as a key resource for COPD management. This is a true direction, especially in consideration of the paradigm shift from a paternalistic and physician-centered to a patient-centered view of healthcare, in which patient engagement - as well as the patient rights exploitation - becomes more and more a vital node of care outcomes.

REFERENCES

Ahleit, B. D. (1995). Interventions for clients with lower respiratory problems. In D. D. Ignatavicius, M. L. Workman, & M. A. Mishler (Eds.), *Medical surgical nursing: a nursing process approach* (2nd ed., pp. 673–728). Philadelphia: Saunders WB.

Aldred, H., Gott, M., & Gariballa, S. (2005). Advanced heart failure: Impact on older patients and informal carers. *Journal of Advanced Nursing*, *49*(2), 116–124. doi:10.1111/j.1365-2648.2004.03271.x PMID:15641944

Alwan, A., MacLean, D. R., Riley, L. M., d'Espaignet, E. T., Mathers, C. D., Stevens, G. A., & Bettcher, D. (2010). Monitoring and surveillance of chronic noncommunicable diseases: Progress and capacity in high-burden countries. *Lancet*, *376*(9755), 1861–1868. doi:10.1016/S0140-6736(10)61853-3 PMID:21074258

Badcott, D. (2005). The expert patient: Valid recognition or false hope? *Medicine, Health Care, and Philosophy*, *8*(2), 173–178. doi:10.1007/s11019-005-2275-7 PMID:16215797

Bao, H., Wang, J., Zhou, D., Han, Z., Zhang, Y., Su, L., & Li, Q. et al. (2015). Community Physician-Guided Long-Term Domiciliary Oxygen Therapy Combined with Conventional Therapy in Stage IV COPD Patients. *Rehabilitation Nursing*, (Sep): 10. PMID:26354385

Bergs, D. (2002). "The hidden client"- women caring for husbands with COPD: Their experience of quality of life. *Journal of Clinical Nursing*, *11*(5), 613–621. doi:10.1046/j.1365-2702.2002.00651.x PMID:12201888

Bettoncelli, G., Blasi, F., Brusasco, V., Centanni, S., Corrado, A., De Benedetto, F., & Sanguinetti, C. M. et al. (2014). The clinical and integrated management of COPD. *Sarcoidosis, Vasculitis, and Diffuse Lung Diseases*, *31*, 3–21. PMID:24820963

Bourbeau, J. (2004). Self-management interventions to improve outcomes in patients suffering from COPD. *Expert review of pharmacoeconomics & outcomes research*, 4(1), 71-7.

Bourbeau, J. (2010). Making pulmonary rehabilitation a success in COPD. *Swiss Medical Weekly*, *140*, w13067. PMID:20809435

Bourbeau, J., Julien, M., Maltais, F., Rouleau, M., Beaupré, A., & Bégin, R. et al. & Chronic Obstructive Pulmonary Disease axis of the Respiratory Network Fonds de la Recherche en Santé du Québec. (. (2003). Reduction of hospital utilization in patients with chronic obstructive pulmonary disease: A disease-specific self-management intervention. *Archives of Internal Medicine*, *163*(5), 585–591. doi:10.1001/archinte.163.5.585 PMID:12622605

Buffum, M. D., & Brod, M. (1998). Humor and well-being in spouse caregivers of patients with Alzheimer's disease. *Applied Nursing Research*, *11*(1), 12–18. doi:10.1016/S0897-1897(98)80031-1 PMID:9549154

Cain, J. C., & Wicks, M. N. (2006). Caregivers attributes as correlates of burden in family caregivers coping with chronic obstructive pulmonary disease. *Journal of Family Nursing*, *6*(1), 46–68. doi:10.1177/107484070000600104

Candy, B., Taylor, S. J., Ramsay, J., Esmond, G., Griffiths, C. J., & Bryar, R. M. (2007). Service implications from a comparison of the evidence on the effectiveness and a survey of provision in England and Wales of COPD specialist nurse services in the community. *International Journal of Nursing Studies*, *44*(4), 601–610. doi:10.1016/j.ijnurstu.2005.12.007 PMID:16504198

Carlucci, A., Guerrieri, A., & Nava, S. (2012). Palliative care in COPD patients: Is it only an end-of-life issue? *European Respiratory Review*, *21*(126), 347–354. doi:10.1183/09059180.00001512 PMID:23204123

Carone, M., Bertolotti, G., Cerveri, I., De Benedetto, F., Fogliani, V., Nardini, S., ... & Edu-Care Working Group. (2002). EDU-CARE, a randomised, multicentre, parallel group study on education and quality of life in COPD. Monaldi archives for chest disease = Archivio Monaldi per le malattie del torace/Fondazione clinica del lavoro, IRCCS [and] Istituto di clinica tisiologica e malattie apparato respiratorio, Università di Napoli. *Secondo ateneo, 57*(1), 25-29.

Casale, G., & Calvieri, A. (2014). Palliative care in Italy: A historical perspective. *MEDIC*, *22*(1), 21–26.

Casas, A., Troosters, T., Garcia-Aymerich, J., Roca, J., Hernández, C., Alonso, A., & Decramer, M. (2006). Integrated care prevents hospitalisations for exacerbations in COPD patients. *The European Respiratory Journal*, *28*(1), 123–130. doi:10.1183/09031936.06.00063205 PMID:16611656

Chavannes, N. H., Grijsen, M., van den Akker, M., Schepers, H., Nijdam, M., Tiep, B., & Muris, J. (2009). Integrated disease management improves one-year quality of life in primary care COPD patients: A controlled clinical trial. *Primary Care Respiratory Journal*, *18*(3), 171–176. doi:10.3132/pcrj.2009.00003 PMID:19142557

Cockram, J., Cecins, N., & Jenkins, S. (2006). Maintaining exercise capacity and quality of life following pulmonary rehabilitation. *Respirology (Carlton, Vic.)*, *11*(1), 98–104. doi:10.1111/j.1440-1843.2006.00791.x PMID:16423209

Curtis, J. R. (2008). Palliative and end-of-life care for patients with severe COPD. *The European Respiratory Journal*, *32*(3), 796–803. doi:10.1183/09031936.00126107 PMID:17989116

Curtis, J. R., Engelberg, R., Young, J. P., Vig, L. K., Reinke, L. F., Wenrich, M. D., & Back, A. L. et al. (2008). An approach to understanding the interaction of hope and desire for explicit prognostic information among individuals with severe chronic obstructive pulmonary disease or advanced cancer. *Journal of Palliative Medicine*, *11*(4), 610–620. doi:10.1089/jpm.2007.0209 PMID:18454614

Curtis, J. R., Engelberg, R. A., Nielsen, E. L., Au, D. H., & Patrick, D. L. (2004). Patient-physician communication about end-of-life care for patients with severe COPD. *The European Respiratory Journal*, *24*(2), 200–205. doi:10.1183/09031936.04.00010104 PMID:15332385

Dal Negro, R. W., & Goldberg, A. I. (Eds.). (2005). *Home Long-term oxygen treatment in Italy. The additional value of telemedicine* (pp. 71–85). Springer Publ. doi:10.1007/88-470-0448-9

Dodaro, A., & Recchia, V. (2011). Inappropriateness in ionizing imaging. The central node of the informed consent: From "event" model to "process" model. *Recenti Progressi in Medicina*, *102*, 421–431. PMID:22120778

Fagerlin, A., & Schneider, C. E. (2004). Enough: The failure of the living will. *The Hastings Center Report*, *34*(2), 30–42. doi:10.2307/3527683 PMID:15156835

Fried, T. R., & O'Leary, J. R. (2008). Using the experiences of bereaved caregivers to inform patient- and caregiver-centered advance care planning. *Journal of General Internal Medicine*, *23*(10), 1602–1607. doi:10.1007/s11606-008-0748-0 PMID:18665427

Fromer, L. (2011). Implementing chronic care for COPD: Planned visits, care coordination, and patient empowerment for improved outcomes. *International Journal of Chronic Obstructive Pulmonary Disease*, *6*, 605–614. doi:10.2147/COPD.S24692 PMID:22162647

Garlo, K., O'Leary, J. R., Van Ness, P. H., & Fried, T. R. (2010). Burden in caregivers of older adults with advanced illness. *Journal of the American Geriatrics Society*, *58*(12), 2315–2322. doi:10.1111/j.1532-5415.2010.03177.x PMID:21087225

Giacomini, M., DeJean, D., Simeonov, D., & Smith, A. (2012). Experiences of living and dying with COPD: A systematic review and synthesis of the qualitative empirical literature. *Archive of. Ontario Health Technology Assessment Series*, *12*(13), 1–47. PMID:23074423

Gillick, M. R. (2004). Advance care planning. *The New England Journal of Medicine*, *350*(1), 7–8. doi:10.1056/NEJMp038202 PMID:14702421

Glasgow, R. E., Toobert, D. J., Riddle, M., Donnelly, J., Mitchell, D. L., & Calder, D. (1989). Diabetes-specific social learning variables and self-care behaviors among persons with type II diabetes. *Health Psychology*, *8*(3), 285–303. doi:10.1037/0278-6133.8.3.285 PMID:2767020

Global Initiative for Chronic Obstructive Lung Disease (GOLD). (2015). *Global Strategy for the Diagnosis, Management, and Prevention of Chronic Obstructive Lung Disease*. Updated 2015. Global Initiative for Chronic Obstructive Lung Disease, Inc. Retrieved from http://www.goldcopd.org/uploads/users/files/GOLD_Report_2015_Sept2.pdf

Global Initiative for Chronic Obstructive Lung Disease (GOLD). (2015). *Strategia globale per la diagnosi, il trattamento e la prevenzione della broncopneumopatia cronica ostruttiva. Updated 2015*. Global Initiative for Chronic Obstructive Lung Disease, Inc. Retrieved from http://www.goldcopd.it/materiale/2015/GOLD_workshop_report_2015.pdf

Gore, J. M., Brophy, C. J., & Greenstone, M. A. (2000). How well do we care for patients with end stage chronic obstructive pulmonary disease (COPD)? A comparison of palliative care and quality of life in COPD and lung cancer. *Thorax*, *55*(12), 1000–1006. doi:10.1136/thorax.55.12.1000 PMID:11083884

Gott, M., Gardiner, C., Small, N., Payne, S., Seamark, D., Barnes, S., & Ruse, C. et al. (2009). Barriers to advance care planning in chronic obstructive pulmonary disease. *Palliative Medicine*, *23*(7), 642–648. doi:10.1177/0269216309106790 PMID:19648222

Graffigna, G., Barello, S., & Triberti, S. (2015). Giving (Back) a Role to Patients in the Delivery of Healthcare Services: Theoretical Roots of Patient Engagement. In G. Graffigna, S. Barello, & S. Triberti (Eds.), *Patient Engagement. A Consumer-Centered Model to Innovate Healthcare* (pp. 13–26). Berlin: De Gruyter Open. doi:10.1515/9783110452440-003

Grant, M., Cavanagh, A., & Yorke, J. (2012). The impact of caring for those with chronic obstructive pulmonary disease (COPD) on carers' psychological well-being: A narrative review. *International Journal of Nursing Studies*, (Mar): 2. PMID:22386988

Gruman, J., Rovner, M. H., French, M. E., Jeffress, D., Sofaer, S., Shaller, D., & Prager, D. J. (2010). From patient education to patient engagement: Implications for the field of patient education. *Patient Education and Counseling*, *78*(3), 350–356. doi:10.1016/j.pec.2010.02.002 PMID:20202780

Gulati, M. (2011). Diagnostic assessment of patients with interstitial lung disease. *Primary Care Respiratory Journal*, *20*(2), 120–127. doi:10.4104/pcrj.2010.00079 PMID:21509417

Hibbard, J. H., Mahoney, E. R., Stock, R., & Tusler, M. (2007). Do increases in patient activation result in improved self-management behaviors? *Health Services Research*, *42*(4), 1443–1463. doi:10.1111/j.1475-6773.2006.00669.x PMID:17610432

Hudson, B. (2005). Sea change or quick fix? Policy on long term conditions in England. *Health & Social Care in the Community*, *13*(4), 378–385. doi:10.1111/j.1365-2524.2005.00579.x PMID:15969709

Janssen, D. J., Engelberg, R. A., Wouters, E. F., & Curtis, J. R. (2012). Advance care planning for patients with COPD: Past, present and future. *Patient Education and Counseling*, *86*(1), 19–24. doi:10.1016/j.pec.2011.01.007 PMID:21316899

Johnson, M. O. (2011). The shifting landscape of health care: Toward a model of health care empowerment. *American Journal of Public Health*, *101*(2), 265–270. doi:10.2105/AJPH.2009.189829 PMID:21164096

Knauft, E., Nielsen, E. L., Engelberg, R. A., Patrick, D. L., & Curtis, J. R. (2005). Barriers and facilitators to end-of-life care communication for patients with COPD. *Chest*, *127*(6), 2188–2196. doi:10.1378/chest.127.6.2188 PMID:15947336

Kruis, A. L., & Chavannes, N. H. (2010). Potential benefits of integrated COPD management in primary care. *Monaldi Archives for Chest Disease*, *73*(3), 130–134. PMID:21214043

Lacasse, Y., Brosseau, L., Milne, S., Martin, S., Wong, E., Guyatt, G. H., & Goldstein, R. S. (2002). Pulmonary rehabilitation for chronic obstructive pulmonary disease. *Cochrane Database of Systematic Reviews*, (3): CD003793. PMID:12137716

Lafata, J. E., Morris, H. L., Dobie, E., Heisler, M., Werner, R. M., & Dumenci, L. (2013). Patient-reported use of collaborative goal setting and glycemic control among patients with diabetes. *Patient Education and Counseling*, *92*(1), 94–99. doi:10.1016/j.pec.2013.01.016 PMID:23433777

Lavorini, F., Levy, M. L., Corrigan, C., & Crompton, G.ADMIT Working Group. (2010). The ADMIT series–Issues in Inhalation Therapy. 6) Training tools for inhalation devices. *Primary Care Respiratory Journal*, *19*(4), 335–341. doi:10.4104/pcrj.2010.00065 PMID:21049263

Levinson, W., Roter, D. L., Mullooly, J. P., Dull, V. T., & Frankel, R. M. (1997). Physician-patient communication. The relationship with malpractice claims among primary care physicians and surgeons. *Journal of the American Medical Association*, *277*(7), 553–559. doi:10.1001/jama.1997.03540310051034 PMID:9032162

Lopez, A. D., & Murray, C. C. (1998). The global burden of disease, 1990–2020. *Nature Medicine*, *4*(11), 1241–1243. doi:10.1038/3218 PMID:9809543

Lusuardi, M., De Benedetto, F., Paggiaro, P., Sanguinetti, C. M., Brazzola, G., Ferri, P., & Donner, C. F. (2006). A Randomized Controlled Trial on Office Spirometry in Asthma and COPD in Standard General Practice. *Chest*, *129*(4), 844–852. doi:10.1378/chest.129.4.844 PMID:16608929

Maglie, R. (in press). Can you read this leaflet? User-friendliness of Patient Information Leaflets in the UK and in Italy.*Proceedings of the International Conference hosted by CERLIS, The language of Medicine: Science, Practice and Academia*, University of Bergamo.

Mallampalli, A. (2004). Nutritional management of the patient with chronic obstructive pulmonary disease. *Nutrition in Clinical Practice*, *19*(6), 550–556. doi:10.1177/0115426504019006550 PMID:16215153

Maurer, J., Rebbapragada, V., Borson, S., Goldstein, R., Kunik, M. E., Yohannes, A. M., & Hanania, N. A. (2008). Anxiety and depression in COPD: current understanding, unanswered questions, and research needs. *Chest Journal, 134(4_suppl)*, 43S-56S.

Messano, G. A., Spaziani, E., Turchetta, F., Ceci, F., Corelli, S., Casciaro, G., & Stagnitti, F. et al. (2013). Risk management in surgery. *Il Giornale di Chirurgia -. The Journal of Surgery*, *34*(7-8), 231–237.

Ministero della Salute. (2010). *Piano nazionale della prevenzione 2010–2012*.

Monninkhof, E., van der Valk, P., van der Palen, J., van Herwaarden, C., & Zielhuis, G. (2003). Effects of a comprehensive self-management programme in patients with chronic obstructive pulmonary disease. *The European Respiratory Journal*, *22*(5), 815–820. doi:10.1183/09031936.03.00047003 PMID:14621090

Moore, P. J., Adler, N. E., & Robertson, P. A. (2000). Medical malpractice: The effect of doctor-patient relations on medical patient perceptions and malpractice intentions. *The Western Journal of Medicine*, *173*(4), 244–250. doi:10.1136/ewjm.173.4.244 PMID:11017984

Murphy, K., Casey, D., Devane, D., Cooney, A., McCarthy, B., Mee, L., & O'Shea, E. et al. (2011). A cluster randomised controlled trial evaluating the effectiveness of a structured pulmonary rehabilitation education programme for improving the health status of people with chronic obstructive pulmonary disease (COPD): The PRINCE study protocol. *BMC Pulmonary Medicine*, *11*(1), 4. doi:10.1186/1471-2466-11-4 PMID:21244668

Murray, S. A., Kendall, M., Boyd, K., & Sheikh, A. (2005). Illness trajectories and palliative care. *BMJ (Clinical Research Ed.)*, *330*(7498), 1007–1011. doi:10.1136/bmj.330.7498.1007 PMID:15860828

Osterlund Efraimsson, E., Klang, B., Larsson, K., Ehrenberg, A., & Fossum, B. (2009). Communication and self-management education at nurse-led COPD clinics in primary health care. *Patient Education and Counseling*, *77*(2), 209–217. doi:10.1016/j.pec.2009.03.033 PMID:19414234

Pander Maat, H., & Lentz, L. (2010). Improving the Usability of Patient Information Leaflets. *Patient Education and Counseling*, *80*(1), 113–119. doi:10.1016/j.pec.2009.09.030 PMID:19854022

Pasqua, F., Biscione, G. L., Crigna, G., Gargano, R., Cardaci, V., Ferri, L., & Clini, E. et al. (2009). Use of functional independence measure in rehabilitation of inpatients with respiratory failure. *Respiratory Medicine*, *103*(3), 471–476. doi:10.1016/j.rmed.2008.09.007 PMID:18977645

Patel, K., Janssen, D. J., & Curtis, J. R. (2012). Advance care planning in COPD. *Respirology (Carlton, Vic.)*, *17*(1), 72–78. doi:10.1111/j.1440-1843.2011.02087.x PMID:22008225

Pauwels, R. A., Buist, A. S., Calverley, P. M. A., Jenkins, C. R., & Hurd, S. S.NHLBI/WHO. (2001). NHLBI/WHO global strategy for the diagnosis, management, and prevention of chronic obstructive pulmonary disease. *American Journal of Respiratory and Critical Care Medicine*, *163*(5), 1256–1276. doi:10.1164/ajrccm.163.5.2101039 PMID:11316667

Payne, S., Smith, P., & Dean, S. (1999). Identifying the concerns of informal carers in palliative care. *Palliative Medicine*, *13*(1), 37–44. doi:10.1191/026921699666872524 PMID:10320874

Plastina, A. F. (in press). Patient (Mis)understanding of Prescription Drug Ads in Social Media: Multimodal Discourse Analysis of eDTCA. *Proceedings of the International Conference hosted by CERLIS, The language of Medicine: Science, Practice and Academia*, University of Bergamo.

Raynor, D. K. (2007). The Importance of Medicines Information for Patients. *Prescriber*, *18*(2), 60–62. doi:10.1002/psb.15

Recchia, V., Dodaro, A., & Braga, L. (2013). Event-based versus process-based informed consent to address scientific evidence and uncertainties in ionising medical imaging. *Insights into Imaging*, *4*(5), 647–653. doi:10.1007/s13244-013-0272-6 PMID:23904249

Rich, M. W., Beckham, V., Wittenberg, C., Leven, C. L., Freedland, K. E., & Carney, R. M. (1995). A multidisciplinary intervention to prevent the readmission of elderly patients with congestive heart failure. *The New England Journal of Medicine*, *333*(18), 1190–1195. doi:10.1056/NEJM199511023331806 PMID:7565975

Sabato, E., Leo, C. G., & Sabina, S. (2009). Continuity of health care in patients with chronic respiratory insufficiency: A macro-model of care integration between hospital and home. *Multidisciplinary Respiratory Medicine*, *4*, 112–120.

Sabato, E., Sabina, S., & Leo, C. G. (2014). Standard Care. In R. W. Dal Negro & R. V. Hodder (Eds.), *Long-Term Oxygen Therapy New Insights and perspectives* (pp. 161–170). Springer-Verlag Italia Srl.

Santus, P., Picciolo, S., Proietto, A., Falcone, F., Mangiacavallo, A., Pellegrino, G., & Centanni, S. et al. (2012). Doctor-patient relationship: A resource to improve respiratory diseases management. *European Journal of Internal Medicine*, *23*(5), 442–446. doi:10.1016/j.ejim.2012.04.004 PMID:22726373

Seamark, D., Blake, S., Seamark, C., Hyland, M. E., Greaves, C., Pinnuck, M., ... & East Devon Respiratory Research Group. (2012). Is hospitalisation for COPD an opportunity for advance care planning? A qualitative study. *Primary care respiratory journal: journal of the General Practice Airways Group*, 21(3), 261-266.

Sexton, D. L., & Munro, B. H. (1985). Impact of a husband's chronic illness (COPD) on the spouse's life. *Research in Nursing & Health*, *8*(1), 83–90. doi:10.1002/nur.4770080115 PMID:3846320

Sharma, G., Kuo, Y. F., Freeman, J. L., Zhang, D. D., & Goodwin, J. S. (2010). Outpatient follow-up visit and 30-day emergency department visit and readmission in patients hospitalized for chronic obstructive pulmonary disease. *Archives of Internal Medicine*, *170*(18), 1664–1670. doi:10.1001/archinternmed.2010.345 PMID:20937926

Shipman, C., White, S., Gysels, M., & White, P. (2009). Access to care in advanced COPD: Factors that influence contact with general practice services. *Primary Care Respiratory Journal*, *18*(4), 273–278. doi:10.4104/pcrj.2009.00013 PMID:19333517

Spence, A., Hasson, F., Waldron, M., Kernohan, G., McLaughlin, D., Cochrane, B., & Watson, B. (2008). Active carers: Living with chronic obstructive pulmonary disease. *International Journal of Palliative Nursing*, *14*(8), 368–372. doi:10.12968/ijpn.2008.14.8.30771 PMID:19023952

Spruit, M. A., Singh, S. J., Garvey, C., ZuWallack, R., Nici, L., Rochester, C., & Wouters, E. F. et al. (2013). An official American Thoracic Society/European Respiratory Society statement: Key concepts and advances in pulmonary rehabilitation. *American Journal of Respiratory and Critical Care Medicine*, *188*(8), e13–e64. doi:10.1164/rccm.201309-1634ST PMID:24127811

Stewart, M. A. (1995). Effective physician–patient communication and health outcomes: A review. *Canadian Medical Association Journal*, *152*, 1423–1433. PMID:7728691

Stoilkova, A., Janssen, D. J., & Wouters, E. F. (2013). Educational programmes in COPD management interventions: A systematic review. *Respiratory Medicine*, *107*(11), 1637–1650. doi:10.1016/j.rmed.2013.08.006 PMID:24012387

Sullivan, M. (2003). The new subjective medicine: Taking the patient's point of view on health care and health. *Social Science & Medicine*, *56*(7), 1595–1604. doi:10.1016/S0277-9536(02)00159-4 PMID:12614708

Terranova, G., Ferro, M., Carpeggiani, C., Recchia, V., Braga, L., Semelka, R. C., & Picano, E. (2012). Low quality and lack of clarity of current informed consent forms in cardiology: How to improve them. *JACC: Cardiovascular Imaging*, *5*(6), 649–655. doi:10.1016/j.jcmg.2012.03.007 PMID:22698536

The SUPPORT Principal Investigators. (1995). A controlled trial to improve care for seriously ill hospitalized patients: The study to understand prognoses and preferences for outcomes and risks of treatments (SUPPORT). *Journal of the American Medical Association*, *274*, 1591–1598. doi:10.1001/jama.1995.03530200027032 PMID:7474243

Thomas, C. (2014). The role of the social worker. *Nephrology News & Issues*, *28*(2), 23–24. PMID:24649752

Tiep, B., & Carter, R. (2008). Oxygen conserving devices and methodologies. *Chronic Respiratory Disease*, *5*(2), 109–114. doi:10.1177/1479972308090691 PMID:18539725

Tunsäter, A., Moutakis, M., Borg, S., Persson, U., Strömberg, L., & Nielsen, A. L. (2007). Retrospective incremental cost analysis of a hospital-based COPD Disease Management Programme in Sweden. *Health Policy (Amsterdam)*, *81*(2-3), 309–319. doi:10.1016/j.healthpol.2006.05.013 PMID:16904788

Van Boven, J. F. M., Vegter, S., Van Der Molen, T., & Postma, M. J. (2013). COPD in the working age population: The economic impact on both patients and government. *COPD: Journal of Chronic Obstructive Pulmonary Disease*, *10*(6), 629–639. doi:10.3109/15412555.2013.813446 PMID:23845002

Vermylen, J. H., Szmuiowicz, E., & Kalhan, R. (2015). Palliative care in COPD: An unmet area for quality improvement. *International Journal of Chronic Obstructive Pulmonary Disease*, *10*, 1543–1551. doi:10.2147/COPD.S74641 PMID:26345486

Visse, M. A., Teunissen, T., Peters, A., Widdershoven, G. A., & Abma, T. A. (2010). Dialogue for air, air for dialogue: Towards shared responsibilities in COPD practice. *Health Care Analysis*, *18*(4), 358–373. doi:10.1007/s10728-009-0139-7 PMID:20063199

Vitacca, M., & Comini, L. (2012). How do patients die in a rehabilitative unit dedicated to advanced respiratory diseases? *Multidisciplinary Respiratory Medicine*, *7*(1), 18. doi:10.1186/2049-6958-7-18 PMID:22958591

Voelkel, N. F. (2000). Raising awareness of COPD in primary care. *Chest*, *117*(5), 372s–375s. doi:10.1378/chest.117.5_suppl_2.372S PMID:10843979

Wagner, E. H. (2000). The role of patient care teams in chronic disease management. *British Medical Journal, 320*(7234), 569–572. doi:10.1136/bmj.320.7234.569 PMID:10688568

Walters, J. (2010). COPD - Diagnosis, management and the role of the GP. *Australian Family Physician, 39*(3), 100–103. PMID:20369108

Walters, J. A., Turnock, A. C., Walters, E. H., & Wood-Baker, R. (2010). Action plans with limited patient education only for exacerbations of chronic obstructive pulmonary disease. *Cochrane Database of Systematic Reviews, 5*, CD005074. PMID:20464737

WHO World Health Organization. (2008a). *World Health Statistics*. Switzerland: World Health Organization.

WHO World Health Organization. (2008b). The global burden of disease: 2004 update. Geneva.

Winzelberg, G. S., Hanson, L. C., & Tulsky, J. A. (2005). Beyond autonomy: Diversifying end-of-life decision-making approaches to serve patients and families. *Journal of the American Geriatrics Society, 53*(6), 1046–1050. doi:10.1111/j.1532-5415.2005.53317.x PMID:15935032

Yawn, B. P., & Kaplan, A. (2008). Co-morbidities in people with COPD: A result of multiple diseases, or multiple manifestations of smoking and reactive inflammation? *Primary Care Respiratory Journal, 17*(4), 199–205. doi:10.3132/pcrj.2008.00021 PMID:18338090

Zwerink, M., Brusse-Keizer, M., van der Valk, P. D., Zielhuis, G. A., Monninkhof, E. M., van der Palen, J., & Effing, T. et al. (2014). Self management for patients with chronic obstructive pulmonary disease. *Cochrane Database of Systematic Reviews, 3*, CD002990. PMID:24665053

KEY TERMS AND DEFINITIONS

Actors: They are all the individuals - both laypeople and healthcare providers - involved in communication and education processes in the management of a disease.

Advance Care Planning: The process that facilitates patients' identification and clarification of their personal values and goals about health and medical treatment. Ideally, it is a process of structured discussion and documentation entwined with the regular process of healthcare that should be reviewed and updated on a regular basis. It is conceived to guarantee that a patient's wishes will be honored in the event that the patient is unable to take part in decision making.

Chronic Obstructive Pulmonary Disease (COPD): A long-term lung disease that causes multiple disease-related symptoms (e.g. shortness of breath and coughing, pain, fatigue, loss of appetite, dyspnoea, phlegm, chest tightness, exercise intolerance, sleep disorders as well as loneliness and restriction of social activities). Being COPD a chronic and not fully reversible disease, its treatment requires further development of new healthcare models intended for chronic conditions (new models of patient activation, participation and self-management).

Exacerbation: It refers to an increase in the severity of a disease or in any of its signs or symptoms. In particular, COPD exacerbation is connected with acute and general impairment of the functioning of respiratory and peripheral skeletal muscles.

Informed Consent: The process whereby the patient and the healthcare professional enter into a constructive dialogue about a proposed medical diagnostic or therapeutic technique with respect to its nature, consequences, harms, benefits, risks, and alternatives.

Integrated Care: It is the result of a constant communication and interpersonal relationship on clinical activities and provided assistance, which should always be coordinated among the contexts of the hospital, the territory and the patient's home.

Patient Autonomy: Mostly, patient autonomy is theorized as the patients' right to make informed decisions about their own care without unnecessary influence or manipulation from others. A central principle of autonomy is that, given suitable information and personal freedom, individuals should be able to make decisions concordant with their own value, preferences, circumstances and opinions. Patient autonomy enhances patient engagement to achieve the best available health outcomes.

Self-Management: It refers to any formal patient education program that highlights the patients' central role in managing the symptoms, treatments, physical and psychosocial consequences and life style changes inherent in living with a chronic condition. Specifically, the program is aimed at improving skills needed to carry out medical interventions specific to the disease, health behavior change, and emotional support for patients to control their disease and functional lives.

Chapter 3
The Power of Words: Deliberation Dialogue as a Model to Favor Patient Engagement in Chronic Care

Sarah Bigi
Catholic University of the Sacred Heart, Italy

Giulia Lamiani
University of Milan, Italy

ABSTRACT

The concept of patient engagement is attracting growing attention from scholars working on doctor-patient interactions. It refers to the condition in which patients are fully aware of their medical condition and willing to be active both in the relationship with their caregivers and towards the health care institutions. However, the operative steps necessary to achieve patient engagement have not yet been fully described. This chapter focuses on the communicative dimension of engagement. Communication is shown to be a pivotal means to improve patient self-efficacy and commitment, both fundamental components of engagement. In particular, the authors take a closer look at the process of decision making in chronic care settings, and propose a normative model to analyze and evaluate the quality of decision making in consultations. It is argued that the model can also be used as a blueprint to create training materials for clinicians.

DOI: 10.4018/978-1-5225-0663-8.ch003

INTRODUCTION

Chronic illnesses such as diabetes, hypertension, and asthma - just to name a few - are nowadays common occurrences in the lives of many individuals. Modern Western lifestyle and the aging population will lead, in the next decades, to an increase in the number of people suffering from chronic diseases (Visser, 2000). Chronicity imposes new challenges to the clinician-patient relationship. As chronic diseases are by nature treatable but not curable, it becomes essential for healthcare providers to engage patients in their care and promote patients' self-management and compliance to treatment in order to maintain a good health (Assal, 1999; Coleman, Austin, Brach, & Wagner, 2009; Nuño, Coleman, Bengoa, & Sauto, 2012).

Recently, the literature on chronic care has focused on the concept of patient engagement. Patient engagement has been generally described as a result of the relationship between patients and health care providers as they work together to "support active patient and public involvement in health and healthcare and to strengthen their influence on healthcare decisions, at both the individual and collective levels" (Coulter, 2011, p. 10). Engagement has also been described as a complex process of exchanges that occur between the patient and the health care system (Graffigna, Barello, Riva, & Bosio, 2014, p. 87), capable of producing positive psychosocial changes in patients and better quality of life (Barello & Graffigna, 2014). A recent model developed by Graffigna et al. (2014) defined patient engagement as a dynamic process, in which patients experience four phases (blackout, arousal, adhesion and eudaimonic project), each encompassing emotional, cognitive and behavioral dimensions. According to this model, engagement is the final outcome of a series of emotional, cognitive and behavioral reframing of the patient's health condition (Barello & Graffigna, 2014). Specifically, fully engaged patients are able to integrate the disease into their identity and life, manage their own care and mobilize healthcare services proactively if needed. As characterized by the literature, patient engagement can be described as an emotional, cognitive and behavioral change. Patient engagement therefore implies a greater ability and motivation to solve health-related problems, the exchange of relevant information with clinicians, shared decision-making, the capacity to cope with complications and follow through with treatment (Barello & Graffigna, 2014).

In the literature, engagement has been mainly described at an individual level in terms of patient's experience and patient's behaviors. However, engagement is promoted and sustained in the verbal day-by-day interactions between the patient and the healthcare providers (Thompson, 2007). More specifically, as a process supporting a proactive role of patients regarding their own health, patient engagement is promoted in the relationships between patients and clinicians within the consultations (Charles, Gafni, & Whelan, 1997, 1999; Epstein & Street, 2011; Street, Elwyn, & Epstein, 2012).

The process of patient engagement, as proposed in the literature, seems to include at least three dimensions that can only be dealt with through communicative processes: motivation, the exchange of relevant information with clinicians, and shared decision-making (Barello & Graffigna, 2014). Several strategies have been identified for clinicians to help patients move along the process of engagement, such as offering clear information on their condition, strengthening motivation to adopt healthy lifestyles, promoting self-efficacy, reinforcing healthy behaviors, and valuing patients' responsibility towards their own health (Graffigna et al., 2014). However, little is known about what specific clinician-patient communicative behaviors could sustain engagement in clinical consultations. In this contribution, we propose the model of the deliberation dialogue (Walton & Krabbe, 1995; Walton, 2006; Walton, Toniolo, & Norman, 2014) as a tool for the analysis of clinician-patient verbal interactions that can help distinguish and assess the components of engagement-oriented dialogues within chronic care consultations.

Previous studies have taken into account different aspects of the challenge of supporting patients' engagement. The present contribution will focus on the aspects of this challenge pertaining to the dimension of verbal communication, particularly to the process of deliberation. Specifically, in this chapter we will first offer a theoretical background on the studies that have addressed the issue of communication and behavior change in chronic care. Then we will describe the model of the deliberation dialogue as a tool to deepen and specify the analysis of medical consultations, which may lead to a better understanding of the communicative processes that are relevant to achieve patient engagement and behavior change. Finally we will offer examples of the application of this model within the setting of chronic care encounters.

BACKGROUND

In this section we provide a brief overview of studies addressing the complex issue of achieving behavior change by highlighting in particular the factors that have been found to have a significant impact on commitment and task performance.

Among the vast literature on behavior change, our intention is to point out a few significant studies that are helpful to understand which are the factors at play in the complex process of eliciting and sustaining behavior change. More specifically, we will focus on those factors that are communicative in nature (e.g., information sharing) or are realized at least in part through communicative exchanges (e.g., self-efficacy). We address first the literature referring to communication and behavior change in the medical encounter and, following, a few studies that have focused on the connection between goals and commitment.

Communication and Behavior Change

The literature addressing the issue of behavior change in the medical encounter is quite concordant in stressing the pivotal role of participatory communication, collaborative goal setting and shared decision-making.

Proactive, participatory patient-provider communication styles have been acknowledged in the literature as pivotal for the improvement of patient outcomes (Lafata et al., 2013). Studies across several chronic settings - such as diabetes, hypertension, cancer and lupus - suggest that patients who are more communicatively involved in their consultations, who express their concerns and who interact with more patient-centered and informative clinicians experience better outcomes (Street et al., 1993).

Studies also suggest that the most relevant moments in constructing effective patient-provider collaboration are collaborative definition of problems, goal setting and planning (Heisler, Bouknight, Hayward, Smith, & Kerr, 2002). Heisler et al. (2003) show that patients who shared in treatment decision-making and discussed the relevant content areas with their physicians were more likely to display agreement with the physicians. Such agreement is positively correlated with health outcomes. However, it is not clear which are the factors that favor or impede patient-provider agreement on treatment goals and strategies. Moreover, it also looks like collaborative goal setting is not equally beneficial under certain conditions: if, for example, the communication exchanges do not facilitate a positive patient-clinician rapport or patients' confidence to achieve goals set during the exchange (Lafata et al., 2013).

Scholars have also highlighted the importance of involving patients in their health management through the concept of shared decision-making (Epstein & Street, 2011; Elwyn et al., 2012). Addressing more specifically the components of decision-making, Epstein and Gramling (2013) highlight the crucial role of exploring patients' preferences, which in the clinical practice are often contextual, conditional and provisional. Empirical evidence has also shown that patients involved in shared decision-making consultations, where clinicians and patients negotiated a treatment regimen that accommodated patient goals and preferences, reported better adherence and clinical outcomes than patients involved in clinician decision-making consultations (Wilson et al., 2010).

In summary, it seems that more active involvement of all participants in the consultation may achieve better results, both at the clinical level and at the level of participants' satisfaction. However, it is not clear whether this is true under all circumstances, nor how to achieve practically more participatory interaction styles. In order to answer these questions, it is probably useful to take a short detour and take into consideration a few studies from the literature on decision-making and behavior change developed since the late 1950s'.

From Goals to Commitment

Ever since the late 1950s' a growing body of studies developed, which addressed the issue of decision-making and behavior change, trying to explain the processes and factors at play in the formation of goals and in the passage from goals to intentions to actual behavior. Many of these studies suggest that behavior change can be cultivated and sustained. The question is therefore what allows to cultivate and sustain behavior change.

According to the theory of planned behavior (Ajzen, 1988, 1991, 2002; Glanz, Rimer, & Viswanath, 2008), human behavior is guided by three kinds of considerations: positive or negative attitudes towards a certain behavior, which are determined by beliefs about the likely consequences or other attributes of the behavior (behavioral beliefs); perceived social pressure, or subjective norm, which is determined by beliefs about the normative expectations of other people (normative beliefs); and perceived behavioral control, which is caused by beliefs about the presence of factors that may further or hinder performance of the behavior (control beliefs). These three elements in combination give rise to behavioral intention, which is considered to be the immediate antecedent to behavior.

In this description, intention is a concept similar to the idea of commitment, i.e. the decision to allocate resources for the achievement of a goal. However, both intention and commitment need to be triggered and supported through time, especially if the aim is to move from a temporary behavior change to consistent new behaviors (such as is the goal of chronic care, when it comes to the issue of patients' lifestyles) (Becker, 1960; Prochaska, Di Clemente, & Norcross, 1992).

Among the relevant dimensions to take into consideration in order to understand the strength of commitment is the system of values in which individuals form their decisions (Becker, 1960), which is the underlying system that sustains the formation of preferences (Boyd et al., 2012, pp. 32-33). It can sometimes happen that individuals express preferences that deviate from their value system. This happens especially in cases of uncertainty and lack of correct or complete information (Epstein & Gramling, 2013, p. 102S).

Other studies discuss how much the process of goal-setting can impact on task performance. Specifically, studies found that the quality of goal-setting can impact on performance, meaning that goal specificity makes a difference in how a task is carried out (Baca-Motes, Brown, Gneezy, Keenan, & Nelson, 2013). Also the degree of self-efficacy was found to have an impact on goal-setting, so that when the goals are self-set, people with higher self-efficacy will set higher goals, will be more committed to the set goal, find and use better strategies to reach them, and will respond better to negative feedback than people with lower self-efficacy (Locke & Latham, 2002).

Finally, participatory goal-setting does not seem to impact directly on the performance of tasks, but rather via self-efficacy. In other words, the fact that people are given the possibility to self-set their goals has an impact more at a cognitive level than at the motivational one, because it stimulates the exchange of information. Exchanging information appears to be an important element in the quality of performance, because in a number of experiments people who could *self-set* their goals performed much better than people who had been *assigned* goals *only* in the cases in which the latter had received no explanations regarding the goals, i.e. when there had been no exchange of relevant information regarding the goals. This leads to believe that one relevant component of self-efficacy is having relevant information and training regarding the problem and possible solutions to it (Locke & Latham, 2002).

Summing up and considering only the factors that are relevant on the communicative level: goal specificity; self-setting goals or having goals assigned together with explanations about them; and, information exchanges seem to be pivotal elements around which decision-making develops and, with it, commitment and behavior change. These factors indicate a procedural hierarchy in the steps that lead from the formation of a goal to consistent behavior. First, a value system seems to be the context within which goals are defined according to evaluations of situations or hypothesized outcomes of an action (Becker, 1960). For example, I might decide to stop smoking because I consider good health to be a high value; on the contrary, my friend might refuse to do the same, because she values more highly the pleasure that smoking can give her. Second, self-efficacy seems to play a significant role for the process of goal-setting, for the degree of commitment once the goal has been set or assigned, and for the quality of the effort a person will put into achieving it. One relevant component of self-efficacy seems to be the possession of adequate information to understand the issue at hand, the goal and the resources needed to achieve it. This should also be relevant for the definition of attitudes and perceived behavioral control (Ajzen, 2002). Finally, the possibility to set one's own goals – as opposed to having goals assigned – seems to be more effective only if there is a high degree of self-efficacy.

Open Problems and Possible Pathways to Solutions

The discussion conducted in the previous sections has helped us define more clearly the problem we are addressing: two elements at the core of patient engagement are information sharing and shared decision-making between clinicians and patients. Indeed, literature indicates that better health outcomes are obtained when values and information are shared and specific goals are assigned, or set. These are goals that can be reached through verbal communication, but it is necessary to be able to characterize the dialogical dimension of information sharing and decision-making in order to plan interventions. Therefore it is crucial to proceed from an adequate theoretical model, able to explain the dialogical complexity of chronic care consultations.

In what follows, we will refer to dialogue and not to communication in general because we are addressing, first of all, the dimension of *verbal communication*, and secondly, the structure of the interaction intended as a communicative action, performed with the aim to reach a precise goal and following specific steps to achieve the goal (Grice, 1975; van Eemeren & Grootendorst, 2004). Moreover, the focus of this chapter on the dialogue structure is motivated by the need to address the higher level components first, and then move into the specificities of communication strategies and techniques.

In the following sections, we will first introduce the theoretical approach to the analysis of dialogues we adopted; we will then focus on the deliberation dialogue as a specific type of dialogue, useful to better understand the dialogical process that leads to patient engagement.

DIALOGUE TYPES AND DIALOGUE PROFILES

When we talk about dialogues, we refer to communicative intentions, or aims, like information giving, or deliberation, that have the same value of the aims we have when we want to obtain something, like for example, to build a house. In both cases, we will have to initiate a chain of actions that will lead us to the achievement of the final goal. Depending on the aims that people have when they interact in different contexts, there are different dialogue types. The main dialogue types are: information-seeking, persuasion, deliberation, inquiry, negotiation, and eristics (Table 1) (Walton & Krabbe, 1995).

The single 'acts' to be performed in order to reach one of these goals are the dialogue moves within a dialogue type and they can be represented as 'profiles of dialogue': "a profile of dialogue is a connected sequence of moves and countermoves in a conversational exchange of a type that is goal-directed and can be represented

Table 1. Types of dialogue and their characteristics

T ype	Initial Situation	Main Goal	Participants' Aims	Side Benefits
Persuasion Dialogue	Conflicting points of view	Resolution of such conflicts by verbal means	Persuade the other(s)	Develop and reveal positions Build up confidence Influence onlookers, Add to prestige
Negotiation	Conflict of interests & need for cooperation	Making a deal	Get the best out of it for oneself	Agreement, Build up confidence Reveal position Influence onlookers Add to prestige
Inquiry	General ignorance	Growth of knowledge & agreement	Find a "proof" or destroy one	Add to prestige Gain experience Raise funds
Deliberation	Need for action	Reach a decision	Influence outcome	Agreement Develop & reveal positions Add to prestige, Vent emotions
Information-seeking	Personal Ignorance	Spreading knowledge and revealing positions	Gain, pass on, show, or hide personal knowledge	Agreement Develop & reveal positions Add to prestige, Vent emotions
Eristics	Conflict & antagonism	Reaching a (provisional) accommodation in a relationship	Strike the other party & win in the eyes of onlookers	Agreement Develop & reveal positions Gain experience, Amusement Add to prestige, Vent emotions

(Walton & Krabbe, 1995)

in a normative model of dialogue" (Walton, 1999, p. 53). The profiles of dialogue map out the moves that are dialogically relevant in order to achieve a specific dialogical aim. The notion of *relevance* refers here to the possibilities that each move opens up for the interlocutor and that are most appropriate to reach the dialogical goal. If we look at Figure 1, the profile of an information-seeking dialogue, we notice that the first question by A opens up to B the possibility for only two alternative relevant moves: 'yes' or 'no'. Technically, no other moves (answers) are possible, unless B decided to not reply by either changing the topic ('I surely have a nice doggie') or by a meta-dialogical refusal of the question ('I don't want to talk about this now'). Reading the development of the profile in Figure 1, we could imagine a police officer interrogating a suspect for abusive behavior. The first question and the options it opens up for B are relevant in this context because the final aim of the dialogue is to gain information that will lead to the identification of the culprit. It wouldn't make much sense here to use dialogical moves that could lead, for example, to the suspect talking about his opinions on the advantages of having a spouse.

Figure 1. Information seeking dialogue

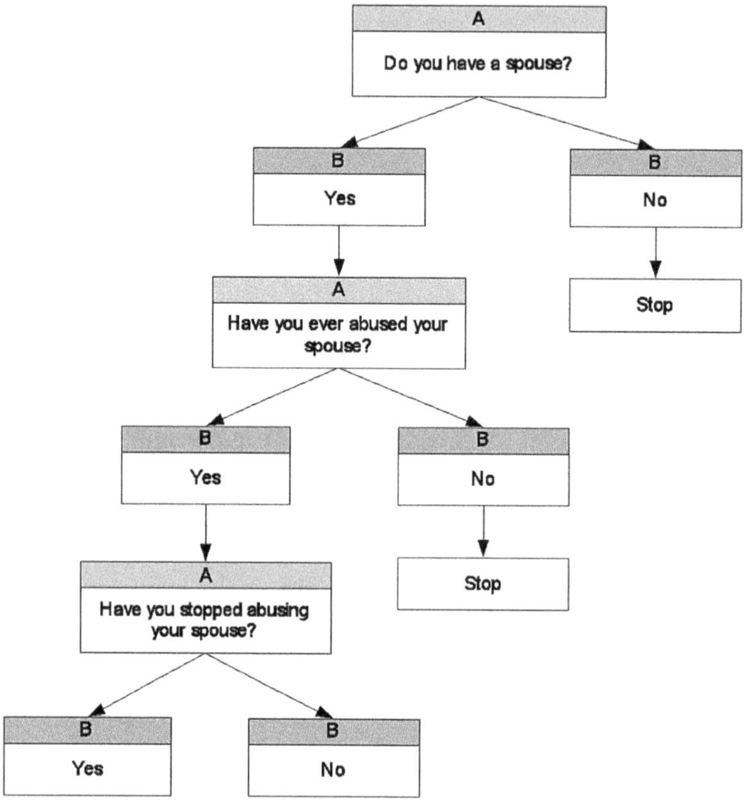

THE DELIBERATION DIALOGUE

As shown in Table 1, deliberation dialogues are abstract patterns that outline the most effective dialogical moves aimed at finding an acceptable course of action to achieve a certain goal (Walton, Atkinson, Bench-Capon, Wyner, & Cartwright, 2010; Walton, 2010). Deliberation dialogues usually take place when there is not a compelling objective way of coping with a problem and parties discuss their reasons for proposing a certain solution.

This is the first relevant feature of this dialogue type that, we think, makes it an adequate model for the analysis of decision-making in chronic care encounters (Bigi, 2014). Indeed, in these consultations the discussions that arise are not about conflicts of opinion *stricto sensu*. In other words, it is seldom the case that clinicians and patients discuss about conflicting opinions in the same way as it could happen during, for example, a dinner, when ideas, interpretations of facts, evaluations are exchanged, which do not have an objective foundation and are different, often non-exclusive, ways of interpreting phenomena.

What happens in chronic care consultations is more often that clinicians and patients may find themselves having one basic kind of discussion about what to do next, given the general health situation of the patient. While trying to answer this question, other kinds of discussions may arise, regarding: wrong or partial information patients have regarding their condition and how to cope with it; different interpretations of symptoms; criteria for preferring one course of action or another.

Secondly, the premise of deliberation dialogues is that parties are out to reach a collective goal, which can be contrary to or different from the individuals' personal goals. In the medical encounter, the patient's health can be construed as a collective goal because it is the only reason for physician and patient to come together in the interaction field of the hospital or outpatient clinic. The discussion is 'task oriented', because the final aim of the relationship between clinicians and patients is to achieve a better health for the latter. In this respect, opinions need to be evaluated against the goal of improved health. In this sense, these discussions are not the same as discussions regarding opinions in a general sense. Chronic patients accumulate lived knowledge on their disease and construct their opinions drawing from their experience and context. As patients' opinions influence their health behavior and lifestyles, it becomes important for clinicians to explore them in order to address possible reasons that support non-healthy behaviors and formulate feasible therapeutic goals. At the same time, it is important that clinicians, who have medical knowledge and more appropriate criteria for evaluation, lead the consultations and, often, the discussions arising within them.

Finally, the dialogical aim of the deliberation dialogue is particularly relevant in the care of chronic patients, where the principle of patient autonomy has partially given back to patients the decisional power regarding their own health and treatment decisions. As mentioned above, clinicians and patients often discuss health goals and treatment options taking into consideration not only clinical evidence but also patients' preferences and values that are usually co-constructed and discovered in the interaction (Truog et al., 2015).

The Structure of Deliberation Dialogues

The structure and development of deliberation dialogues are reported in Figure 2. Deliberation dialogues usually develop in three stages: the opening stage, the argumentation stage and the closing stage. In the case of the medical consultation, we could consider these stages as the "communicative bricks" of the shared decision-making process. It is important to notice that the stages' names do not necessarily refer to the timeline of the consultation but rather to the communicative content discussed.

Figure 2. Stages of deliberation dialogue
(Walton et al., 2014)

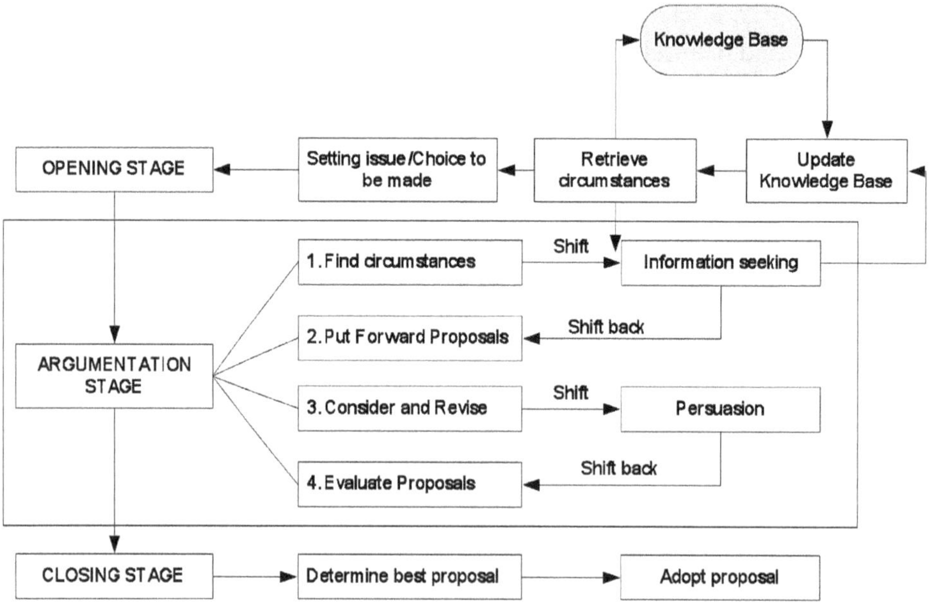

Probably the most interesting characteristic of this model, and the one that makes it particularly appropriate for our discussion, is that the deliberation dialogue is represented as a 'hybrid' dialogue, which develops through the intersection with an information seeking and a persuasion dialogue.

Opening Stage and the Role of Information Sharing

In the opening stage the parties become aware that there is a problem and a choice needs to be made (for example, that it is necessary for the patient to lose weight). A process begins in which the parties need to figure out what are the available options for action. In order to do this, they must engage in an information seeking type of dialogue, in which the final aim is to share information regarding the issue. Therefore the pattern of the information seeking dialogue comes into play almost immediately in the deliberation process.

This moment is particularly relevant for the whole deliberation process, for various reasons. When it is conducted effectively, i.e. when the dialogical moves are relevant, it allows the parties to share important information regarding the abilities of the parties to carry out an intended course of action, the values or beliefs behind choices, and any new event that might have changed the configuration of previously shared knowledge between the two. The set of information that is shared during this phase adds to the previously shared knowledge and provides the foundation for the core part of deliberation, in which the parties will put forward actual proposals for action.

The relevance of this process of information is greater than what might be imagined at first. An ongoing study on a corpus of real life interactions between clinicians and patients in an Italian diabetes care setting is revealing that when the information seeking phase is more thorough, the outcome of the deliberation process – i.e. the indication for action – becomes much more specific than in other cases (Bigi, Macagno, & Mayweg-Paus, submitted). This observation can be explained by the fact that, once the relevant information regarding options, ability and criteria for action has been shared, it is much easier for both clinicians and patients to become more specific about the behavior to follow. This finding is interesting because it is coherent with the studies on commitment and goal setting mentioned above, in which goal specificity seemed to be a moderator for commitment (Baca-Motes et al., 2013).

Another reason to stress the importance of the process of information sharing realized through the pattern of the information seeking dialogue is the impact it can have on self-efficacy. As mentioned above, self-efficacy can be bolstered by providing the interlocutor with appropriate information regarding the problem at issue (the disease) and the ways to cope with it (self-management training) (Locke & Latham, 2002). It is worthwhile to work on the strengthening of self-efficacy because it has been shown that, when the difficulty of a goal is controlled, the fact of self-setting the goal or having it assigned does not impact on the quality of performance if the level of self-efficacy is high in both cases (Locke & Latham, 2002). This is a very interesting observation for those patients who need or prefer a more paternalistic and directive relationship, i.e. those who would prefer to have goals assigned to them, rather than self-setting their own goals (Barello & Graffigna, 2014). In these cases, it looks like a well conducted information sharing phase would have the potential to make up – in terms of degree of commitment – for the less participatory style of interaction.

Argumentation Stage and Relevant Persuasion as the Key to Stronger Commitment

Once the problem is clear and relevant information has been shared, the argumentation stage begins, in which the parties actually put forward alternative proposals for the solution of the problem. In chronic care consultations, it means that the clinician and the patient start a discussion about the changes that the patient could adopt in order to achieve a health improvement.

At this point, the most important effect of having shared the information is that both parties are aware of all the circumstances that can have an impact on the proposals they make. Therefore, it will be easier to avoid proposing impossible behaviors or behaviors that the patient will refuse.

The act of proposing is the most relevant move at this stage of the deliberation and the one that calls into play the pattern of the persuasion dialogue. 'Persuasion' is intended here in a neutral sense and it refers to the act of putting forward arguments for or against a certain proposal for action with the aim of finding an agreement on the one that both satisfies the parties and reaches the aim of solving the problem identified at the beginning of the deliberation (on the acceptability of persuasion dialogue within the medical consultation, see Rubinelli, 2013).

Persuasion dialogues are made up of proposals and the arguments to support them, or counter-arguments to oppose a proposal that the interlocutor has put forward. The typical argument scheme (Walton, Reed, & Macagno, 2008) used in deliberations is the one from consequences, because the criteria for deciding on one course of action instead of another are fundamentally the positive effects (consequences) that should ensue from it. The argument from consequences, however, can be off the mark and very weak if the interlocutors do not share the same criteria for considering an outcome as positive or negative. Here, again, we notice how relevant a good information sharing at the beginning of a deliberation can be. We also find a connection with the studies mentioned previously that stress the relevance of the value system within which decisions are made in order to understand commitment (Becker, 1960).

In the argumentation stage of deliberation, clinicians may want to leave room for patients to self-set their goals if possible or desirable. As argued elsewhere (Bigi et al., 2015), asking patients to self-set their goals can even be used as a training strategy by clinicians, to exercise and develop patients' interpretive abilities and skills for self-management. In all cases, this is the stage of deliberation in which the previously shared information is translated into practical indications for action and in which patients' preferences and therapeutic goals are attuned and aligned. This is possible precisely through the combination of the information seeking and persuasion dialogues as components of the deliberation process.

Closing Stage and Patient Commitment

The closing stage, precisely because it comes last, plays a fundamental role for the effectiveness of the whole deliberation. It is at this point that the parties converge on a proposal that best fits the aims of the interaction, regardless of individual goals and desires. A patient may not desire to go on a diet, but may agree to it because during the argumentation stage the positive consequences of losing weight have effectively emerged. At the same time, a physician may want a patient to start treatment with interferon, but may agree to postpone it if the patient during the argumentation phase refused to start the treatment at that moment because of family reasons. However, as mere agreement is not enough, deliberation is effective when patients make an explicit commitment to the agreed course of action (see on this topic, Amrhein, Miller, Yahne, Palmer, & Fulcher, 2003).

APPLICATION OF DELIBERATION DIALOGUE TO CHRONIC CARE ENCOUNTERS

Given its aim, the model of deliberation dialogues can be fruitfully applied to actual clinician-patient conversations where there is a health related problem that calls for action and where there is a decision to be made. As deliberation dialogue is a theoretical model of "best practice", in actual clinical conversations it may happen that only some stages are present. For example, it may happen that the opening stage and the definition of the problem remain implicit, or that the argumentation is missing or is carried out only by one party. It can also happen that there is no closing stage, nor patient commitment. The analysis of the consultations according to the deliberation dialogue model is particularly interesting as it allows the identification of sub-optimal realizations of deliberation and therefore shared decisions within the consultations. The lack of some stages may influence the effectiveness of communication and may hinder patient engagement and adherence. The model can be used to make hypotheses regarding the dialogical components of deliberation dialogues that are more likely to have an impact on patients' commitment, thus also allowing a tentative definition of the pathways that lead from the communication styles used within the consultation to the dimensions of patient engagement and adherence.

To describe the potential of the model, in this section we discuss examples of the application of the deliberation dialogue in the field of hemophilia. Hemophilia is an inherited bleeding disorder, treated by replacing a missing protein responsible for correct coagulation by intravenous injections. The excerpts reported are taken from a set of video-recorded physician-patient consultations collected as a part of a larger multicenter study on patient adherence (Lamiani et al., 2015). The excerpts are extracted from longer check-up visits between different physicians (Md) and patients (Pt). The examples reported in the following sections show two deliberation dialogues where some stages are missing, and one complete deliberation dialogue. The phases of deliberation dialogues are indicated in the left column. The dialogues, which are reported in the right column, are sequential, unless specified.

Incomplete Argumentation and Closing Stage

In excerpt 1 (Table 2), we can observe an incomplete argumentative stage (performed only by the physician) and closing stage.

In this dialogue, we can observe an opening stage where the problem of the patient's suboptimal adherence to treatment is brought up by the physician, but the patient does not seem to be aware of its severity ("Why?"). The physician puts forward a proposal ("3.000 units twice a week") and tries to reach an early closure. As the patient's agreement ("Yes, yes") seems not an actual commitment, a new argumentative stage begins a little later, where the physician argues in favor of a behavior change without asking information regarding the reasons for the patient's non adherence. The dialogue ends without a proper closing stage in which we can find an explicit commitment from the patient. A possible reason for not achieving an effective deliberation, and therefore a closure, could be the lack of information regarding the patient's behavior (information seeking dialogue), and the lack of patient engagement in the argumentation stage.

Table 2. Incomplete argumentation and closing stage

Opening Stage	Md: What have you been doing? Pt: Why? Md: 4000 units once a week, no…stop it!
Argumentation Stage	Pt: Eh, little by little now we'll start again... Md: No, no we should do 3.000 units twice a week, always Pt: Ok
Closing Stage	Md: Do you promise me? Pt: Yes, yes, as I did before Md: Do I have to make you swear? Pt: Eh..by your head?!
Argumentation Stage	Md: No, no by *your* head… It has been proved that once a week is not enough to protect you and you risk that… Pt: ...something happens... Md: Moreover, it has been proved that whoever has had such an hemorrhage is more likely to have another one, so no fooling around and no wild experiments Pt: No ok, but it has only been this time. Up until two months ago, we have always being doing the treatment Md: Now you be good, because all the rest is fine. Why should you go looking for trouble? Moreover, also your joints will benefit from it.
	Md: Now we'll let you go....did you stop by the reception for the new appointment? Pt: Yes

Lack of Closing Stage

In the second excerpt (Table 3), we can observe a deliberation dialogue where the closing stage is missing.

In this dialogue a problem regarding smoking is raised in the opening stage and both the physician and the patient enter the argumentation stage. In this stage it is interesting to notice that the physician and the patient share a different hierarchy of values. At the top of the physician's priorities is the patient's health and everything else is subordinated to achieving this goal; on the other hand, the patient minimizes the risks of smoking due to the pleasure of it, thus almost implying that this pleasure is more important to him than his own health. The proposals for action they put forward in the argumentation stage ("You can do without it"; "No because it is a pleasure") are based on these different hierarchies. In spite of this, the physician does not explore the reasons behind the patient's apparent disregard for his own health and the patient is not given the opportunity to self-set his goal. As the argumentation stage develops more into a dispute than a deliberation, the closing stage is avoided and the physician moves forward on an easier ground with another medical exam.

Complete Deliberation Dialogue

Excerpt 3 (Table 4) offers a good example of a complete deliberation dialogue where the physician and the patient reach a shared goal regarding the therapeutic regimen that is different from the individual goals.

In this excerpt, all the stages of the deliberation dialogue are present in the communication flow. In the opening stage, the problem regarding treatment adherence

Table 3. Lack of a closing stage

Opening Stage	Md: Do you smoke? Pt: Something now and then Md: How much? Pt: Three cigarettes a day Md: Well, this is not "now and then"…it is regularly Pt: Well, compared to people who smoke a packet a day, for me it is now and then …. Yeah, well, you are right though...
Argumentation Stage	Md: You know, I am almost more sympathetic with people who smoke 20 cigarettes a day because it is really an addiction and it's difficult to quit… three cigarettes, you can do without them Pt: No because it is a pleasure! Md: Yes, but you can do without them Pt: Yes, yes, I mean, if I do without them I don't die...I agree…but it's a pleasure!
	Md: Did you take the pill for your pressure today? [Taking the blood pressure]

Table 4. Complete deliberation dialogue

Opening Stage	Md: The medicine intake is good? Do you have any problems? Pt: Yes, it is good but...Doc, I am not doing the prophylaxis anymore… Md: Why? is the prophylaxis not going well? Pt: The problem is that I have few venous accesses left, so I try to preserve those I've left for when I really need them. When I see I have some bruises then I understand that that is the time for treatment Md: So let's say that you are doing a "customized" prophylaxis Pt: You got it...
Argumentation Stage	Md: Yes, I understand that you are adjusting your prophylaxis. However, you have to keep in mind that as you are not protected by the drug, then you'll end up moving less and less and you'll give up doing things. You won't feel confident to be doing anything more than what you feel sure about… So I am not saying you must do the prophylaxis three times a week, because now we know that every patient reaches his optimal regimen… however, this does not mean that the patient gives up doing the prophylaxis alltogether. Pt: So, Doc, instead of doing 3000 units three times a week, we could do 3000 units twice a week. Md: I think this is the bare minimum for a person like you who still has an active lifestyle.
Closing stage	Pt: Yes, absolutely, I need to go to work. So, ok we can do like that: 3000 units twice a week (They talk about other issues) Md: Ok, then. Shall we try to do the prophylaxis twice a week? Pt: I'll try it, Doc

is explicitly expressed by the patient ("I am not doing the prophylaxis anymore"). Instead of immediately entering the argumentation stage, the physician explores the reasons of the patient's sub-optimal adherence engaging the patient in an information seeking dialogue ("Why? is the prophylaxis not going well?"). In the argumentative stage, the physician and the patient put forward some proposals to solve the problem and find a compromise. The physician can argue in favor of not giving up prophylaxis based on the knowledge of the patient's lifestyle. The patient is enabled to self-set his therapeutic goal, which is agreed upon by the physician. As the deliberation stage has been conducted effectively, in the closing stage we can observe the patient's commitment ("Ok, we can do like that, 3000 units twice a week").

SOLUTIONS AND RECOMMENDATIONS

As shown in the examples above, applying the model of the deliberation dialogue to chronic care consultations may help analyze the dialogical structure of the decision-making phases, identifying suboptimal realizations and indicating pathways for interventions.

One of the advantages of this model is that it seems possible to integrate it with one of the most known and used methods of analysis for medical consultations, such as the Roter Interaction Analysis System (RIAS). The RIAS takes as the minimal unit of analysis the utterance (Roter & Larson, 2002). By coding each utterance according to categories that describe the 'verbal action' performed by each speaker, the researcher is able to obtain a 'measure' of the degree of patient-centerdness of a consultation[1]. This method however does not allow to reconstruct larger inferential patterns of meaning. On the other hand, an analysis of consultations performed by using the components of the deliberation dialogue allows a description of the macro-structure of the interaction (Bigi & Macagno, submitted). At this point, the two levels of analysis could be combined to gain useful insights into what kind of utterances can more successfully achieve the goal of effective deliberation. An assessment of the effectiveness of the deliberation would be supported by the patient-centerdness evaluation of the consultation obtained through the RIAS coding. This kind of integration between the analysis of the utterance level through the RIAS system and the analysis of the dialogue level through an operationalization of the model of deliberation dialogue is being developed through a joint effort between researchers at the Dept. of Linguistic Sciences of the Catholic University of Milano and colleagues at the Dept. of Health Sciences at the University of Milano, San Paolo Hospital.

From a practical point of view, the results of an analysis conducted by using the model of the deliberation dialogue could enhance the understanding and effectiveness of approaches for behavior change already used in the clinical practice.

For example, the motivational interview suggests a number of techniques to encourage active patient participation and strengthening of commitment (Burke, Arkowitz, & Menchola, 2003; Miller & Rollnick, 2002). These techniques however are not set within a description of the dialogical structure of the consultation and the appropriateness of their use is not related to specific dialogical moves nor to the larger dialogical patterns that typically occur during consultations. We believe that the value of these techniques would not be obliterated if they were observed and reconsidered within a description of the consultation obtained through the analysis conducted at the dialogical level. On the contrary, they could be more easily combined with dialogical goals and stages and become even more focused and effective.

In this sense, the structure of the deliberation dialogue could actually become the blueprint for a 'communication protocol' to conduct more effective decision-making phases and thus be used for clinicians' training. This hypothesis is currently being tested in the framework of an ongoing research project based at Milano's Catholic University (www.unicatt.it/healthyreasoning-eng).

At a more general level, the pattern of the deliberation dialogue constitutes a response to the perplexity that is sometimes expressed by clinicians, that communication skills cannot be taught because they cannot be 'standardized', given the fact that patients are all different one from the other (Bigi & Rossi, 2015). We believe this model shows very well the possibility for a 'standardized' approach able at the same time to incorporate the individual characteristics of every patient. Clinical conversations will vary depending on the information collected in the information sharing stage and the argumentation stage will focus on different arguments based on the patient's individuality.

Finally, the approach to shared decision-making based on the deliberation dialogue is compatible with the most recent formulations of patient-centered care, which values patient autonomy that is expressed in the interaction with clinicians and is not an end to itself (Duggan, Geller, Cooper, & Beach, 2006). Indeed, the ethical preoccupations of respecting patients' individuality and decisional autonomy are matched in this analytical approach with the practical preoccupation of conducting an effective consultation that will have a positive effect on patients. The patient-centered model defines the dialogical objectives of the consultation, but not the dialogical structures that can realize them. The model of the deliberation dialogue outlines the dialogical steps the parties can and should take in order to reach consensus on a behavior by foreseeing 'room' for the expression of both parties' views and reasons.

In conclusion, clinicians' training based on the structure of the deliberation dialogue could improve clinicians' effectiveness in promoting patient engagement and adherence.

FUTURE RESEARCH DIRECTIONS

Elwyn and Miron-Shatz (2009) have convincingly discussed the unsoundness of establishing correlations between the quality of decision-making practices and clinical outcomes. Instead, they argue that decision-making should be assessed based on the quality of deliberation, which ultimately means favoring the definition of the problem and the outline of the different options for its solution. Therefore, their proposal is to link the assessment of the quality of decision-making to the patient's perception about and recall of the deliberation steps. If the model of the deliberation dialogue were used as a blueprint for conducting decision-making phases within consultations, the approach proposed by Elwyn and Miron-Shatz (2009) could be used to test for better recall of and perceptions about the deliberation steps in the consultation.

Further, deliberation dialogue only offers the structural components within which an effective deliberation can occur. It does not explicitly suggest specific communication skills that can be used to achieve the single stages of deliberation dialogues. It should be paired with existing approaches based on specific communication skills in order to create comprehensive and usable training materials for clinicians.

Finally, we know from the literature that, beyond communication skills, relational qualities, such as curiosity, respect, emotional availability and partnership, are essential for a good clinician-patient relationship (Lamiani, Barello, Browning, Vegni, & Meyer, 2012), especially in the field of chronic care where clinicians build long-term relationship with their patients. These qualities are often conveyed by clinicians through the tone of voice, intonation, and non-verbal communication, more than specific words. For this reason, future research could explore the emotional tone of deliberation dialogues in chronic care by assessing whether or not the global degree of affect of the clinician leading the conversation (e.g. dominance, friendliness, respectfulness, interest, anger etc.) impacts on effective deliberation and patient outcomes.

CONCLUSION

The chapter has taken into consideration the concept of patient engagement from the point of view of its dialogical component. Patient engagement refers to a status in which individuals are willing to behave in active and responsible ways with regard to the management of their health conditions. Such status can be fostered, improved and maintained in particular by conscious efforts on the part of clinicians within the boundaries of the medical consultations. It is, however, a complex condition that is achieved by attuning the cognitive, emotional and behavioral levels. Studies on patient engagement are at an early stage and we do not have yet a full-fledged description of the components that contribute to supporting and improving patient engagement. Especially at a practical level, there is still lack of specific and evidence based indications to guide interventions and training for clinicians.

One factor that has been described as fundamental for the achievement of patient engagement is effective communication between clinicians and patients. Moreover, the condition of being fully engaged requires that patients change their attitudes and behaviors with regard to the management of their health, and this is particularly true for chronic conditions. The relevance of the communicative dimension in relation to behavior change calls into play interdisciplinary competences, which are necessary to analyze in particular the dialogical structure and dynamics within the consultation.

In this chapter, we have focused on shared decision-making in chronic care consultations, considered as a pivotal moment for the achievement of patient engagement. We have proposed to consider the dialogical structure of decision-making by the adoption of a normative model – the model of the deliberation dialogue – which was developed within the research field of Argumentation Theory and has already been applied in the domain of AI. This model formalizes the dialogical intention of deliberation through the dialogical moves that are considered the most effective to reach consensus on a solution to a problem. This kind of dialogue seems to be particularly frequent in chronic care setting, where consultations often have the aim to support motivation for behavior change or to find agreement on a therapeutic prescription. In the chapter, the model has been presented on the backdrop of its theoretical setting and explained in its fundamental features. Three examples have been provided to show the analytical potential of this model to guide the scholar to identify suboptimal realizations of decision-making phases in the consultation. It has also been argued that the results of such analyses could be well integrated with results from more traditional analyses of consultations, such as the RIAS coding. Moreover, the same results could be used to improve our understanding and use of techniques such as the ones proposed within the framework of the motivational interview.

We believe that this model is an effective tool for the analysis of real life cases and to provide evidence that could support the design and implementation of interventions to improve clinicians' decision-making skills.

REFERENCES

Ajzen, I. (1988). *Attitudes, personality, and behavior*. Chicago, IL: Dorsey.

Ajzen, I. (1991, December). (1991). The theory of planned behavior. *Organizational Behavior and Human Decision Processes*, *50*(2), 179–211. doi:10.1016/0749-5978(91)90020-T

Ajzen, I. (2002). Perceived Behavioral Control, Self-Efficacy, Locus of Control, and the Theory of Planned Behavior. *Journal of Applied Social Psychology*, *32*(4), 665–683. doi:10.1111/j.1559-1816.2002.tb00236.x

Amrhein, P. C., Miller, W. R., Yahne, C. E., Palmer, M., & Fulcher, L. (2003). Client Commitment Language During Motivational Interviewing Predicts Drug Use Outcomes. *Journal of Consulting and Clinical Psychology*, *71*(5), 862–878. doi:10.1037/0022-006X.71.5.862 PMID:14516235

Assal, J. P. (1999). Revisiting the approach to treatment of long-term illness: From the acute to the chronic state. A need for educational and managerial skills for long-term follow-up. *Patient Education and Counseling*, *37*(2), 99–111. doi:10.1016/S0738-3991(98)00109-8 PMID:14528538

Baca-Motes, K., Brown, A., Gneezy, A., Keenan, E. A., & Nelson, L. D. (2013). Commitment and Behavior Change: Evidence from the Field. *The Journal of Consumer Research, 39*(5), 1070–1084. doi:10.1086/667226

Barello, S., & Graffigna, G. (2014). Engaging patients to recover life projectuality: an Italian cross-disease framework. *Quality of Life Research,* 24(5), 1087-1096. doi:10.1007/s11136-014-0846-x

Becker, H. S. (1960). Notes on the Concept of Commitment. *American Journal of Sociology, 66*(1), 32–40. doi:10.1086/222820

Bigi, S. (2014). Key components of effective collaborative goal setting in the chronic care encounter. *Communication & Medicine, 11*(2), 103–115. doi:10.1558/cam.v11i2.21600 PMID:26596119

Bigi, S., & Macagno, F. (Manuscript submitted for publication). From types of dialogue to dialogue moves - The case of doctor-patient interaction as a communicative practice. *Discourse Processes.*

Bigi, S., Macagno, F., & Mayweg-Paus, L. (Manuscript submitted for publication). Medical consultation as a type of dialogical practice. *Patient Education and Counseling.*

Bigi, S., & Rossi, M. G. (2015). Comunicare (nel)la cronicità [Communicating (within) chronic care]. *MeDIA. Aggiornamento e Formazione in Diabetologia e Malattie Metaboliche, 15*(3).

Bigi, S., Rossi, M. G., Barello, S., Graffigna, G., Mulas, M. F., & Musacchio, N. (2015). *Speaking wisely: pratiche dialogiche appropriate in diabetologia* [Speaking wisely: appropriate dialogical practices in diabetes care]. Paper presented at XX Congresso Nazionale AMD, L'Evoluzione della Diabetologia alla luce del Piano Nazionale Diabete, Genova, Italy.

Boyd, C. M., Singh, S., Varadhan, R., Weiss, C. O., Sharma, R., Bass, E. B., & Puhan, M. A. (2012). *Methods for Benefit and Harm Assessment in Systematic Reviews. Methods Research Report. (Prepared by the Johns Hopkins University Evidence-based Practice Center under contract No. 290-2007-10061-I). AHRQ Publication No. 12(13)-EHC150-EF.* Rockville, MD: Agency for Healthcare Research and Quality.

Burke, B. L., Arkowitz, H., & Menchola, M. (2003). The efficacy of motivational interviewing: A meta-analysis of controlled clinical trials. *Journal of Consulting and Clinical Psychology, 71*(5), 843–861. doi:10.1037/0022-006X.71.5.843 PMID:14516234

Charles, C., Gafni, A., & Whelan, T. (1997). Shared decision-making in the medical encounter: What does it mean? (or it takes at least two to tango). *Social Science & Medicine*, *44*(5), 681–692. doi:10.1016/S0277-9536(96)00221-3 PMID:9032835

Charles, C., Gafni, A., & Whelan, T. (1999). Decision-making in the physician-patient encounter: Revisiting the shared treatment decision-making model. *Social Science & Medicine*, *49*(5), 651–661. doi:10.1016/S0277-9536(99)00145-8 PMID:10452420

Coleman, K., Austin, B. T., Brach, C., & Wagner, E. H. (2009). Evidence On The Chronic Care Model In The New Millennium. *Health Affairs*, *28*(1), 75–85. doi:10.1377/hlthaff.28.1.75 PMID:19124857

Coulter, A. (2011). *Engaging patients in healthcare*. New York: McGraw-Hill Education.

Duggan, P. S., Geller, G., Cooper, L. A., & Beach, M. C. (2006). The moral nature of patient-centeredness: Is it "just the right thing to do"? *Patient Education and Counseling*, *62*(2), 271–276. doi:10.1016/j.pec.2005.08.001 PMID:16356677

Elwyn, G., Frosch, D., Thomson, R., Joseph-Williams, N., Lloyd, A., Kinnersley, P., & Barry, M. et al. (2012). Shared Decision-making: A Model for Clinical Practice. *Journal of General Internal Medicine*, *27*(10), 1361–1367. doi:10.1007/s11606-012-2077-6 PMID:22618581

Elwyn, G., & Miron-Shatz, T. (2009). Deliberation before determination: The definition and evaluation of good decision-making. *Health Expectations*, *13*(2), 139–147. doi:10.1111/j.1369-7625.2009.00572.x PMID:19740089

Epstein, R., & Street, R. L. (2011). Shared Mind: Communication, Decision-making, and Autonomy in Serious Illness. *Annals of Family Medicine*, *9*(5), 454–461. doi:10.1370/afm.1301 PMID:21911765

Epstein, R. M., & Gramling, R. E. (2013). What is shared in shared decision-making? Complex decisions when the evidence is unclear. *Medical Care Research and Review. Supplement to*, *70*(1), 94S–112S.

Glanz, K., Rimer, B. K., & Viswanath, K. (2008). *Health Behavior and Health Education: Theory, Research, and Practice* (4th ed.). San Francisco: Jossey-Bass.

Graffigna, G., Barello, S., Riva, G., & Bosio, A. C. (2014). Patient engagement: The key to redesign the exchange between the demand and supply for healthcare in the era of active ageing. In G. Riva, P. Ajmone Marsan, & C. Grassi. (Eds.), Active Ageing and Healthy Living (pp. 85-95). Amsterdam: IOS Press.

Grice, H. P. (1975). Logic and conversation. In P. Cole & J. L. Morgan (Eds.), Syntax and Semantics (Vol. 3, pp. 41-58). New York: Academic Press.

Heisler, M., Bouknight, R. R., Hayward, R. A., Smith, D. M., & Kerr, E. A. (2002). The relative importance of physician communication, participatory decision-making, and patient understanding in diabetes self-management. *Journal of General Internal Medicine*, *17*(4), 243–252. doi:10.1046/j.1525-1497.2002.10905.x PMID:11972720

Heisler, M., Vijan, S., Anderson, R. M., Ubel, P. A., Bernstein, S. J., & Hofer, T. P. (2003). When do patients and their physicians agree on diabetes treatment goals and strategies, and what difference does it make? *Journal of General Internal Medicine*, *18*(11), 893–902. doi:10.1046/j.1525-1497.2003.21132.x PMID:14687274

Lafata, J. E., Morris, H. L., Dobie, E., Heisler, M., Werner, R. M., & Dumenci, L. (2013). Patient-reported use of collaborative goal setting and glycemic control among patients with diabetes. *Patient Education and Counseling*, *92*(1), 94–99. doi:10.1016/j.pec.2013.01.016 PMID:23433777

Lamiani, G., Barello, S., Browning, D. M., Vegni, E., & Meyer, E. C. (2012). Uncovering and validating clinicians' experiential knowledge when facing difficult conversations: A cross-cultural perspective. *Patient Education and Counseling*, *87*(3), 307–312. doi:10.1016/j.pec.2011.11.012 PMID:22196987

Lamiani, G., Strada, I., Mancuso, M. E., Coppola, A., Vegni, E., & Moja, E. A. (2015). Factors influencing illness representations and perceived adherence in haemophilic patients: A pilot study. *Haemophilia*, *21*(5), 598–604. doi:10.1111/hae.12654 PMID:25684356

Locke, E. A., & Latham, G. P. (2002). Building a practically useful theory of goal setting and task motivation. *The American Psychologist*, *57*(9), 705–717. doi:10.1037/0003-066X.57.9.705 PMID:12237980

Miller, W., & Rollinck, S. (2002). *Motivational interviewing: preparing people to change*. New York: Guilford Press.

Nuño, R., Coleman, K., Bengoa, R., & Sauto, R. (2012). Integrated care for chronic conditions: The contribution of the ICCC Framework. *Health Policy (Amsterdam)*, *105*(1), 55–64. doi:10.1016/j.healthpol.2011.10.006 PMID:22071454

Ong, L. M. L., Visser, M. R. M., Kruyver, I. P. M., Bensing, J. M., Van Den Brink-Muinen, A., Stouthard, J. M. L., & De Haes, J. C. J. M. et al. (1998). The Roter Interaction Analysis System (RIAS) in oncological consultations: Psychometric properties. *Psycho-Oncology*, *7*(5), 387–401. doi:10.1002/(SICI)1099-1611(1998090)7:5<387::AID-PON316>3.0.CO;2-G PMID:9809330

Prochaska, J. O., Di Clemente, C. C., & Norcross, J. C. (1992). In search of how people change. Applications to addictive behaviors. *The American Psychologist*, *47*(9), 1102–1114. doi:10.1037/0003-066X.47.9.1102 PMID:1329589

Roter, D. L. (2002). *The Roter Method for Interaction Process Analysis*. RIAS Manual.

Roter, D. L., & Larson, S. (2002). The Roter interaction analysis system (RIAS): Utility and flexibility for analysis of medical interactions. *Patient Education and Counseling*, *46*(4), 243–251. doi:10.1016/S0738-3991(02)00012-5 PMID:11932123

Rubinelli, S. (2013). Rational versus unreasonable persuasion in doctor-patient communication: A normative account. *Patient Education and Counseling*, *92*(3), 296–301. doi:10.1016/j.pec.2013.06.005 PMID:23830240

Street, R. L. Jr. (2013). How clinician-patient communication contributes to health improvement: Modeling pathways from talk to outcome. *Patient Education and Counseling*, *92*(3), 286–291. doi:10.1016/j.pec.2013.05.004 PMID:23746769

Street, R. L., Elwyn, G., & Epstein, R. (2012). Patient preferences and health care outcomes: An ecological perspective. *Expert Review of Pharmacoeconomics & Outcomes Research*, *12*(2), 167–180. doi:10.1586/erp.12.3 PMID:22458618

Street, R. L., Piziak, V. K., Carpentier, W. S., Herzog, J., Hejl, J., Skinner, G., & McLellan, L. (1993). Provider-patient communication and metabolic control. *Diabetes Care*, *16*(5), 714–721. doi:10.2337/diacare.16.5.714 PMID:8495610

Thompson, A. G. H. (2007). The meaning of patient involvement and participation in health care consultations: A taxonomy. *Social Science & Medicine*, *64*(6), 1297–1310. doi:10.1016/j.socscimed.2006.11.002 PMID:17174016

Truog, R. D., Brown, S. D., Browning, D., Hundert, E. M., Rider, E. A., Bell, S. K., & Meyer, E. C. (2015). Microethics: The ethics of everyday clinical practice. *The Hastings Center Report*, *45*(1), 11–17. doi:10.1002/hast.413 PMID:25600383

van Eemeren, F. H., & Grootendorst, R. (2004). *A systematic theory of argumentation*. Cambridge, MA: Cambridge University Press.

Visser, A. (2000). Chronic diseases, aging, and dementia: Implications for patient education and counseling. *Patient Education and Counseling*, *39*(2-3), 293–309. doi:10.1016/S0738-3991(99)00002-6

Walton, D. (1999). Profiles of Dialogue for Evaluating Arguments from Ignorance. *Argumentation*, *13*(1), 53–71. doi:10.1023/A:1007738812877

Walton, D. (2006). How to make and defend a proposal in a deliberation dialogue. *Artificial Intelligence and Law, 14*(3), 177–239. doi:10.1007/s10506-006-9025-x

Walton, D. (2010). Types of dialogues and burdens of proof. In P. Baroni, F. Cerutti, M. Giacomin, & G. R. Simari (Eds.). *Computational Models of Argument: Proceedings of COMMA 2010* (13-24). Amsterdam: IOS Press.

Walton, D., Atkinson, K., Bench-Capon, T., Wyner, A., & Cartwright, D. (2010). Argumentation in the framework of deliberation dialogue. In C. Bjola, & M. Kornprobst (Eds.), Arguing Global Governance (pp. 201-230). London: Routledge.

Walton, D., & Krabbe, E. (1995). *Commitment in Dialogue: Basic Concepts of Interpersonal Reasoning*. Albany, NY: State University of New York Press.

Walton, D., Reed, C., & Macagno, F. (2008). *Argumentation Schemes*. Cambridge, MA: Cambridge University Press. doi:10.1017/CBO9780511802034

Walton, D., Toniolo, A., & Norman, T. (2014). Missing phases of deliberation dialogue for real applications.*Proceedings of the 11th International Workshop on Argumentation in Multi-Agent Systems,* 1-20.

Wilson, S. R., Strub, P., Buist, A. S., Knowles, S. B., Lavori, P. W., Lapidus, J., & Vollmer, W. M. (2010). Shared treatment decision making improves adherence and outcomes in poorly controlled asthma. *American Journal of Respiratory and Critical Care Medicine, 181*(6), 566–577. doi:10.1164/rccm.200906-0907OC PMID:20019345

KEY TERMS AND DEFINITIONS

Adherence: Extent to which the patient's behavior (e.g. taking medicines, following healthy lifestyles, attending the check-ups) coincides with the recommendations shared with clinicians.

Chronic Care: Care of patients who suffer from chronic diseases. Chronic diseases are treatable, but not curable. They usually have a slow onset, a progressive development and require a complex treatment. When not managed correctly, they can cause acute episodes. On the other hand, badly treated acute conditions may develop into chronic ones.

Deliberation Dialogue: Type of dialogue pattern that takes place when there is a situation that calls for action and the parties aim to reach an optimal collective decision. It is characterized by the combination between the information seeking and the persuasion dialogues.

Dialogical Move: Any of the minimal meaningful units of a dialogue, which contribute to the achievement of the dialogue's aim.

Goal Setting: The specific phase during decision-making in which, after collecting information on the patient's health, it is necessary to decide on the best therapy and behaviors the patient should follow until the next visit.

Patient Engagement: It refers to the condition in which patients have integrated their disease into their identity and are active participants both in the relationship with their caregivers and towards the health care institutions.

Patient-Centered Care: Model of care that takes into account both the patient's disease and the illness experience (e.g. feelings, expectations, interpretations and context). The patient-centered clinical method indicates the communicative aims useful to achieve a patient-centered care.

Persuasion: Used here as a general term to refer to the process of presenting arguments in favor of or against a certain standpoint, also referred to as 'argumentation'. There can be different kinds of persuasion; what usually takes place within medical consultations is not a truth-oriented kind of persuasion process, but rather a pragmatic one, aimed at grounding the acceptability of an opinion on the benefits that can be derived from it.

Shared Decision-Making: Within the healthcare setting, it indicates the process to follow in order to come to a shared decision on therapies and lifestyles. In its early definitions, shared decision-making implied a physician providing medical information and a patient sorting out that information and making choices based on his/her values and preferences. More recent approaches consider it as a process in which both the criteria for choice and decisions are co-constructed in the consultation via a sharing of information and preferences. These recent approaches do not consider physicians as neutral individuals, with no preferences nor biases. Because of this, shared decision-making phases should first of all favor the discussion and sharing of values and preferences before decisions are outlined and assessed.

ENDNOTES

1 The RIAS assigns each utterance to a predefined category. Physician communication is classified according to 34 categories, while patient communication to 28. Examples of categories are: Gives information – medical condition; Empathy statements; Asks for opinion (physician only) (Roter, 2002; Ong et al., 1998).

Chapter 4
Patient and Family Engagement in THE Conversation:
Pathways from Communication to Care Outcomes

Jennifer Freytag
Texas A&M University, USA

Richard L. Street Jr.
Texas A&M University, USA

ABSTRACT

This chapter uses a patient-centered communication framework to examine observational studies of patient and family engagement in communication about end-of-life care. It analyzes how the literature has connected communication with health outcomes in end-of-life care. Within this analysis, it brings together three main ideas. First, family plays an important and overlooked role in communication about end-of-life care. Second, the literature describes communication that serves multiple functions, and it describes the special challenges presented by end-of-life care communication. Finally, it links these communicative functions with health outcomes and outlines directions for future research.

DOI: 10.4018/978-1-5225-0663-8.ch004

INTRODUCTION

In this chapter, we focus on patient and family engagement what is often called the conversation: when physicians, patients, and families discuss healthcare at the end of life. Indeed, movements in advance care planning such as The Conversation Project and Angelo Volandes' popular work The Conversation: A Revolutionary Plan for End-of-Life Care (2015) underscore the idea that conversations about this kind of care are perhaps the most important of our lives. Those who have experienced and studied the conversation know that the word "conversation," which paints a simple picture of two people talking, perhaps looking one another in the eye and nodding knowingly, does not describe the complexity of the circumstances in end-of-life care (See, e.g., Barnes et al., 2012). In reality, communication about end-of-life care involves many important people in addition to the patient and her physician, such as nurses, social workers, and other caregivers. Additionally, it involves members of the patient's family who will ultimately become surrogate decision-makers, using communicative behaviors that are difficult to unravel because they are informed by a tangle of individual experiences, beliefs, and goals (See, e.g., Gance-Cleveland, 2005). Thus the conversation is ongoing talk involving a clutter of people who sometimes cannot connect. Thus, to improve the effect of these conversations on patient care, our focus must shift from merely advocating for these conversations to critically studying how they work, what they accomplish, how they affect health outcomes, and how to engage all stakeholders.

Current literature describes the importance of patient, physician, and family engagement in a patient-centered approach to end-of-life care communication (See, e.g., Tang et al., 2014; Weeks et al., 2012). A patient-centered approach emphasizes the importance of considering patients' needs and experiences; encouraging patients to actively engage in their healthcare; and enhancing the patient-physician relationship (Epstein & Street, 2007; Stewart, 2003). The overall goal of this approach is to improve healthcare quality for individual patients. Patient-centeredness, then, changes the image of the conversation to one in which all participants are situated around the patient (who is both subject and participant), attending to one another for the purpose of improving the patient's well-being and quality of life.

In other clinical settings, the patient-centered approach has positively impacted patient satisfaction with their care, the quality of healthcare patients' received, and can contribute to improved health outcomes (Stewart, 2003; Epstein & Street, 2007; Hibbard & Greene, 2013). Some studies involving end-of-life care communication indicate similar results (See, e.g., White, Braddock, Bereknyei, & Curtis, 2007a). Unfortunately, results from large-scale studies show an ongoing disconnect between patients' wishes for end-of-life care and their experiences, which means we need to further examine how patient-centered communication could work in this context

(Hall, Levant, & DeFrances, 2013). What we lack is a broad picture of exactly how patient-centered communication about end-of-life care functions and what health outcomes it produces. To that end, our goal in this chapter is to reexamine existing literature involving observational studies of patient-physician communication about end-of-life care so that we more clearly see how patient-centered communication functions in this context, how it affects health outcomes, and how future research might target gaps in this area. We frame the literature reviewed in a patient-centered communication framework so that we can more clearly see how different types of communication have been linked to health outcomes.

To accomplish this goal, we bring together three main ideas. First, we examine the important role of family engagement in patient-centered communication generally and in end-of-life care communication specifically. Previous studies have reported mixed results on the effects of family presence in healthcare encounters on health outcomes (Wolff & Roter, 2011), but models of patient-centered communication acknowledge that family plays a critical role in achieving the goals of patient-centered care (Epstein & Street, 2007; White et al., 2007a). We argue that family engagement is uniquely important in end-of-life care communication because families often transition from stakeholders in the patient's care to surrogate decision makers.

Second, we use a patient-centered communication framework to describe the challenges of end-of-life care communication. Using Epstein and Street's (2007) model of patient-centered communication, we analyze existing studies in terms of the communicative functions they target. These functions include engaging in information exchange, responding to emotion, managing uncertainty, fostering relationships, making decisions, and enabling self-management. For example, some studies focus on informational aspects of communication such as the need to educate patients on their choices near end of life (e.g., Barnes et al., 2012), while others focus on coping with emotions and uncertainty (e.g., Clayton et al., 2013). Epstein and Street argue that these functions are "neither independent nor hierarchical. Rather they overlap and interact to produce communication that can affect important health outcomes" (p. 17).

Identifying communicative functions emerging from this literature not only provides a way of understanding the challenges of patient-centered end-of-life care communication; it also allows us to connect communication with health outcomes in the final part of the chapter. Using a pathway model that links communication to health outcomes (Street, Makoul, Arora, & Epstein, 2009; Wolff & Roter, 2011), we review existing research to identify the routes through which patient-family-clinician communication contributes to improved healthcare. For end-of-life care, some of these health outcomes include less pain experienced, better functional ability, and healthier emotional well-being. Ultimately, we will use this analysis to discuss future directions for research in this area.

FAMILY ENGAGEMENT IN PATIENT-CENTERED COMMUNICATION

Families play multiple, important roles in achieving the goals of patient-centered care, especially in end-of-life care communication. Patient-centered care is comprehensively defined as "patients, families, their representatives, and health professionals working in active partnership at various levels across the healthcare system direct care, organizational design and governance, and policy making to improve health and health care" (Carman et al., 2013, p. 224). Families engage in different ways throughout a patient's healthcare experience; they can be caregivers, surrogates, advocates, and a filter through which patients review health information (Spoth & Redmond, 2000). Families also influence understanding and attitudes toward health; and they reflect demographic and cultural barriers to care (Maurer, Dardess, Carman, Frazier, & Smeeding, 2012).

These characteristics of family involvement in patient-centered care are the foundation for two key ways family is particularly influential in patient-centered communication about end-of-life care. First, family engagement in patient-centered communication undoubtedly affects health outcomes in all health contexts, but it is particularly important at the end-of-life. Zolfaghari, Asgari, Bahramnezhad, AhmadiRad, & Haghani (2015) offer a clear example of family influence on outcomes in maintenance of a chronic disease. In a study of dialysis patients, they found increased patient adherence when families were educated about the treatment along with the patient, compared to an education program that only involved the patient. Families emphasized to the patient the value of adherence, and they helped the patient monitor his or her condition.

The effect of communication with family on healthcare outcomes is particularly important in end-of-life care because as the end of life approaches, family members become increasingly involved in both decision-making and caregiving. At the end of life, patients often shift to palliative options from curative options. Choosing palliative care options over curative options involves difficult emotional and intellectual decisions. While curative treatments can also involve these difficulties, these decisions require the negotiation of heightened emotions, an urgency to make decisions, and, the involvement of family, especially as the patient's ability to function declines (Faulkner, 1998). Families have the added burden of negotiating their own wishes for the patient as well as honoring the patient's wishes when these two positions conflict (Morrison & Meier, 2004).

Examples of family decision-making that directly affects healthcare outcomes can be found most clearly in literature involving two end-of-life care contexts: when families make care decisions for intensive care unit (ICU) patients and when parents shift from curative to palliative treatment for children. ICU family meetings are an important context for family involvement in end-of-life care communication because patients are often too sick to make care decisions independently (Pham, Thornton, Engelberg, Jackson, & Curtis, 2008). Many deaths involving the withdrawal of life support take place in hospital ICUs. Families frequently report dissatisfaction with the level of communication they have with ICU care providers (Weaver, Bradley, & Brasel, 2012). A cause of this dissatisfaction is the inability of family members to comprehend the extent of the patient's diagnosis, prognosis, and the nature of the decisions they would be asked to make (Azoulay et al., 2012).

When parents of dying children are put in the position of choosing palliative treatment over curative treatment, they face a nearly opposite effect; parents are informed, but sometimes they are shielded from making difficult choices by physicians (deVos et al., 2015). In these situations, families are engaged in care, but must negotiate their role in the decision-making process. A study of parent involvement in palliative care for children, for example, reported that although parents were given a great deal of information, they were rarely asked to participate in actual decision-making (deVos et al., 2015).

A second way in which families are influential in patient-centered communication about end-of-life care is that the presence of families changes the communication dynamic among patients and physicians. One study found that physicians actually gave more prognostic information to families when the patient was not present (Gramling et al., 2013a). Physicians in these instances also incorporated more information that would make decision-making more complicated; that is, they revealed more of the actual ambiguities of the treatment options. A study of hospice team meetings that sometimes included family members found that social workers and chaplains participated more and engaged in more socio-emotional talk when family was present (Wittenberg-Lyles et al., 2013). The meetings that included families also focused more on relationship-building with family members, as well as more biomedical education for family members and non-medical staff.

Of course, family members bring their own sets of issues to the conversation about end-of-life care (Hseih, Shannon, & Curtis, 2006). While the overarching tension is often whether or not to use life-saving treatments, the underlying tensions include whether foregoing treatment is "allowing the patient to die" or killing her, whether death is a benefit or burden; whether to honor the patients' or the family's wishes, whether the patient gave contradictory indications of their preferences, and whether the family or a chosen representative should even be making the decision in the first place. Hseih, Shannon and Curtis (2006) found that physicians employed two different communication strategies for dealing with these tensions: a directed decision-centered strategy or an information-seeking strategy. With directed decision-making strategies, the physician presents options and elicits a choice from the family. With information-seeking strategies, the physician asks the family questions about patient goals and checks their understanding of the patient's situation. The information-seeking strategies were found to be the most successful because they promoted not only conversation between the family and the physician, but also important conversations among family members.

Whether these tensions come to the surface in interactions with clinicians or not, they become part of the fabric of the communication among stakeholders. These relationships are not dyadic because they necessarily involve multiple participants, and they are subject not only to the involvement of family, but must meet the family's communicative needs as well (Pham et al., 2008).

FUNCTIONS OF END-OF-LIFE CARE COMMUNICATION

To recognize and pinpoint the challenges facing patient-centered communication in end-of-life care, it is important to first understand how this communication works in measurable terms. That is, we need to articulate what the communication actually *does* in a way that can be empirically studied. As mentioned earlier, the communication framework conceptual framework adopted for this review (Epstein & Street, 2007) describes six patient-centered communicative functions: fostering relationships, exploring information, responding to emotions, managing uncertainty, making decisions, and enabling patient self-management. In order to unknot the interplay of these functions, we first define the functions and then describe the challenges these functions present using three themes from the literature, communicating about death, communicating about treatment options, and communicating decisions.

Communicative functions describe the communication goals and outcomes physicians, patients, and families try to achieve in their interactions. It is important to note that communication among these participants is mutually influenced. That is, the way any one participant communicates affects the others, and participants will adjust how they communicate based on the way others do. If a physician encourages a patient and her family to ask questions, for example, the patient and family might do more information seeking than they otherwise would (Street, Gordon, Ward, Krupat, & Kravitz, 2005). On the other hand, a patient or family member might seek information by interrupting a physician who has not solicited questions (Eggly et al., 2006).

Because we focus on communication among patients, physicians and families about end of life care, perhaps the most important of the communicative functions is building relationships. Effective patient-physician relationships involve building trust, creating rapport, and defining the roles among patients, physicians, and their families (Epstein & Street, 2007). Out of this relationship comes a rapport among the participants, a sense of connection that is fostered through behaviors such as listening attentively to one another's concerns.

Information exchange is the most widely discussed of the functions and has historically been the subject of much of the observational research involving patient-physician communication (Street, 1991). Physicians, patients, and their families can alternately seek and provide information that is crucial to the encounter. Conversations about palliative and end-of-life care necessarily involve the exchange of difficult, ambiguous, and sometimes confusing information. Because of this difficulty, responding to emotion is an important function that can affect a patient's overall health (Dean & Street, 2014). In fact, the response to emotion has an impact not only on the wellbeing of patients, but on families and physicians themselves.

Both patients and physicians deal with uncertainties in treatment in regular medical care, but management of uncertainty is particularly important in discussions of end-of-life care. The uncertainty involved in death brings to bear existential questions that cannot be answered. Additionally, disease trajectories can be unpredictable, and life expectancy estimates are often incorrect (See, e.g., Chow et al., 2001). Despite this uncertainty, patients, physicians, and their families must continually make decisions. Communication involving decision-making typically involves information exchange, deliberation, and final decisions. Finally, enabling self-management involves recommendations and advocacy by companion that help the patient cope with her health, her prognosis, and her eventual death (Wollf & Roter, 2008). This type of communication involves both discovering ways others can help the patient and ways the patient can contribute to his or her healthcare.

Communicating about Death

The nature of end-of-life care and dealing with the idea of death is the first and perhaps the most prominent of the challenges to patient-centered communication in these situations. In a healthcare system dedicated to curing disease and helping patients live longer, managing the topic of death is challenging for physicians, patients, and families. In some patient-physician conversations about end-of-life care, death becomes the proverbial elephant in the room. Rodriguez, Gambino, Butow, Hagerty and Arnold (2007) found that patients and their physicians often avoided direct verbal references to death, despite their focus on end-of-life care. Of the oncologist-terminal patient interactions described in their study, only half involved a direct reference to death. In fact, patients and their families only explicitly referred to death in an emotional context—to express concern or anxiety about a prognosis, rather than to discuss their health status or treatment. Most other times, patients and families mentioned death indirectly, through common euphemisms such as "pushing up daisies."

This avoidant behavior stems in part from an unwillingness or inability to confront the emotional response to death. When emotions are addressed, however, a door may open to more frank and direct communication about death. Anderson, Kools and Lyndon (2013) found that physicians who coaxed patients by probing patients' emotional distress and acknowledging the possibility of death with the patient opened the conversation to more clear conversations about patient goals and desires for their care. The frank discussion of death, as well as talking about patient emotions, were found to be the critical turning points in patient-physician encounters that determined whether more specific discussion of patient preferences would be discussed.

However, the physician's response to patient and family emotions about death is among the most missed opportunities in a clinical encounter (Curtis et al., 2005). Lidén, Öhlén, Hydén and Friberg (2010) found that physicians generally "respond more often to informational than emotional cues" (p. 406). They classified avoidance strategies according to a communicative frame. Physicians tended to respond to a patient's emotional expression by redirecting the conversation or by avoiding the topic. For example, a physician might deflect a patient's expression of fear by redirecting the conversation to their physical symptoms. In the "patient-professional frame", the patient makes an emotional revelation and the physician, in her capacity as an expert, responds to the patient's feelings using "toning-down strategies" to steer the conversation to medically explain their feelings. The physician might, for example, explain a burst of tears or sadness as a result of fatigue. Thus, the physician effectively avoids responding to the patient's emotions. Avoiding emotion about death contributes to a climate that discourages patients and families from expressing their emotions in the encounter (Detmar, Muller, Wever, Schornagel, & Aaronson, 2001).

Although avoidant behavior leads to less direct discussion of death and the emotions surrounding it, some research suggests that talk about subject matter outside of healthcare may help patients and physicians develop a relationship that leads to more direct discussions. Lidén et al. (2010) describe a person-person frame in which the patient and physician communicate without the imposition of the power differences that normally affect patient-physician communication. In a person-person frame, patients and physicians build a relationship using talk that is outside of medical discourse. Talk that fosters person-person relationships can be collegial, in which the physician and patient treat one another as distant equals; playful, in which the physician and patient use humor to introduce ideas outside of the clinical; or existential, in which the physician and patient engage in talk about the meaning of life and death. Participants can engage this frame at various times during the encounter. Lidén et al. (2010) argue that this kind of talk contributes to the shared creation of a narrative of the patient's experience, which not only fosters a stronger patient-physician relationship in which more direct conversation can occur, but can be therapeutic for the patient as well. This narrative benefits the patient, who not only has a shared experience of their illness with someone with whom they share a relationship, but it also helps them process their own experience of their illness.

Communicating Options

Understanding treatment options is an important aspect of any healthcare encounter, but the palliative treatments involved in end-of-life care present communication challenges. These challenges stem from multiple causes, but they primarily involve the way physicians, patients, and families deal with complicated medical knowledge and the uncertainty associated with treatments. Exchange of information is essential for building understanding of medical information in a clinical setting (Epstein & Street, 2007). This exchange involves shoring up differences in medical knowledge by checking for understanding. For example, Friberg, Lidén, Håkanson and Öhlén (2014) found that physicians and patients can engage patient knowledge using visualization strategies, such as using readily available items for demonstration, and contrasting strategies, such as comparing the patient's subjective experiences with less serious illnesses, to help patients understand changes to their bodies. Using metaphor and common language, as well as patient experience, to understand health conditions also helps patients and physicians build rapport and develop mutual understanding.

However, checking for understanding is more difficult and often does not occur when families are involved. White et al. (2007a) found that physicians routinely did not check for understanding in families or patients. That is, they delivered information, but did not solicit from the family what the family internalized or understood. Encounters involving self-management also lack in checks for understanding. In conversations about adherence to anti-retroviral treatment for patients with advanced HIV, providers asked five times as many questions, rarely engaged in problem-solving dialogue, and made more directive statements to patients (Laws et al., 2013). In other words, physicians used dictatorial strategies for discussing compliance, as opposed to checking patient understanding of strategies for compliance. Racial disparities have also been observed in adherence encounters, with physicians of all races and ethnicities telling Black and Hispanic patients about adherence more, but not soliciting strategies for adherence from patients or engaging in dialogue that probed their knowledge (Laws et al., 2014).

Uncertainty also presents challenges in patient and physician communication about end-of-life care. Although physicians are often comfortable discussing symptoms and the course of disease, alternatives to curative treatments are more difficult to explain and may not be discussed (Koedoot et al., 2004). In palliative radiation consultations, for example, none involved an explanation of "watchful waiting", an alternative treatment in which symptoms are monitored and cared for prior to treatment. Any information on this type of treatment was avoided, perhaps because patients had prepared for the radiation treatment. Timmermans et al. (2005) also observed that patients who had decided to undergo palliative radiation treatment outside of the clinical encounter were not asked how they arrived at their decision. For example, once a patient made the decision to pursue radiation with their oncologist, their radiologist did not further inquire about how that decision was made or what kind of conversation they had with their oncologist.

Uncertainty is most acute and sometimes avoided in conversations about advance care planning. This type of planning involves making decisions about the level of care a patient wishes in different circumstances, which is mediated by factors such as the level of pain they can tolerate and the level of disability they are willing to endure. The level of prognostic information given has been found to vary with family's education level, with less information-giving associated with a lower level of family education (White, Engelberg, Wenrich, Lo, & Curtis, 2007b). That is, physicians do not engage in more complicated discussions involving more uncertainty with less educated people. In a study of clinical encounters involving advance directives, the majority of the conversations, which averaged five minutes, did not address uncertain situations (Tulsky, Fischer, Rose, & Arnold, 1998). These uncertain situations included more complicated treatment choices that would lead to less certain health outcomes. Rather, in the overwhelming majority of the encounters, physicians chose to present patients with a dire situation in which they would not survive with any level of curative care. Only in a smaller number of the encounters did physicians also present patients with circumstances in which their condition was potentially reversible, the kinds of circumstances in which patient preferences can be ambiguous, leading to greater uncertainty.

These decisions are further complicated by the consideration of quality of life issues. Detmar et al. (2001) noted that although patients wanted to discuss ways to improve their health-related quality of life (HRQOL), which involves factors such as fatigue and emotional distress, equally as much as technical or other medical issues, physicians were considerably less likely to address HRQOL strategies for self-management. On average, less than a quarter of the encounter was spent on these issues. And of the quality of life issues discussed, physicians were more likely to focus on management of pain and daily activity, to the detriment of managing emotional issues and fatigue. The discussion of HRQOL is often couched in treatment discussion, and even when patients have greatly advanced disease, the focus of these conversations is still on treatment and physical symptoms (Rodriguez et al., 2010).

Communicating Decisions

A final challenge to end-of-life care is the communication around making decisions among patients, families, and physicians. These decisions are limited by time. Patients at the end of life can actively participate in decision making for a limited amount of time. Thus, timing is crucial to determining whether patients can participate in decision-making because of the functional limitations caused by their deteriorating health (Bélanger et al., 2014). The way these conversations are initiated depends on the urgency of the situation and the nearness of death, but engaging the patient in the initiation of the conversation is the most effective strategy. Bélanger et al. (2014) observed that while physicians could initiate decision-making regarding symptoms and impending treatments, a more successful strategy was to segue into conversations about death by probing patient understanding of their condition.

After initiating the conversation about end-of-life care decision-making, physicians frame choices for patients. This framing can influence patient and family engagement in decision-making. One way physicians can frame these choices is through a technique called signposting (Norton et al., 2013). With signposting, the physician defines a condition or change in health status that is cause for further decision-making or for revisiting a decision that has been made. When a patient reaches a signpost, the physician uses other techniques to facilitate decision making, such as closing off a goal, or narrating the fact that a hoped-for outcome had not been reached, and by using a technique called clarifying the current path, which involves narrating the best and worst-case outcomes for the patient. In describing paths and signposts, physicians also can take opportunities to align possible outcomes with patient goals. That is, when a patient is considering a possible path, the physician defines paths in terms of their consistency with previously expressed goals.

OUTCOMES OF PALLIATIVE CARE COMMUNICATION

If the goal of patient-centered communication is to ultimately improve the quality of care a patient receives, then communication functions must be empirically linked to health outcomes. Although communication can sometimes directly affect health outcomes, more often than not, communication leads to outcomes that are proximal or intermediate. That is, while communication does not directly affect health most of the time, it very often affects outcomes along the way to improved health. The inability to link communication to these proximal or intermediate outcomes and ultimately to health outcomes is borne out by inconsistent results in communication-related studies (Street et al., 2009). Without an established pathway from communication to health outcomes, a causal connection cannot be made.

Thus patient-centered communication can be linked to proximal and intermediate outcomes, which in turn link communication to health outcomes in a pathways model (Street et al., 2009). Proximal outcomes mediate the relationship between communication processes and intermediate outcomes and health outcomes. Proximal outcomes tend to immediately follow the interaction and include patient understanding, patient satisfaction, clinician-patient agreement, trust, feeling "known" or understood, a patient's feeling of involvement, rapport, and motivation. Intermediate outcomes include access to care, quality medical decision, commitment to treatment, trust in the healthcare system, social support, self-care skills, and emotional management. These outcomes in turn can lead to health outcomes such as survival, lessening of suffering, emotional wellbeing, pain control, and functional ability (Street et al., 2009).

It is important to note that these pathways are contextual; the links to better outcomes depend on the circumstances in which the patient-centered communication occurs (Street et al., 2009). For palliative and end-of-life care, the circumstances are such that health outcomes do include physical outcomes such as pain control, but more often, in the absence of curative treatments, the target outcomes more often than not focus the emotional wellbeing of the patient and family members.

Several studies involving palliative care communication focused on have focused on proximal and intermediate outcomes that could contribute to better emotional well-being. For example, Casarett et al. (2010) found that patients whose physicians used metaphor and analogy felt they had received more information than patients whose physicians did not. They were also more likely to feel that their physician made sure that they understood their condition. The increased use of metaphor and analogy did not correspond to patients' feeling heard, though. Nor did it correspond to a patient's feeling that they had enough time to be heard by their oncologist.

Patient understanding can also be used as a vehicle for discussing more difficult aspects of end-of-life care. Bélanger et al. (2014) observed that while physicians could initiate decision-making regarding symptoms and impending treatments, a more successful strategy was to segue into conversations about death by probing patient understanding of their condition. This interactive approach, one that emphasized and incorporated the patient's understanding actually led to deeper and more meaningful conversation about end-of-life choices. However, the study also found that the rhetorical strategies used by physicians still largely relied on patient initiation of the discussion of death. That is, they concluded that physicians still place the onus on patients to directly discuss death. Patients did this by asking questions as well as directly bringing up their future.

Another circumstance involving patient understanding is the management of uncertainty, which was perceived as successful by patients, though these encounters often did not involve more ambiguous possibilities for treatment. In their study of advance care planning discussions by Tulsky et al. (2008), the vast majority of participants who were later surveyed about the encounter found the conversation worthwhile, and it adequately helped address their uncertainty. However, researchers noted that while almost all conversations discussed the direst of circumstances, only a little more than half dealt with the kinds of medical situations typically faced in end-of-life care, such as treatments that have an unknown or untested prognosis.

Finally, a successful strategy for getting patients involved in the conversation is to broach the subject of death by starting the conversation by probing a patient's emotional state. Anderson et al. (2013) found that physicians who coaxed patients by asking questions about patients' emotional distress and acknowledging with the patient the possibility of death opened the conversation to talking about patient goals and desires for their care. The frank discussion of death, as well talking about patient emotions, were found to be the critical turning points in patient-physician encounters that determined whether more specific discussion of patient preferences would be discussed.

Studies dealing with proximal outcomes involved the engagement and satisfaction of families in end-of-life care planning. For families, higher levels of shared decision-making were associated with higher levels of satisfaction with the process of communicating with physicians about palliative care options (White et al., 2007a). This kind of involvement can also lead to more effective decision-making. Additionally, families that were involved in ICU conversations in which physicians both asked questions and facilitated question-asking from families were more engaged in decision-making. Information-seeking strategies such as checking for understanding and soliciting family characteristics were found to be the most successful because they promoted not only conversation between the family unit and the physician, but important conversation among the family members (Hseih et al., 2006). This family engagement outside of the clinical environment also bolsters intermediate outcomes such as social support, as it activates the patient's social connections in their care.

Despite these positive findings, it is important to return to the difficulty of measuring outcomes for families, especially as they deal with the death of a loved one. Under these circumstances, communication methods that are effective in other contexts may not be useful. Gramling et al. (2013b) describe circumstances in which physicians must negotiate between their knowledge of impending death and family's holding onto hope for a better prognosis. In these cases, physicians were observed to acknowledge the family's beliefs, but assert their experience in the hopes of better preparing the family for the patient's death. Despite attempts to achieve meaningful family engagement, the family's beliefs in these cases may be insurmountable. In a study of the parents of 19 critically ill children, the majority of parents agreed when physicians expressed that their child should discontinue curative treatment. Although many agreed, their emotions expressed at this suggestion were understandably strong. During final consultations, when their children were very close to the end of life, all parents expressed a desire for their children to not suffer, but some still hoped for a miracle, in some cases asking whether their child could be brought back to consciousness so that they could say goodbye (de Vos et al., 2015).

FUTURE RESEARCH DIRECTIONS

Organizing the literature into this framework reveals many areas for future research in each of the three topics discussed, the role of family in end-of-life care communication, the functions of this communication, and related health outcomes. First, the complex role of family bears much more in-depth exploration. While there is some observational research on family engagement in ICU and pediatric palliative care contexts (e.g., Pham et al., 2008), the communicative roles of family in other contexts, such as hospice, routine provider visits, and conversations regarding advance care planning should be explored. Additionally, observational research can target other communicative functions of families, which extend beyond their decision-making responsibilities. These targets could include promoting patient self-efficacy, managing emotions, and the development of rapport with physicians. Finally, family communication should also be considered further as it affects intermediate and health outcomes. Although one study focused indirectly on social support as an outcome, the quality of health decisions, access to care options, should also be considered. Studies should also target health outcomes for both patients and families in an effort to connect communication outcomes to overall emotional and physical health of all stakeholders involved in these interactions.

Future research should also broaden the exploration of the functions of communication in palliative and end-of-life care. Although some studies deal with patient understanding, more work can be done in other areas. Communication involving self-management and managing uncertainty are ripe for more work. Although self-management becomes limited toward the end of life, this function could be studied in conjunction with pain management early on in the end-of-life process. Better pain management has been associated with positive health outcomes involving emotional wellbeing as well as survival rates (Temel, et al., 2010).

Finally, observational studies in palliative and end-of-life care communication should, despite the inherent difficulties involved in studying end-of-life care, attempt to connect health outcomes to intermediate and proximal outcomes. These studies must be conducted delicately, negotiating the considerable ethical challenges of any intrusion into a patient's end-of-life experience. Still, they are needed to be able to fully associate palliative and end-of-life care communication with improvements in pain control, emotional wellbeing, and even survival rates. These studies might include scales that measure well-being, records of pain levels, and an inspection of days in palliative care programs.

CONCLUSION

THE conversation is much more complex and emotionally charged than many ordinary conversations. Reviewing the literature of patient, family, and physician communication about end-of-life care using a patient-centered communication framework shows that more work can be done in this area to improve patients' quality of care. The challenge lies in effectively engaging patients, physicians, and families in this communication. Effective engagement can be achieved with attention to the three main ideas presented in this review. First, the important role of family in end-of-life care communication should be taken into consideration in the development of interventions and future studies. Additionally, a functional approach that can link specific types of communication to health outcomes should be used so that the types of communication that influence better quality care can be targeted and enhanced.

REFERENCES

Anderson, W. G., Kools, S., & Lyndon, A. (2013). Dancing Around Death Hospitalist–Patient Communication About Serious Illness. *Qualitative Health Research*, *23*(1), 3–13. doi:10.1177/1049732312461728 PMID:23034778

Azoulay, E., Chevret, S., Leleu, G., Pochard, F., Barboteu, M., Adrie, C., & Schlemmer, B. et al. (2000). Half the families of intensive care unit patients experience inadequate communication with physicians. *Critical Care Medicine*, *28*(8), 3044–3049. doi:10.1097/00003246-200008000-00061 PMID:10966293

Barnes, S., Gardiner, C., Gott, M., Payne, S., Chady, B., Small, N., & Halpin, D. et al. (2012). Enhancing patient-professional communication about end-of-life issues in life-limiting conditions: A critical review of the literature. *Journal of Pain and Symptom Management*, *44*(6), 866–879. doi:10.1016/j.jpainsymman.2011.11.009 PMID:22819438

Bélanger, E., Rodríguez, C., Groleau, D., Légaré, F., Macdonald, M. E., & Marchand, R. (2014). Initiating decision-making conversations in palliative care: An ethnographic discourse analysis. *BMC Palliative Care*, *13*(1), 63. doi:10.1186/1472-684X-13-63 PMID:25859161

Carman, K. L., Dardess, P., Maurer, M., Sofaer, S., Adams, K., Bechtel, C., & Sweeney, J. (2013). Patient and family engagement: A framework for understanding the elements and developing interventions and policies. *Health Affairs*, *32*(2), 223–231. doi:10.1377/hlthaff.2012.1133 PMID:23381514

Casarett, D., Pickard, A., Fishman, J. M., Alexander, S. C., Arnold, R. M., Pollak, K. I., & Tulsky, J. A. (2010). Can metaphors and analogies improve communication with seriously ill patients? *Journal of Palliative Medicine*, *13*(3), 255–260. doi:10.1089/jpm.2009.0221 PMID:19922170

Chow, E., Harth, T., Hruby, G., Finkelstein, J., Wu, J., & Danjoux, C. (2001). How accurate are physicians' clinical predictions of survival and the available prognostic tools in estimating survival times in terminally ill cancer patients? A systematic review. *Clinical Oncology*, *13*(3), 209–218. PMID:11527298

Clayton, J. M., Butow, P. N., Waters, A., Laidsaar-Powell, R. C., O'Brien, A., Boyle, F., & Tattersall, M. H. et al. (2013). Evaluation of a novel individualised communication-skills training intervention to improve doctors' confidence and skills in end-of-life communication. *Palliative Medicine*, *27*(3), 236–243. doi:10.1177/0269216312449683 PMID:22711714

Curtis, J. R., Engelberg, R. A., Wenrich, M. D., Shannon, S. E., Treece, P. D., & Rubenfeld, G. D. (2005). Missed opportunities during family conferences about end-of-life care in the intensive care unit. *American Journal of Respiratory and Critical Care Medicine*, *171*(8), 844–849. doi:10.1164/rccm.200409-1267OC PMID:15640361

de Vos, M. A., Bos, A. P., Plötz, F. B., van Heerde, M., de Graaff, B. M., Tates, K., ... & Willems, D. L. (2015). Talking With Parents About End-of-Life Decisions for Their Children. Pediatrics, peds-2014.

Dean, M., & Street, R. L. Jr. (2014). A 3-stage model of patient-centered communication for addressing cancer patients' emotional distress. *Patient Education and Counseling*, *94*(2), 143–148. doi:10.1016/j.pec.2013.09.025 PMID:24169023

Detmar, S. B., Muller, M. J., Wever, L. D., Schornagel, J. H., & Aaronson, N. K. (2001). Patient-physician communication during outpatient palliative treatment visits: An observational study. *Journal of the American Medical Association*, *285*(10), 1351–1357. doi:10.1001/jama.285.10.1351 PMID:11255393

Eggly, S., Penner, L. A., Greene, M., Harper, F. W., Ruckdeschel, J. C., & Albrecht, T. L. (2006). Information seeking during "bad news" oncology interactions: Question asking by patients and their companions. *Social Science & Medicine, 63*(11), 2974–2985. doi:10.1016/j.socscimed.2006.07.012 PMID:16962218

Epstein, R. M., & Street Jr, R. L. Patient-Centered Communication in Cancer Care: Promoting Healing and Reducing Suffering. *National Cancer Institute, NIH Publication* (07-6225).

Faulkner, A. (1998). ABC of palliative care. Communication with patients, families, and other professionals. *BMJ: British Medical Journal, 316*(7125), 130–132. doi:10.1136/bmj.316.7125.130 PMID:9462321

Friberg, F., Lidén, E., Håkanson, C., & Öhlén, J. (2014). Communicating bodily changes: Physicians' ways of enabling patient understanding in gastrointestinal cancer consultations. *Palliative & Supportive Care*, 13(3), 661-671. PMID:24784141

Gance-Cleveland, B. (2005). Family-Centered Care. *Journal for Specialists in Pediatric Nursing, 10*(3), 151–155. doi:10.1111/j.1744-6155.2005.00028.x PMID:16083436

Gramling, R., Norton, S., Ladwig, S., Winters, P., Metzger, M., Quill, T., & Alexander, S. (2013b). Latent Classes of Prognosis Conversations in Palliative Care: A Mixed-Methods Study. *Journal of Palliative Medicine, 16*(6), 653–660. doi:10.1089/jpm.2012.0381 PMID:23659459

Gramling, R., Norton, S. A., Ladwig, S., Metzger, M., DeLuca, J., Gramling, D., & Alexander, S. (2013a). Direct observation of prognosis communication in palliative care: A descriptive study. *Journal of Pain and Symptom Management, 45*(2), 202–212. doi:10.1016/j.jpainsymman.2012.02.004 PMID:22652135

Hall, M. J., Levant, S., & DeFrances, C. J. (2013). Trends in inpatient hospital deaths: National Hospital Discharge Survey, 2000-2010. *NCHS data brief*, (118), 1.

Hibbard, J. H., & Greene, J. (2013). What the evidence shows about patient activation: Better health outcomes and care experiences; fewer data on costs. *Health Affairs, 32*(2), 207–214. doi:10.1377/hlthaff.2012.1061 PMID:23381511

Hsieh, H. F., Shannon, S. E., & Curtis, J. R. (2006). Contradictions and communication strategies during end-of-life decision making in the intensive care unit. *Journal of Critical Care, 21*(4), 294–304. doi:10.1016/j.jcrc.2006.06.003 PMID:17175415

Koedoot, C. G., Oort, F. J., De Haan, R. J., Bakker, P. J. M., De Graeff, A., & de Haes, J. C. J. M. (2004). The content and amount of information given by medical oncologists when telling patients with advanced cancer what their treatment options are: Palliative chemotherapy and watchful-waiting. *European Journal of Cancer*, *40*(2), 225–235. doi:10.1016/j.ejca.2003.10.008 PMID:14728937

Laws, M. B., Beach, M. C., Lee, Y., Rogers, W. H., Saha, S., Korthuis, P. T., & Wilson, I. B. et al. (2013). Provider-patient adherence dialogue in HIV care: Results of a multisite study. *AIDS and Behavior*, *17*(1), 148–159. doi:10.1007/s10461-012-0143-z PMID:22290609

Laws, M. B., Lee, Y., Rogers, W. H., Beach, M. C., Saha, S., Korthuis, P. T., & Wilson, I. B. et al. (2014). Provider–Patient Communication About Adherence to Anti-retroviral Regimens Differs by Patient Race and Ethnicity. *AIDS and Behavior*, *18*(7), 1279–1287. doi:10.1007/s10461-014-0697-z PMID:24464408

Lidén, E., Öhlén, J., Hydén, L. C., & Friberg, F. (2010). Ways of talking about illness and prognosis in palliative cancer care consultations—two interactional frames. *Supportive Care in Cancer*, *18*(4), 399–408. doi:10.1007/s00520-009-0673-8 PMID:19504353

Maurer, M., Dardess, P., Carman, K. L., Frazier, K., & Smeeding, L. (2012). *Guide to patient and family engagement: environmental scan report*. Rockville, MD: Agency for Healthcare Research and Quality.

Morrison, R. S., & Meier, D. E. (2004). Palliative care. *The New England Journal of Medicine*, *350*(25), 2582–2590. doi:10.1056/NEJMcp035232 PMID:15201415

Norton, S. A., Metzger, M., DeLuca, J., Alexander, S. C., Quill, T. E., & Gramling, R. (2013). Palliative Care Communication: Linking Patients' Prognoses, Values, and Goals of Care. *Research in Nursing & Health*, *36*(6), 582–590. doi:10.1002/nur.21563 PMID:24114740

Pham, K., Thornton, J. D., Engelberg, R. A., Jackson, J. C., & Curtis, J. R. (2008). Alterations during medical interpretation of ICU family conferences that interfere with or enhance communication. *CHEST Journal*, *134*(1), 109–116. doi:10.1378/chest.07-2852 PMID:18347204

Rodriguez, K. L., Bayliss, N., Alexander, S. C., Jeffreys, A. S., Olsen, M. K., Pollak, K. I., & Arnold, R. M. (2010). How oncologists and their patients with advanced cancer communicate about health-related quality of life. *Psycho-Oncology*, *19*(5), 490–499. doi:10.1002/pon.1579 PMID:19449348

Rodriguez, K. L., Gambino, F. J., Butow, P., Hagerty, R., & Arnold, R. M. (2007). Pushing up daisies: Implicit and explicit language in oncologist–patient communication about death. *Supportive Care in Cancer, 15*(2), 153–161. doi:10.1007/s00520-006-0108-8 PMID:16969631

Spoth, R., & Redmond, C. (2000). Research on family engagement in preventive interventions: Toward improved use of scientific findings in primary prevention practice. *The Journal of Primary Prevention, 21*(2), 267–284. doi:10.1023/A:1007039421026

Stewart, M. (2003). *Patient-centered medicine: transforming the clinical method.* Radcliffe Publishing.

Street, R. L. Jr. (1991). Information-giving in medical consultations: The influence of patients' communicative styles and personal characteristics. *Social Science & Medicine, 32*(5), 541–548. doi:10.1016/0277-9536(91)90288-N PMID:2017721

Street, R. L. Jr, Gordon, H. S., Ward, M. M., Krupat, E., & Kravitz, R. L. (2005). Patient participation in medical consultations: Why some patients are more involved than others. *Medical Care, 43*(10), 960–969. doi:10.1097/01.mlr.0000178172.40344.70 PMID:16166865

Street, R. L. Jr, Makoul, G., Arora, N. K., & Epstein, R. M. (2009). How does communication heal? Pathways linking clinician–patient communication to health outcomes. *Patient Education and Counseling, 74*(3), 295–301. doi:10.1016/j.pec.2008.11.015 PMID:19150199

Tang, S. T., Liu, T. W., Liu, L. N., Chiu, C. F., Hsieh, R. K., & Tsai, C. M. (2014). Physician–patient end-of-life care discussions: Correlates and associations with end-of-life care preferences of cancer patients—a cross-sectional survey study. *Palliative Medicine, 28*(10), 1222–1230. doi:10.1177/0269216314540974 PMID:24965755

Temel, J. S., Greer, J. A., Muzikansky, A., Gallagher, E. R., Admane, S., Jackson, V. A., & Lynch, T. J. et al. (2010). Early palliative care for patients with metastatic non–small-cell lung cancer. *The New England Journal of Medicine, 363*(8), 733–742. doi:10.1056/NEJMoa1000678 PMID:20818875

Timmermans, L. M., van der Maazen, R. W., Verhaak, C. M., van Roosmalen, M. S., van Daal, W. A., & Kraaimaat, F. W. (2005). Patient participation in discussing palliative radiotherapy. *Patient Education and Counseling, 57*(1), 53–61. doi:10.1016/j.pec.2004.03.016 PMID:15797153

Tulsky, J. A., Fischer, G. S., Rose, M. R., & Arnold, R. M. (1998). Opening the black box: How do physicians communicate about advance directives? *Annals of Internal Medicine*, *129*(6), 441–449. doi:10.7326/0003-4819-129-6-199809150-00003 PMID:9735081

Volandes, A. E. (2015). *The conversation: a revolutionary plan for end-of-life care*. Bloomsbury Publishing USA.

Weaver, J. L., Bradley, C. T., & Brasel, K. J. (2012). Family engagement regarding the critically ill patient. *The Surgical Clinics of North America*, *92*(6), 1637–1647. doi:10.1016/j.suc.2012.08.004 PMID:23153887

Weeks, J. C., Catalano, P. J., Cronin, A., Finkelman, M. D., Mack, J. W., Keating, N. L., & Schrag, D. (2012). Patients' expectations about effects of chemotherapy for advanced cancer. *The New England Journal of Medicine*, *367*(17), 1616–1625. doi:10.1056/NEJMoa1204410 PMID:23094723

White, D. B., Braddock, C. H., Bereknyei, S., & Curtis, J. R. (2007a). Toward shared decision making at the end of life in intensive care units: Opportunities for improvement. *Archives of Internal Medicine*, *167*(5), 461–467. doi:10.1001/archinte.167.5.461 PMID:17353493

White, D. B., Engelberg, R. A., Wenrich, M. D., Lo, B., & Curtis, J. R. (2007b). Prognostication during physician-family discussions about limiting life support in intensive care units*. *Critical Care Medicine*, *35*(2), 442–448. doi:10.1097/01.CCM.0000254723.28270.14 PMID:17205000

Wittenberg-Lyles, E., Oliver, D. P., Demiris, G., Burt, S., & Regehr, K. (2009). Inviting the absent members: Examining how caregivers' participation affects hospice team communication. *Palliative Medicine*. PMID:20007820

Wittenberg-Lyles, E., Oliver, D. P., Kruse, R. L., Demiris, G., Gage, L. A., & Wagner, K. (2013). Family caregiver participation in hospice interdisciplinary team meetings: How does it affect the nature and content of communication? *Health Communication*, *28*(2), 110–118. doi:10.1080/10410236.2011.652935 PMID:22435889

Wolff, J. L., & Roter, D. L. (2011). Family presence in routine medical visits: A meta-analytical review. *Social Science & Medicine*, *72*(6), 823–831. doi:10.1016/j.socscimed.2011.01.015 PMID:21353358

Zolfaghari, M., Asgari, P., & Bahramnezhad, F., AhmadiRad, S., & Haghani, H. (2015). Comparison of two educational methods (family-centered and patient-centered) on hemodialysis: Related complications. *Iranian Journal Of Nursing & Midwifery Research*, *20*(1), 87–92. PMID:25709696

KEY TERMS AND DEFINITIONS

Communicative Function: The purpose of a given type of communication.

End-of-Life Care: Healthcare delivered to a patient that has a prognosis of six months or less to live.

Health Outcome: A medical or health-related result such as survival or quality of life.

Intermediate Outcome: A mediator of the relationships between communication outcomes and health outcomes.

Patient-Centered Communication: Communication between patients and physicians that considers the patient's needs and perspective, gives the patient the opportunity to participate in their own healthcare, and enhances the patient-physician relationship.

Proximal Outcome: A mediator of the relationship between communication processes and intermediate outcomes as well as health outcomes.

Sign-Posting: Framing an event or series of events as an opportunity to make a decision.

Section 2
The Potentiality of New Technologies to Promote Patient's Participation and Engagement in Health Management

Chapter 5
Engaging Patients and Lowering Costs:
Technology to the Rescue

Tony Zordich
Business BenchmaRx, USA

Julia Menichetti
Catholic University of the Sacred Heart, Italy

ABSTRACT

Societies need solutions to achieve the "triple aim" of improved health outcomes, better patient care, and lower costs; and engaging patients in their care by using technological solutions is claimed as a possible strategy to achieve this vital goal. On this basis, the chapter focuses on reviewing, categorizing and synthesizing technological tools currently available in the market today designed to engage patients in their own care process. In particular, the goals of medication adherence, reduced hospital readmission, behavior modification, and health literacy - with related technologies - are assessed, since they are considered todays most expensive health care burdens. The advantages, shortcomings, and potential economic impact of such tools are finally discussed.

INTRODUCTION

Judging by the investment dollars stimulating the digital health industry, the provocative statement that "patient engagement is the blockbuster drug of the century" (Chase, 2012) appears to be on track. Rock health has reported that 2014 venture capital funding into that space exceeded USD $4 billion, nearly equivalent to the

DOI: 10.4018/978-1-5225-0663-8.ch005

prior three years. It is evident how this has moved investments to foster the patient engagement demand without burdening healthcare systems (Graffigna & Barello, 2015). The potential payoff promises to contribute to a triple aim approach, a framework developed by the institute for healthcare improvement (Ihi, 2015) to improve population health and patients' experience of care while reducing costs (Berwick, Nolan, & Whittington, 2008). The reward can be huge. Consequently, tools aimed to activate the patient with a specific health care-related action represent to date one of the top investment categories inside the digital health market (Ricciardi, Mostashari, Murphy, Daniel, & Siminerio, 2013; Wang, 2015). Despite high expectations, the value of technologies for patient engagement in controlling health care costs is still largely unknown.

Moving from these premises, the following paragraphs detail how technologies are developing to reply to the need of improving the patients' experience of care, that is giving them a new more active role in the healthcare path, while lowering costs (Ihi, 2015; Berwick et al., 2008). Thereafter, on this basis, the chapter focuses on reviewing, categorizing and synthesizing technological tools currently available in the market today designed to engage patients in their own care process. In particular, the goals of medication adherence, reduced hospital readmission, behavior modification, and health literacy - with related technologies - are assessed, since they are considered among today's most expensive health care burdens (Iuga & mcguire, 2014; Goetzel et al., 1998). The advantages, shortcomings, and potential economic impact of such tools are finally discussed.

BACKGROUND

Stating that health care costs, especially in the united states, continue to capture an extraordinary amount of the gross domestic product is nothing of news (Levit et al., 2003). A quick assessment of published data in just a few related healthcare categories reveals staggering costs.

The cost of medication non-adherence in the U.S. has been estimated at $100 billion to $300 billion annually (Hagland 2013; pharmaceutical research and manufacturers of america [pharma], 2011) and is directly related to poor clinical outcomes, high health care costs, and lost productivity (Sokol, Mcguigan, Verbrugge, & Epstein, 2005). Approximately 3.3 million adult 30-day hospital readmissions occurred during 2011 in the united states, associated with about $41.3 billion in hospital costs (Hines, Barrett, Jiang, & Steiner, 2011). Estimates from the Institute of Medicine (2012) indicate that a health-literate society could save excess health care costs estimated at $73 billion.

Needless to say, those are too many billions to ignore.

Engaging Patients and Lowering Costs

Societies need solutions to achieve the "triple aim" of improved health outcomes, better patient care, and lower costs. Patient engagement seems to be a possible answer to the economical and organizational issues contemporary societies has to cope with, since it increases individual responsibility and awareness about one's health/wellbeing and the risk of unhealthy behaviors (Graffigna & Barello, 2015). Engaging patients in their own care is claimed as a promising strategy to achieve this vital triple aim goal (Hibbard & Greene, 2013). However, patients are one of the most underutilized resources in the healthcare ecosystem. The enabled patient can assume a starring role in their healthcare journey including involvement in the health plan and decision process, and embrace the growing wave of efforts to improve the quality of health care (Menichetti, Libreri, Lozza, & Graffigna, 2014).

Indeed, a growing body of evidence demonstrates that citizens who are more actively involved in their healthcare experience better health outcomes and incurs lower costs (Hibbard, Greene, & Overton, 2013). As a result, many public and private health organizations are defining and applying strategies to engage their clients. Different efforts have been made to define what engaging patients really mean and how this goal can be accomplished (Barello, Graffigna, Vegni, & Bosio, 2014; Hibbard et al., 2013). Graffigna suggests a comprehensive analysis of patient engagement should be defined as "a processual multi-level experience that results

Figure 1. Patient engagement survey

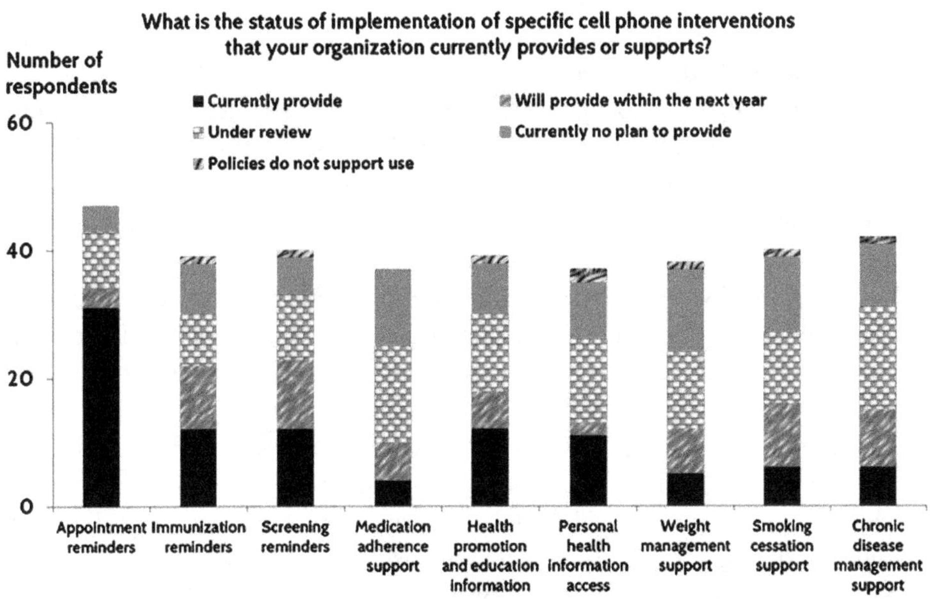

Figure 2.

Study Population	Readmission Costs (as a percentage of total cost of study population readmissions)	Readmission Rate (per 100 admissions)
Medicare (65+ years)	58.2%	17.2
Medicaid (18 to 64 years)	18.4%	14.6
Privately Insured (18 to 64 years)	19.6%	8.7
Uninsured (18 to 64 years)	3.7%	10.6

from conjoint cognitive (think), emotional (feel) and conative (act) orientation of individuals towards their health management" (Graffigna, Barello, Wiederhold, Bosio, & Riva, 2013a).

While early reports suggest medication adherence, behavior modification, and reduced hospital admissions are visible results of having better engaged patients in managing their health condition, only slow progresses in these efforts are occurring and "the task of improving individuals' care is hardly completed" (Berwick, Nolan, & Whittington, 2008, p. 760). Societies are still struggling to make patients aware actors in their health care path and active stakeholders able to optimally manage their health conditions and productively interact with their health providers.

The commonwealth fund (2015), reports lackluster adoption of patient engagement technologies to date. In their survey of 180 responding health care facilities, most reported utilizing cell phone technology for appointment, immunization, and screening reminders yet identify arguably the most health- and cost-effective technologies as projects for the coming year or under review, including chronic disease management, medication adherence, educational health promotion, weight management, and tobacco cessation programs.

Moreover, too few improvement efforts are proven cost-effective and sustainable for healthcare institutions. It is unclear if patient engagement on a large scale and its related costs are positively associated. Although some studies reported that more activated patients help healthcare institutions in reducing costs (Hibbard et al., 2013), the costs of adopting solutions or delivering interventions for this effort are not considered. For this reason, technologies –thanks to their advantages of being convenient, easy to use, and widely diffused – are more and more adopted to help patients in adhering to medications, autonomously manage the health condition, or support lifestyles changes (Mcgrady, Conger, Blanke, & Landry, 2010).

Technology-based solutions can be a rescue. As such, there has been a spread of tracking systems, platforms for patients to share information, portals to safely communicate with health professionals to boost patient engagement along the healthcare journey. Along with these solutions, mobile health solutions, wearable devices and home-based systems have also been adopted to support the engagement of health consumers. It is evident how a wide range of technology-based solutions are now playing a role in engaging patients with their disease management and their health, and consequently in accomplishing the triple aim of having better health outcomes while reducing costs.

TECHNOLOGY TO THE RESCUE?

A spectacular collection of highly creative and problem-solving technologies are now available to patients (consumer), health care providers, and payers to address these costly issues an overview of the technology is presented by condition and intervention type, and divided into the main goals of medication adherence, reduced hospital readmission, behavior modification, and health literacy.

Medication Adherence

Approximately 30 percent of hospital admissions of older adults are drug related, with more than 11 percent attributed to medication non-adherence and 10 to 17 percent related to adverse drug reactions (Marek & Antle, 2008). Medication non-adherence includes patients forgetting to take a prescribed medicine, stopping their medicine earlier than instructed, and taking incorrect amounts (Dayer, Heldenbrand, Anderson, Gubbins, & Martin, 2013). The medication adherence market segment is being vigorously addressed with a variety of patient activation strategies and embraces currently available technologies such as smart phones or dedicated tablets.

Mobile solutions: medication dose reminders, educational resources, and automated refill prompts can be delivered to and accessed from patients' phones to manage their prescriptions digitally (Dayer et al., 2013; Park, Howie-Esquivel, Chung, & Dracup, 2014). The market of mobile solutions for medication adherence is wide and most of the times out of the reach of the published academic literature. As shown in one recent review of medication adherence applications available on the operating systems of apple, android, and blackberry, generally those solutions and their efficacy are untested (Dayer et al., 2013). However, we are recently assisting to a growth of researches aimed to test the efficacy of the different mobile tools available in the market (park et al., 2014). These studies suggest that automated text and short message service (Sms) messaging are among the most commonly used communication formats (Dayer et al., 2013; Park et al., 2014; Vervloet et al., 2012). In particular, personalized or tailored Sms with motivational and educational contents have greater adherence results (Park et al., 2014). Education, prompts, gamification, and awards might well improve medication adherence with an engaging and entertaining patient experience (Cafazzo, Casselman, Hamming, Katzman, & Palmert, 2012; Park et al., 2014; Darlow & Wen, 2015). Early trial outcomes appear favorable, but ongoing creative engagements seem essential to maintain long-term novelty.

Interactive, real-time communications, commonly text messaging, is also available, but early analysis of this method in cardiovascular and diabetes morbidities suggests limited success (Misono et al., 2010). Sms messaging is a reliable text service used by a number of developers engaged in this space, proved to be one of the most feasible and acceptable solutions for health management (park et al., 2014). It does not, however, always meet health insurance portability and accountability act (Hipaa) requirements (Yang & Silverman, 2014). The use of personal health information (Phi) in mobile communication represents a debated and problematic issue (Luxton, Kayl, & Mishkind, 2012). This limitation can compromise communications, especially with health care providers. Generally, the available applications remind the patient when it is time to take their medication with instruction for proper administration of the drug (Dayer et al., 2013; Park et al., 2014). These application reminders are also delivered to family members, friends, and caregivers to monitor patient medication activity remotely (Piette et al., 2015). Progressive reminder systems help patients remember their medication and notify specific caregivers when a medication is missed. Ideally, outreach from the notified caregiver can occur to prevent mishap. Generally, few studies report a cost-analysis of their mobile reminder intervention (Park et al., 2014).

Directly observed therapy: a patented technology utilizing directly observed therapy (dot), including interactive facial recognition and motion-sensing technology, is under review to monitor medication adherence. An observer can remotely visualize actual oral insertion and ingestion of the medication via real-time smart phone video although a relatively failsafe approach to adherence monitoring, dot might be interpreted as intrusive and laborious for ongoing use. Studies to support the long-term viability of this approach are needed.

Presorted medications: several patient-specific presorted medication packs, including multiple prescription fulfillments, are available labeled with the medication names and date and time to use (Bear & Jain, 2011; Burg, Ingalz, Yamashita, & Takarada, 2009). The patients and caregivers can readily identify administration tracking and details about each prescription. Presorted medication packages provide an easy-to-use approach yet is easily subject to overt misuse (Bear & Jain, 2011; Burg et al., 2009).

Smart pill bottles: several unique pill bottles are currently available or under investigation in pharmaceutical and research engagements with integral technology to monitor medication dispensing (Lai, 2006; Passamante, 1998). The smart bottles, programmed to the patient's medication regimen, will glow, flash, and/or beep, and utilizing wireless technology or mobile phone connectivity, sends patients automated phone calls and text messages as reminders. The device also collects and sends adherence data in real time to appropriate support personnel (Lai, 2006; Passamante, 1998).

Electronic monitoring devices: digital health and the inherent ease of tracking provides for concise and convenient monitoring of medication compliance. Dashboard displays from many applications provide real-time information or weekly summaries to pharmacies or health care providers detailing the prescription-history data (Curtis et al., 2008; Farmer, 1999). Monitoring the patient from a professional and family or friend circle of care is achievable and likely to improve outcomes.

Hospital Readmission

The centers for Medicare and Medicaid services defines readmission as an admission to a subsection hospital within 30 days of a discharge from the same or another subsection hospital (CMS, 2014).

The U.S. affordable care act of march 2010 (2011) includes a Medicaid program payment adjustment for provider-preventable conditions that aim to reduce the number of readmissions relate to CMS-authorized payments, including health care-acquired conditions. In October 2012, CMS began reducing Medicare payments for the inpatient prospective payment system to hospitals with excessive readmission rates based initially on several morbidities, with annual incremental morbidity measures (e.g., stroke, pneumonia, heart failure, total hip or knee arthroplasty, chronic obstructive pulmonary disease).

At the time of this writing (April 2015), Medicare penalties for readmission rates affected 2,610 us hospitals for the preceding reporting year. From October 1, 2015, through September 30, 2016, those hospitals will receive lower payments for every Medicare patient stay, not just for those patients who are readmitted. Medicare estimates that over the course of the year, the fines will total about $428 million (Rau, 2014).

Perhaps as no surprise, 30-day readmission rates appear influenced by patient age and location, and socioeconomic status (Weissman, stern, & Epstein 1994). An analysis of Medicare data by the Dartmouth atlas project (2015) revealed that one in five elderly patients, age 65 and over, is readmitted. The report also states, "there are many different reasons for higher readmission rates across certain regions and hospitals including differences in patient health status, the quality of inpatient care, discharge planning and care coordination prior to discharge, and the availability and effectiveness of ambulatory services in the community" (dap, 2015).

Numerous strategies are being adopted to address the readmission issue (Ahmad, Metlay, Barg, Henderson, & Werner, 2013). Early findings of in-home physician visits, staff or contract nurse agency visits, and proactive phone contact with the patient following discharge to ensure appropriate patient compliance is encouraging (rich et al., 1995; blue et al., 2001; Krumholz et al., 2002). The report of national committee for quality assurance (NCQA, 2012) - insights for improvement, reducing readmission: measuring health plan performance - suggests that interventions such as nurse case management, physician follow-up visits, home visits, telephone follow-up, and care in a patient-centered medical home (PCMH) achieved reductions in readmissions ranging from 5 percent to nearly 30 percent with patients experiencing congestive heart failure. Generally, the potential to reduce readmissions is significant given the professional and technical interventions available today.

Mobile apps: as with medication adherence, mobile applications address a variety of disease types and are available for iOS and Droid smart phones and tablets to enhance patient support during the transition of care through recovery (West, 2012). The apps allow patients to maintain a constant and ongoing communication with providers and care transition teams during the critical 30-day period and beyond (West, 2012). Many applications allow patients to add their own vital data manually into the mobile device or by connecting to wearable or connected devices. Patient management and tracking is accomplished through data capture, storage, and sharing with the health care provider. Dashboard-type displays monitored at a caregiver facility display trends and subtle changes in monitored parameters, enabling real-time or episodic monitoring (West, 2012).

Connecting devices: the movement of a patient from one setting of care (hospital, ambulatory primary care practice, ambulatory specialty care practice, long-term care, home health, rehabilitation facility) to another or home presents a disruption in service and creates a condition requiring oversight. Team collaboration is enhanced by connecting provider organizations and ultimately improving outcomes and reducing costs (Coleman, Austin, Brach, & Wagner, 2009). Numerous population management packages allow for efficient health care history and treatment information exchange (electronic medical record) during the patient hand-off from the hospital to an ambulatory or community care setting (Graetz et al., 2009). Indeed, population health management allows health care providers to remotely monitor with tracking technology large groups of patients with the same chronic condition (Graetz et al.,

2009). The inherent power of technology to analyze and compare patient data enables providers to stratify patients into high-risk, low-risk, and rising-risk categories and potentially intervene when needed. Patients essentially maintain contact with their health care provider between regular visits. This proactive approach is economically efficient and can lead to better outcomes and reduced readmissions.

As an economic alternative to in-office or in-home visits, secure video conferencing for routine follow-up is possible for face-to-face communications and interaction (Finkelstein, Speedie, & Potthoff, 2006). Secure conferencing between health providers and patients can serve as a method for dialogue or assistance with disease management, a vehicle for education, or as more contact points for interaction (Gaikwad & Warren, 2009; Perednia & Allen, 1995).

Care management, through a multifaceted approach, should include family caregivers, reminders for post discharge appointments on patients' smart phones, and intervention by case managers and providers to rapidly assess and monitor the patient through dashboard monitoring to prevent hospital readmission.

Phone health coaching: as noted earlier, many health care systems provide nurse or physician house calls to monitor the patient in his or her home setting. Alternatively, direct patient contact is provided by health-connected health coaches (Bennett, Coleman, Parry, Bodenheimer, & Chen, 2010). Health coaches are often nurse credentialed and staff call centers with excellent personal and professional patient support (Bennett et al., 2010). Well-trained non-nurse staff and social workers coach the patient through the care plans with personal phone calls and messages (Holmes-Rovner et al., 2008). Different trials demonstrate how telephone coaching improve health outcomes, medication adherence and reduce hospital readmission (Turner et al., 2008; Vale et al., 2003; Holmes-Rovner et al., 2008) many coach and nurse line services are provided 24/7 (Bennett et al., 2010).

Symptom tracking devices: digital glucose meters, scales, blood pressure cuffs, stethoscopes, and other wearable and connectable activity monitors track daily patterns and record in a rhythm journal normal living patterns by combining activity data – sitting, standing, walking, and lying down – with the location (Swan, 2009). If a change occurs, the patient receives an alert, and it is easier to see the bigger picture and predict whether issues need follow-up.

Behavior Modification

The evolution of novel patient engagement tools and approaches holds great promise to improve health care outcomes and reduce associated costs (Ahern, Phalen, & Eaton, 2008). The efficacy of these efforts will rest largely on the patient's active participation and utilization of such programs.

The barriers to successful compliance are plentiful. Lack of exercise, forgetting to take medication, inability to afford the copayment or read the directions on the medicine bottle, depression/stress/anxiety, and lack of motivation are a few. Technology can help the patient or the caregiver to identify barriers, stratify the patient position, and address and tweak behaviors (Graffigna, Barello, & Riva, 2013b). To date, there is a great availability of evidence-based behavioral change programs supported by a generous number of technology developers (Free et al., 2013).

Monitoring devices: wearable devices and sensors monitor and track patient activity information for continuous monitoring (Swan, 2009). Activity data includes sitting, standing, walking, and lying down (Swan, 2009). Smart algorithms establish life pattern norms for each individual patient. Changes in the patient's daily life patterns can be a precursor to a developing problem, and those in the circle of care can be notified for potential intervention (Swan, 2009).

Technology-based health coaching: health coaches and the delivery of care, cited earlier in the chapter, deserve further attention as related to behavior modification (Bennett et al., 2010). Utilizing interactive and rule-based technology, collaborative health management enables patient-centric support by coaches, physicians, direct caregivers, pharmacists, and family and friends, especially at vulnerable times. Costly errors and complications can potentially be reduced or eliminated through intervention and encouraged behavioral modification.

Games and rewards: rewards and incentives in various sectors of the health care industry have garnered much attention in the past several years. The intent of these rewards and incentives is to motivate consumers to lead healthier lifestyles and are being offered by employers, health plans, and payers.

The U.S. federal government is also heavily engaged in incentive motivation through the Affordable Care Act (ACA) and centers for Medicare and Medicaid services with outcomes-based wellness and cessation programs. A meta-analysis with a pooled study sample of 1,403 participants showed that financial incentives designed using concepts from behavioral economics were effective for promoting health behavior change (Haff et al., 2015).

Although Cass and Sunstein (2015) have cited behavioral scientists who have shown that people are "loss averse" and tend to dislike losses more than they like corresponding gains, patient engagement applications available to date, as known by the author, utilize a rewards and incentive approach. Many mobile apps feature reward systems combined with a gamification strategy, making health care education and engagement more enticing. Apps featuring gamification provide psychological incentives for patients and appeal to their sense of achievement while introducing a series of engaging tasks and challenges in small, achievable steps. A popular medication adherence application awards patients "points" for self-reporting daily medication adherence, taking weekly quizzes, and opening educational content delivered prompts. Points are then redeemable for health-related merchandise at a private shopping site. Motivation through gamification triggers immediate action and, ideally, will result in long-term behavior modification.

Health Literacy

A likely starting point in the assessment of a patient's current and ideal level of active health care participation is understanding his or her level of health care literacy (Smith, Curtis, Wardle, Von Wagner, & Wolf, 2013). The Institute of Medicine (2004) have defined health literacy as "the capacity to obtain, process, and understand basic health information and services needed to make appropriate health decisions", basically how well a patient can understand and act on health information (Sørensen et al., 2012).

Berkman et al. (2004) have stated that limited health literacy is associated with poorer health outcomes and higher health care costs. Patients who are unable to follow medical recommendations because of insufficient understanding face greater risk of noncompliance, readmission, and medical complications. Language and cultural barriers exacerbate the problem (Safeer, Cooke, & Keenan, 2006). As we move toward a patient-centered organization of health care where consumers take an active role in their healthcare plans, patients need more and more strong health information skills (Boren, 2009). Technologies can help interventions to be delivered in a cost-effective way, thus strengthening the information skills of patients (Boren, 2009).

Computerized solutions: recently developed software applications address the health care literacy issue with creative and easy-to-follow tutorials through numerous formats. Most content is developed at a mid-elementary school level for easy consumption and is evaluated for patients with low levels of health literacy (Bickmore & Paasche-Orlow, 2012). Moore et al. (2014) reported "encouraging evidence" (p. 110-122) of assisting the patient as a technology supported apprentice to elevate self-efficacy and empowerment with several disease states. Several developers have also provided on-boarding assessment to identify key patient barriers and creating a literacy baseline prior to the first touch (Bickmore & Paasche-Orlow, 2012). A personalized care plan can then be delivered starting with the area of the patient's interest and expand the plan and knowledge base with clinically validated data. Computerized intervention systems usually link text information to audio, video or graphical displays, and use touch screen so to be developed for people with low computer literacy levels (Gerber et al., 2005). Some recent studies also test the utility of using embodied conversational agents instead than other modalities to support the optimal exchange of health information among patients with low health literacy scores (Bickmore et al., 2010).

Videos: condition-specific educational video streaming is also available for viewing on home computers or mobile devices. Video content can include condition background and management information, and can be delivered on an introductory or scheduled, ongoing basis (Pignone, Dewalt, Sheridan, Berkman, & Lohr, 2005). As well, during in-office visits, physicians can be notified on portable devices or pc about the health literacy skills of their patients to communicate properly and aid in educating and conversing with patients (Seligman et al., 2005).

Phone systems: some telephone solutions are available in the market to overcome computer literacy or computer access barriers. Generally, these systems are interactive voices with a response-based implementation (Bickmore & Paasche-Orlow, 2012). Some studies report how these solutions can help overcoming the health literacy barriers and engaging patients in their care (Shea et al., 2008).

SO CLOSE YET SO FAR

With this chapter, we aimed to provide an overview of the main technologies available on the market to sustain the patient engagement innovation, with a particular emphasis to the goals of medication adherence, behavior modification, reduced hospital readmission, and improved health literacy. The impact of technologies to support behavioral change, improve health literacy levels, and sustain a good long-term recovery may be substantial. As other reviews showed, technologies have the potential to be feasible and well-accepted by patients (Beatty, Fukuoka, & Whooley, 2013). However, best practices and effective strategies for such technology are yet to be established (Beatty, Fukuoka, & Whooley, 2013), and the cost-analysis of such solutions is too often forgotten.

While a great potential of health technologies to support the big global challenge of patient engagement exist today, so too does a lack of systematic and scientific studies around the theme. Too often those solutions are developed by the market and are not inserted into effectiveness trials to evaluate their impact on health and economic outcomes. Combining adequate methodological approaches with rigorous theories may guide the development and delivery of technological solutions truly able to sustain a better engagement of patients in their care. As the study of Greenhalgh and Russell (2010) suggests, market development of technological solution for patient engagement may be moved by goals different than the social, economic, and/or political circumstances in play. Surely, future studies are required to explore topics such as patient engagement, behavioral health outcomes, cost-effectiveness, and theories supporting those goals. Similar studies will allow developing and delivering effective technologies truly grounded on scientific results and patients' needs. Furthermore, the role of technologies in fostering patient engagement efforts need to be determined. Finally, a possible solution to these challenges may be adopting methods involving the different contexts and actors that play a role in the process of constructing the final product (Greenhalgh & Russell, 2010).

We should also not overlook the human touch. Perhaps the most significant potential obstacle to the success of these technologies is the adaptation and capability of the patient (Malkin, 2007). Not only do drugs need to be loaded into dispensers for consumption; the dispensers must be loaded with the correct drugs. Automated coaching and text support is effective only if patients carry their smart phones and read the messaging. Caregiver analysis of data trend can occur only if data are entered or automated collection occurs. Human intervention will continue to be an important ingredient in the implementation and utilization of technology (Newman, Szkodny, Llera, & Przeworski, 2011). Family members, friends, and health caregiver personnel become a vital link in the technology equation. The need for the human touch and support is heightened among persons with mental or physical disabilities, those suffering from depression or facing multiple chronic conditions, and the elderly, might struggle with technology. Peer network support and a highly engaged social community can help one another overcome the numerous challenges associated with modifying life-long behaviors. Finally, large vendors need to step up their technology design / acquisition, and health care providers will need to look beyond their primary it supplier to advance their engagement efforts more rapidly.

SOLUTIONS AND RECOMMENDATIONS

There has been a proliferation of technological solutions aimed to enhance health outcomes and engage patients. However, we are seeing a critical need for research in this field. Surely, patient-centric design in both the technology development and intervention process is mandatory for quick and easy adoption and long-term use. Obviously, system design strengths and weaknesses should be strongly considered when developing and implementing programs.

The big challenge is defining technological solutions that are really aimed to enhance patient engagement (Graffigna et al., 2013a; Barello et al., 2014), and not only partial behavioral outcomes of such a process. The relationship between patient engagement and such outcomes need to be verified, and it is hard by now to understand how technologies are sustaining and supporting patient engagement.

Additionally, the patient engagement is often considered a whole goal without considering and targeting specific critical issues. This is particularly important in the case of technology-based interventions. For example, the aging population presents specific design challenges in addition to application functionality. As an example, does the application require a smart phone or tablet trade-off? Although the larger format display of a tablet might better suit the elderly for improved visualization, smart phones offer the clear advantage of mobility and convenience. Ideal application design offers the user option of either device type.

Furthermore, the largest EHR vendors appear to be lagging in patient engagement technology development. Given the large vendors focus on delivering stable core functionality, a sizable opportunity to potentially improve outcomes and reduce costs gets stuck in longer term product roadmaps. System integrators might be best positioned to bring the variety of third-party apps to reality. Systems integration enables health care systems and consumers to select best-of-breed solutions across disease types and maintain continuity across the EHR platform. These advantages are commonly enjoyed via an accelerated implementation strategy and time frame compared to the slow-moving giants.

FUTURE RESEARCH DIRECTIONS

The path forward to successful technology implementation of effective patient engagement must be followed by many concerned parties. The technology however, cannot stand on its own. Developers should design solutions also suitable for an aging patient who might have comorbidities. Design efforts need to be shaped by their final users including patients, caregivers, professionals, and stakeholders, and its application to real health contexts (Greenhalgh & Russell, 2010). The patient engagement and educational process should start early in the condition diagnosis process and continue through acute condition recovery, and ongoing for chronic condition management. Transitional care tools and procedures are a crucial step and require utilization by all interventional team members. Ultimately, the circle of care needs family, friends, and peer support groups as activated participants throughout condition life cycle (Piette et al., 2015). As reported elsewhere in this chapter, peer-reviewed studies illustrating positive health-related outcomes and cost reduction with the new innovative patient engagement technologies is limited. More evidence-based research is needed to measure effective engagement strategies and establish best practices.

The future of effective patient engagement is indeed very bright.

CONCLUSION

The evolution of technologies in the healthcare field seems to be inevitable in this era and may be a rescue if we consider the global need of improving the quality of care while reducing costs. There is a widespread increase of technological solutions to improve medication adherence, reduce hospital readmission, sustain behavior change, and increase health literacy levels. Those goals are all pivotal factors that have a substantial economic impact on the healthcare market and that result from having engaged patients in their care. However, we found a lack of specific technological solutions for patient engagement and of a rigorous analysis of their cost impact. Furthermore, we suggest the need of interventions developed to target specific disadvantaged populations. As technological solutions for patient engagement have potential to reach and provide practical strategies to patients and the healthcare systems, further explorations and rigorous analysis should follow to understand how patient can be effectively engaged without burdening health systems and how technologies can be used to reach such a goal.

REFERENCES

Ahern, D., Phalen, J. M., & Eaton, C. B. (2008). The role of eHealth in patient engagement and quality improvement. In M. C. Gibbons (Ed.), *eHealth solutions for healthcare disparities* (pp. 75–92). New York: Springer. doi:10.1007/978-0-387-72815-5_9

Ahmad, F. S., Metlay, J. P., Barg, F. K., Henderson, R. R., & Werner, R. M. (2013). Identifying hospital organizational strategies to reduce readmissions. *American Journal of Medical Quality*, *28*(4), 278–285. doi:10.1177/1062860612464999 PMID:23118202

Barello, S., Graffigna, G., Vegni, E., & Bosio, A. C. (2014). The challenges of conceptualizing patient engagement in healthcare: A lexicographic literature review. *Journal of Participatory Medicine*, *6*, e9.

Bear, D. M., & Jain, Y. (2011). *U.S. Patent No. 8060249*. Washington, DC: U.S. Patent and Trademark Office.

Beatty, A. L., Fukuoka, Y., & Whooley, M. A. (2013). Using mobile technology for cardiac rehabilitation: A review and framework for development and evaluation. *Journal of the American Heart Association*, *2*(6), e000568. doi:10.1161/JAHA.113.000568 PMID:24185949

Bennett, H. D., Coleman, E. A., Parry, C., Bodenheimer, T., & Chen, E. H. (2010). Health coaching for patients. *Family Practice Management*, *17*(5), 24–29. PMID:21121566

Berkman, N. D., DeWalt, D. A., Pignone, M. P., Sheridan, S. L., Lohr, K. N., Lux, L., & Bonito, A. J. et al. (2004). *Literacy and health outcomes (AHRQ Publication No. 04-E007-2)*. Rockville, MD: Agency for Healthcare Research and Quality.

Berwick, D. M., Nolan, T. W., & Whittington, J. (2008). The triple aim: Care, health, and cost. *Health Affairs*, *27*(3), 759–769. doi:10.1377/hlthaff.27.3.759 PMID:18474969

Bickmore, T., Pfeifer, L., Byron, D., Forsythe, S., Henault, L., Jack, B., & Paasche-Orlow, M. et al. (2010). Usability of conversational agents by patients with inadequate health literacy: Evidence from two clinical trials. *Journal of Health Communication*, *15*(2), 197–210. doi:10.1080/10810730.2010.499991 PMID:20845204

Bickmore, T. W., & Paasche-Orlow, M. K. (2012). The role of information technology in health literacy research. *Journal of Health Communication*, *17*(3), 23–29. doi:10.1080/10810730.2012.712626 PMID:23030559

Blue, L., Lang, E., McMurray, J. J., Davie, A. P., McDonagh, T. A., Murdoch, D. R., & Morrison, C. E. et al. (2001). Randomised controlled trial of specialist nurse intervention in heart failure. *BMJ (Clinical Research Ed.)*, *323*(7315), 715–718. doi:10.1136/bmj.323.7315.715 PMID:11576977

Boren, S. A. (2009). A review of health literacy and diabetes: Opportunities for technology. *Journal of Diabetes Science and Technology*, *3*(1), 202–209. doi:10.1177/193229680900300124 PMID:20046666

Burg, B., Ingalz, K., Yamashita, M., & Takarada, S. (2009). *U.S. Patent Application 12/415,269*.

Cafazzo, J. A., Casselman, M., Hamming, N., Katzman, D. K., & Palmert, M. R. (2012). Design of an mHealth app for the self-management of adolescent type 1 diabetes: A pilot study. *Journal of Medical Internet Research*, *14*(3), e70. doi:10.2196/jmir.2058 PMID:22564332

Cass, R., & Sunstein, J. D. (2015). Nudging smokers. *The New England Journal of Medicine*, *372*(22), 2150–2151. doi:10.1056/NEJMe1503200 PMID:25970008

Centers for Medicare and Medicaid Services. (2014). *Readmission reduction program*. Retrieved September 29, 2015, from http://www.cms.gov/Medicare/Medicare-Fee-for-Service-payment/AcuteInpatientPPS/Readmissions-Reduction-Program.html

Chase, D. (2012, September 9). Patient engagement is the blockbuster drug of the century. *Forbes.com.* Retrieved from http://www.forbes.com/sites/davechase/2012/09/09/patient-engagement-is-the-blockbuster-drug-of-the-century/

Coleman, K., Austin, B. T., Brach, C., & Wagner, E. H. (2009). Evidence on the Chronic Care Model in the new millennium. *Health Affairs, 28*(1), 75–85. doi:10.1377/hlthaff.28.1.75 PMID:19124857

Commonwealth Fund. (2015). *Mobile health and patient engagement in the safety net: A survey of community health centers and clinics.* Retrieved from http://www.commonwealthfund.org/publications/issue-briefs/2015/may/mobile-health-and-patient-engagement-in-the-safety-net

Curtis, D. W., Pino, E. J., Bailey, J. M., Shih, E. I., Waterman, J., Vinterbo, S. A., & Ohno-Machado, L. et al. (2008). SMART—an integrated wireless system for monitoring unattended patients. *Journal of the American Medical Informatics Association, 15*(1), 44–53. doi:10.1197/jamia.M2016 PMID:17947629

Darlow, S., & Wen, K. Y. (2015). Development testing of mobile health interventions for cancer patient self-management: A review. *Health Informatics Journal.* PMID:25916831

Dartmouth Atlas Project. (2015). *Understanding of the efficiency and effectiveness of the health care system.* Retrieved from http://www.dartmouthatlas.org/

Dayer, L., Heldenbrand, S., Anderson, P., Gubbins, P. O., & Martin, B. C. (2013). Smartphone medication adherence apps: Potential benefits to patients and providers. *Journal of the American Pharmacists Association: JAPhA, 53*(2), 172–181. doi:10.1331/JAPhA.2013.12202 PMID:23571625

Farmer, K. C. (1999). Methods for measuring and monitoring medication regimen adherence in clinical trials and clinical practice. *Clinical Therapeutics, 21*(6), 1074–1090. doi:10.1016/S0149-2918(99)80026-5 PMID:10440628

Finkelstein, S. M., Speedie, S. M., & Potthoff, S. (2006). Home telehealth improves clinical outcomes at lower cost for home healthcare. *Telemedicine Journal and e-Health, 12*(2), 128–136. doi:10.1089/tmj.2006.12.128 PMID:16620167

Free, C., Phillips, G., Galli, L., Watson, L., Felix, L., Edwards, P., & Haines, A. et al. (2013). The effectiveness of mobile-health technology-based health behaviour change or disease management interventions for health care consumers: A systematic review. *PLoS Medicine, 10*(1), e1001362. doi:10.1371/journal.pmed.1001362 PMID:23349621

Gaikwad, R., & Warren, J. (2009). The role of home-based information and communications technology interventions in chronic disease management: A systematic literature review. *Health Informatics Journal*, *15*(2), 122–146. doi:10.1177/1460458209102973 PMID:19474225

Gerber, B. S., Brodsky, I. G., Lawless, K. A., Smolen, L. I., Arozullah, A. M., Smith, E. V., & Eiser, A. R. et al. (2005). Implementation and evaluation of a low-literacy diabetes education computer multimedia application. *Diabetes Care*, *28*(7), 1574–1580. doi:10.2337/diacare.28.7.1574 PMID:15983303

Goetzel, R. Z., Anderson, D. R., Whitmer, R. W., Ozminkowski, R. J., Dunn, R. L., & Wasserman, J.Health Enhancement Research Organization (HERO) Research Committee. (1998). The relationship between modifiable health risks and health care expenditures: An analysis of the multi-employer HERO health risk and cost database. *Journal of Occupational and Environmental Medicine*, *40*(10), 843–854. doi:10.1097/00043764-199810000-00003 PMID:9800168

Graetz, I., Reed, M., Rundall, T., Bellows, J., Brand, R., & Hsu, J. (2009). Care coordination and electronic health records: Connecting clinicians.[). American Medical Informatics Association.]. *AMIA ... Annual Symposium Proceedings / AMIA Symposium. AMIA Symposium*, *2009*, 208. PMID:20351851

Graffigna, G., & Barello, S. (2015). Innovating Healthcare in the Era of Patient Engagement: Challenges, Opportunities & New Trends. In G. Graffigna, S. Barello, & S. Triberti (Eds.), *Patient Engagement: A Consumer-Centered Model to Innovate Healthcare*. Berlin: De Gruyter Open. doi:10.1515/9783110452440-002

Graffigna, G., Barello, S., & Riva, G. (2013b). Technologies for patient engagement. *Health Affairs*, *32*(6), 1172–1172. doi:10.1377/hlthaff.2013.0279 PMID:23733998

Graffigna, G., Barello, S., Wiederhold, B. K., Bosio, A. C., & Riva, G. (2013a). Positive technology as a driver for health engagement. *Studies in Health Technology and Informatics*, *191*, 9–17. PMID:23792833

Greenhalgh, T., & Russell, J. (2010). Why do evaluations of eHealth programs fail? An alternative set of guiding principles. *PLoS Medicine*, *7*(11), 1331. doi:10.1371/journal.pmed.1000360 PMID:21072245

Haff, N., Patel, M. S., Lim, R., Zhu, J., Troxel, A. B., Asch, D. A., & Volpp, K. G. (2015). The role of behavioral economic incentive design and demographic characteristics in financial incentive-based approaches to changing health behaviors: A meta-analysis. *American Journal of Health Promotion*, *29*(5), 314–323. doi:10.4278/ajhp.140714-LIT-333 PMID:25928816

Hagland, M. (2013). CVS Caremark report: Medication non-adherence in U.S. costs up to $290 billion annually. Retrieved from http://www.healthcare-informatics.com/news-item/cvs-caremark-report-medication-non-adherence-us-costs-290-billion-annually

Hibbard, J. H., & Greene, J. (2013). What the evidence shows about patient activation: Better health outcomes and care experiences; fewer data on costs. *Health Affairs*, *32*(2), 207–214. doi:10.1377/hlthaff.2012.1061 PMID:23381511

Hibbard, J. H., Greene, J., & Overton, V. (2013). Patients with lower activation associated with higher costs; delivery systems should know their patients' 'scores'. *Health Affairs*, *32*(2), 216–222. doi:10.1377/hlthaff.2012.1064 PMID:23381513

Hines, A. L., Barrett, M. S., Jiang, H. J., & Steiner, C. A. (2011). *Conditions with the largest number of adult hospital readmissions by payer*. Retrieved from https://www.hcup-us.ahrq.gov/reports/statbriefs/sb172-Conditions-Readmissions-Payer.jsp

Holmes-Rovner, M., Stommel, M., Corser, W. D., Olomu, A., Holtrop, J. S., Siddiqi, A., & Dunn, S. L. (2008). Does outpatient telephone coaching add to hospital quality improvement following hospitalization for acute coronary syndrome? *Journal of General Internal Medicine*, *23*(9), 1464–1470. doi:10.1007/s11606-008-0710-1 PMID:18618189

Institute for Healthcare Improvement. (2015). *Triple aim initiative*. Retrieved from http://www.ihi.org/Engage/Initiatives/TripleAim/pages/default.aspx

Institute of Medicine. (2004). *Health literacy: a prescription to end confusion*. Washington, DC: The National Academies.

Iuga, A. O., & McGuire, M. J. (2014). Adherence and health care costs. *Risk management and healthcare policy, 7*, 35.

Krumholz, H. M., Amatruda, J., Smith, G. L., Mattera, J. A., Roumanis, S. A., Radford, M. J., & Vaccarino, V. et al. (2002). Randomized trial of an education and support intervention to prevent readmission of patients with heart failure. *Journal of the American College of Cardiology*, *39*(1), 83–89. doi:10.1016/S0735-1097(01)01699-0 PMID:11755291

Lai, J. (2006). *U.S. Patent No. 7081807*. Washington, DC: U.S. Patent and Trademark Office.

Levit, K., Smith, C., Cowan, C., Lazenby, H., Sensenig, A., & Catlin, A. (2003). Trends in US health care spending, 2001. *Health Affairs*, *22*(1), 154–164. doi:10.1377/hlthaff.22.1.154 PMID:12528847

Luxton, D. D., Kayl, R. A., & Mishkind, M. C. (2012). mHealth data security: The need for HIPAA-compliant standardization. *Telemedicine Journal and e-Health*, *18*(4), 284–288. doi:10.1089/tmj.2011.0180 PMID:22400974

Malkin, R. A. (2007). Design of health care technologies for the developing world. *Annual Review of Biomedical Engineering*, *9*(1), 567–587. doi:10.1146/annurev.bioeng.9.060906.151913 PMID:17430083

Marek, K. D., & Antle, L. (2008). Patient safety and quality: An evidence-based handbook for nurses. In R. G. Hughes (Ed.), *Medication management of the community-dwelling older adult*. Rockville, MD: Agency for Healthcare Research and Quality.

McGrady, E., Conger, S., Blanke, S., & Landry, B. J. (2010). Emerging technologies in healthcare: Navigating risks, evaluating rewards. *Journal of Healthcare Management*, *55*(5), 353. PMID:21077584

Menichetti, J., Libreri, C., Lozza, E., & Graffigna, G. (2014). Giving patients a starring role in their own care: A bibliometric analysis of the on-going literature debate. *Health Expectations*, November, 1–11. PMID:25369557

Misono, A. S., Cutrona, S. L., Choudhry, N. K., Fischer, M. A., Stedman, M. R., Liberman, J. N., & Shrank, W. H. et al. (2010). Healthcare information technology interventions to improve cardiovascular and diabetes medication adherence. *The American Journal of Managed Care*, *16*(12), 82–92. PMID:21314228

Moore, J. O., Marshall, M. A., Inch, B. C., Judge, D. C., Moss, F. H., Gilroy, S. J., & Zusman, R. M. et al. (2014). Technology-supported apprenticeship in the management of hypertension: A randomized control trial. *Journal of Clinical Outcomes Management*, *21*(3), 110–122.

National Committee for Quality Assurance. (2012). Insights for Improvement. Reducing Readmission: Measuring Health Plan Performance. Retrieved from http://www.ncqa.org/portals/0/Publications/2012%20BI_NCQA%20ReAdMi%20_Pub.pdf

Newman, M. G., Szkodny, L. E., Llera, S. J., & Przeworski, A. (2011). A review of technology-assisted self-help and minimal contact therapies for anxiety and depression: Is human contact necessary for therapeutic efðcacy? *Clinical Psychology Review*, *31*(1), 89–103. doi:10.1016/j.cpr.2010.09.008 PMID:21130939

Park, L. G., Howie-Esquivel, J., Chung, M. L., & Dracup, K. (2014). A text messaging intervention to promote medication adherence for patients with coronary heart disease: A randomized controlled trial. *Patient Education and Counseling*, *94*(2), 261–268. doi:10.1016/j.pec.2013.10.027 PMID:24321403

Passamante, A. P. (1998). *U.S. Patent No. 5752621*. Washington, DC: U.S. Patent and Trademark Office.

Perednia, D. A., & Allen, A. (1995). Telemedicine technology and clinical applications. *Journal of the American Medical Association*, *273*(6), 483–488. doi:10.1001/jama.1995.03520300057037 PMID:7837367

Pharmaceutical Research and Manufacturers of America. (2011). *Improving prescription medicine adherence is key to better health care*. Retrieved from http://www.phrma.org/sites/default/files/pdf/PhRMA_Improving%20Medication%20Adherence_Issue%20Brief.pdf

Piette, J. D., Striplin, D., Marinec, N., Chen, J., Trivedi, R. B., Aron, D. C., & Aikens, J. E. et al. (2015). A Mobile Health Intervention Supporting Heart Failure Patients and Their Informal Caregivers: A Randomized Comparative Effectiveness Trial. *Journal of Medical Internet Research*, *17*(6), e142. doi:10.2196/jmir.4550 PMID:26063161

Pignone, M., DeWalt, D. A., Sheridan, S., Berkman, N., & Lohr, K. N. (2005). Interventions to improve health outcomes for patients with low literacy. *Journal of General Internal Medicine*, *20*(2), 185–192. doi:10.1111/j.1525-1497.2005.40208.x PMID:15836553

Rau, J. (2014). *Medicare fines 2,610 hospitals in third round of readmission penalties*. Retrieved from http://khn.org/news/medicare-readmissions-penalties-2015

Ricciardi, L., Mostashari, F., Murphy, J., Daniel, J. G., & Siminerio, E. P. (2013). A national action plan to support consumer engagement via e-health. *Health Affairs*, *32*(2), 376–384. doi:10.1377/hlthaff.2012.1216 PMID:23381531

Rich, M. W., Beckham, V., Wittenberg, C., Leven, C. L., Freedland, K. E., & Carney, R. M. (1995). A multidisciplinary intervention to prevent the readmission of elderly patients with congestive heart failure. *The New England Journal of Medicine*, *333*(18), 1190–1195. doi:10.1056/NEJM199511023331806 PMID:7565975

Safeer, R. S., Cooke, C. E., & Keenan, J. (2006). The impact of health literacy on cardiovascular disease. *Vascular Health and Risk Management*, *2*(4), 457–464. doi:10.2147/vhrm.2006.2.4.457 PMID:17323600

Seligman, H. K., Wang, F. F., Palacios, J. L., Wilson, C. C., Daher, C., Piette, J. D., & Schillinger, D. (2005). Physician notification of their diabetes patients' limited health literacy. A randomized, controlled trial. *Journal of General Internal Medicine, 20*(11), 1001–1007. doi:10.1111/j.1525-1497.2005.00189.x PMID:16307624

Shea, J., Guerra, C., Weiner, J., Aguirre, A., Ravenell, K., & Asch, D. (2008). Adapting a patient satisfaction instrument for low literate and Spanish-speaking populations: Comparison of three formats. *Patient Education and Counseling, 73*(1), 132–140. doi:10.1016/j.pec.2008.03.026 PMID:18486414

Smith, S. G., Curtis, L. M., Wardle, J., von Wagner, C., & Wolf, M. S. (2013). Skill set or mind set? Associations between health literacy, patient activation and health. *PLoS ONE, 8*(9), e74373. doi:10.1371/journal.pone.0074373 PMID:24023942

Sokol, M. C., McGuigan, K. A., Verbrugge, R. R., & Epstein, R. S. (2005). Impact of medication adherence on hospitalization risk and healthcare cost. *Medical Care, 43*(6), 521–530. doi:10.1097/01.mlr.0000163641.86870.af PMID:15908846

Sørensen, K., Van den Broucke, S., Fullam, J., Doyle, G., Pelikan, J., Slonska, Z., & Brand, H. (2012). Health literacy and public health: A systematic review and integration of definitions and models. *BMC Public Health, 12*(1), 80. doi:10.1186/1471-2458-12-80 PMID:22276600

Swan, M. (2009). Emerging patient-driven health care models: An examination of health social networks, consumer personalized medicine and quantified self-tracking. *International Journal of Environmental Research and Public Health, 6*(2), 492–525. doi:10.3390/ijerph6020492 PMID:19440396

The U. S. Affordable Care Act of March 2010. (2011). U.S. Federal Register, *76*(108), 32331. Retrieved from http://www.gpo.gov/fdsys/pkg/FR-2011-06-06/pdf/2011-13801.pdf

Turner, B. J., Weiner, M., Berry, S. D., Lillie, K., Fosnocht, K., & Hollenbeak, C. S. (2008). Overcoming poor attendance to first scheduled colonoscopy: A randomized trial of peer coach or brochure support. *Journal of General Internal Medicine, 23*(1), 58–63. doi:10.1007/s11606-007-0445-4 PMID:18030540

Vale, M. J., Jelinek, M. V., Best, J. D., Dart, A. M., Grigg, L. E., Hare, D. L., & McNeil, J. J. et al. (2003). Coaching patients On Achieving Cardiovascular Health (COACH): A multicenter randomized trial in patients with coronary heart disease. *Archives of Internal Medicine, 163*(22), 2775–2783. doi:10.1001/archinte.163.22.2775 PMID:14662633

Vervloet, M., Linn, A. J., van Weert, J. C., De Bakker, D. H., Bouvy, M. L., & Van Dijk, L. (2012). The effectiveness of interventions using electronic reminders to improve adherence to chronic medication: A systematic review of the literature. *Journal of the American Medical Informatics Association*, *19*(5), 696–704. doi:10.1136/amiajnl-2011-000748 PMID:22534082

Wang, T. (2015). Digital health funding tops $4.1B: 2014 year in review. Retrieved September 15, 2015, from: http://rockhealth.com/2015/01/digital-health-funding-tops-4-1b-2014-year-review/

Weissman, J. S., Stern, R. S., & Epstein, A. M. (1994). The impact of patient socioeconomic status and other social factors on readmission: A prospective study in four Massachusetts hospitals. *Inquiry*, 31(2), 163–172. PMID:8021022

West, D. (2012). How mobile devices are transforming healthcare. *Issues in technology innovation*, 18(1), 1-11.

Yang, Y. T., & Silverman, R. D. (2014). Mobile health applications: The patchwork of legal and liability issues suggests strategies to improve oversight. *Health Affairs*, *33*(2), 222–227. doi:10.1377/hlthaff.2013.0958 PMID:24493764

KEY TERMS AND DEFINITIONS

Digital Health: An overarching term used to describe a collection of services to help healthcare providers and consumers' better monitor health and disease progression through wireless devices, smart phone applications, remote monitoring services, and other computer based actions.

Electronic Health Record (EHR): Similar to an Electronic Medical Record, an Electronic Health Record typically extends health related information beyond primary care givers to include, laboratory reports, specialist's activity, nursing care, and other support services.

Electronic Medical Record (EMR): A digital file of a patient's health history containing clinical information relevant to diagnosis and treatment of the patient.

Gamification: The process of compelling people to engage in an activity through interesting and fun techniques.

Medicaid: A United States federal government health insurance program for certain people and families with limited income.

Medicare: A United States federal government health insurance program for certain people who are 65 years or older, or have certain disabilities.

On-Boarding: A process where an individual's knowledge and skills are assessed, then fortified with new and advanced lessons.

Personal Health Record (PHR): Similar to an Electronic Health Record, a PHR is typically maintained by a patient in a secure environment for information share with interested parties.

Transition of Care: The movement of a patient from one healthcare setting to another.

Chapter 6
Meeting Patients Where They Are:
Using Multimedia and Interactive Voice Technology to Humanize Communication and Engage Patients

Geri Lynn Baumblatt
Emmi Solutions, LLC, USA

ABSTRACT

In this chapter the author describes the challenges of engaging and communicating with patients and how technology can improve communication, elicit honest patient disclosure, and create more productive conversation and help patients engage and partner in their care. The author will also discuss how research with multimedia programs reveals it can help reduce anxiety, improve knowledge, help low health literacy audiences, and contribute to improved outcomes. This chapter will also examine how multimedia decision aid programs can help patients understand their options and complex risk information, while helping them consider their values and preferences so they can truly engage in shared decision making.

DOI: 10.4018/978-1-5225-0663-8.ch006

INTRODUCTION

Each of us becomes a patient when we interact with the healthcare system. We all want to avoid pain and suffering, feel better, and have a good quality of life. Beyond that, we also want to avoid adverse events, infections, procedures, and unnecessary costly treatments that drive up the cost of care for everyone. And people definitely do not want to accrue medical bills that put them or their family in serious financial jeopardy (Himmelstein, Warren, Thorne, & Woolhandler, 2005).

Yet, despite the high stakes and their own wellbeing, "patients are the most underutilized resource" in healthcare (Safran, 2004). Why is this?

Unfortunately, even in the best circumstances, patient-provider relationships are beset with challenges. Over the course of a year, clinicians only have the opportunity to spend mere minutes interacting with patients and family caregivers. The challenges are compounded by the patient-clinician power dynamic, health literacy and literacy challenges, as well as, social, economic, emotional and physical stress, not to mention any pain, fatigue, or challenges caused by an illness.

Many people end up at the mercy of poor health, feeling anything but competent and in control. Illness and disease often robs us of our autonomy and diminishes our volition. The process of seeking treatment or getting diagnosed can also be unnerving. For example, if you have chest pain, are you over-reacting or under-reacting if you go to the emergency department? We often lack the knowledge to evaluate the situation and act. In the face of a diagnosis or procedure we want to feel in control and capable of dealing with our circumstances. Instead, even physicians report feeling carried along by a system that makes it harder instead of easier to act or question events.

As kidney cancer patient and Society of Participatory Medicine board member Peggy Zuckerman explains, "Patients would be more likely to communicate with their doctors, whether electronically or otherwise, if there was real encouragement in communication. Right now, much of it is one-way, physician-to-patient, with the physician setting the rules and the agenda. In most other personal encounters, there is a bit of time to create a tone of collaboration. In a medical setting, the time constraints, the culture of paternalism, and the complexity of information to be dispersed and/or shared makes communication more difficult" (personal communication, April 30, 2015).

Yet, each day patients need to take medications, make challenging lifestyle and behavior changes, remember how to do their physical therapy exercises, and show up for important but intimidating procedures, like colonoscopies.

This chapter will explore how poor communication, knowledge gaps and incomplete understanding (the realm of health literacy) and communication affects the ability, interest and motivation of patients to engage in self-care, even at the most basic level.

Then it will look at how technology such as web-based multimedia programs and interactive voice response (IVR) calls, can empower patients to participate and partner in their care and become owners of their health and wellbeing. These tools create an easy, low effort, and less stressful way for patients and families to understand their health conditions and procedures, ask honest and even embarrassing questions, and create the competency and understanding they need to participate in shared decision making. It will also describe research showing these programs can reduce anxiety and improve knowledge as well as clinical outcomes.

BACKGROUND

The term "patient" stems from Old French *pacient or "patience"* meaning: "quality of being willing to bear adversities, calm endurance of misfortune, suffering, etc." To be "patient" is to "endure without complaint" (Harper, 2001). This is a historical definition, but it connotes deference, powerlessness, and passivity as well as a need to be firm and unyielding, as if to say: do as caregivers say, but do not give in to pain or despair. Only fairly recently do patients no longer see themselves as passive recipients of care or those who are acted upon, but as motivated partners, or even as advocates who must intervene in their care.

As many have noted, the term "patient engagement" implies patients must be activated to engage. Yet, in this fundamentally mutual enterprise, we often fail to provide patients with the most essential tools to participate: a real understanding of their condition, how it will affect their life over time, their treatment options, and the time, ability, and a safe and unintimidating setting to ask meaningful questions about their care.

Leaving Patients to Connect the Dots

Too often, we presume patients know and understand their condition at least at a very basic level. We assume people were previously educated — that there was a moment of level setting, candor, knowledge transfer, and teach-back to confirm understanding. However, in most cases, that either never took place, or the patient, still reeling from the news of a diabetes or cancer diagnosis, simply could not absorb it. Other times, a silent condition like hypertension may not register as important or even real. And the information is often provided at a level many people cannot fully understand, or in a way that leaves it to patients to "connect the dots."

For example, when a patient is diagnosed with type 2 diabetes, simply understanding the concept of blood sugar is new. And when we talk about "sugar", how many people understand this is not limited to refined sugar, desserts, and sugary drinks? Do we truly help them understand how what they eat and their ability to manage diabetes will affect their body over time? It is fairly easy for patients to understand what it means when we say that over time diabetes will affect their eyes and vision. And it can even be fairly straightforward to explain how diabetes affects the nerves in their feet to help them understand why they may not feel a cut or injury that can become infected. But while some people understand an infection can lead to the loss of a foot, or may know of family members this happened to, other times this potential outcome is inferred and not made explicit. This is not to suggest we should frighten people into action, but to ensure they understand what is at stake so their actions are moored in that knowledge.

To go a step further, if a patient is told that over time, diabetes will affect their kidneys and can lead to kidney disease, what does that mean to them? Kidney disease sounds bad, but for most people it is largely an abstraction — organs that sound important but do not confer the same type of immediately understandable benefit like eyesight. How many people understand that "kidney problems" may eventually lead to dialysis, surgery to create a fistula in their arm so they can receive dialysis, or to a potential kidney transplant? And how often is there a clear conversation about how their condition and treatment will affect their longevity?

In the United States, nephrologists often find that a large number of people with diabetes and hypertension never show up when they are referred to a nephrologist. Patients often have no understanding why they are being referred or how important it is. It seems unfair to assume they simply do not care. Instead, patients often reach a point where they need to make decisions about their renal care, and when they hear how their condition has progressed, they often feel blind-sided by a conversation about dialysis.

It is extremely challenging to be candid with people about this kind of information. And these messages need to be repeated multiple times and in various ways to ensure people take it in and know what it means for their day-to-day life. When these dots are not connected to create a unified picture, people *appear* un-engaged. In reality, they are not acting because they do not recognize how their condition, medication, or procedure will affect (or is already affecting) them.

The Challenge of Low Health Literacy

Numerous studies bear out the health literacy gaps that create failures in what should be a smooth connection between knowledge, activation, and action. The study of Fang, Panguluri, Machtinger and Schillinger (2009) measured the health literacy of 183 patients who were taking warfarin (most of them for many years) to prevent a stroke. "When questioned about the drug, however, only 9.3% of the study participants understood that the purpose of their taking warfarin was to prevent stroke. Perhaps even more shocking was the fact that more than 40% of patients surveyed did not know what a stroke was" (Fang et al., 2009). Of course, without basic health education, most people do not know what a stroke is or the diversity of problems it can cause.

When people do not get the knowledge and information about their health in a way they can understand — and what it means in the near and long term — how can we expect them to be activated to engage?

Health literacy research shows that avoiding medical jargon and communicating with patients in plain language is essential. Yet, even when information is understandable, working memory (the ability to remember, process and comprehend information) fails. Pain and illness adds additional burdens to focus, attention, and comprehension. It is no wonder research shows by time patients walk out the door they have already forgotten anywhere from 40% to 80% of what they were told; and much of what is remembered is often incorrect (Kessels, 2003).

Power Dynamics at Play

Patients both rely on and are intimidated by clinicians. Many clinicians make meaningful efforts to mitigate this power dynamic; but patients are often embarrassed to ask questions or voice concerns (Katz, Jacobson, Veldar, & Kripalani, 2007). People often nod their heads as though in agreement, afraid or unable to articulate their concerns. Other times, people silently choose not to take a medication because it previously gave a relative or friend a side effect, like leg pain. As a VP of Clinical Care Management for a U.S. health system explained, "You're asking for personal information from people… But I knew people were leaving medications at the pharmacy and not picking them up. And I knew people wouldn't tell you things like that" (Gerr, Saulsberry, Clark, & Kerns, 2014, p. 25).

Whether consciously or unconsciously, patients often do not respond honestly or withhold information because they want to be viewed positively and create a good impression. This "impression management" (also called "self presentation") means that as patients, we are not reliable (Leary & Kowalski, 1990). Unfortunately, clinicians get a less accurate picture of what patients are and are not willing and able to do. This causes communication gaps, especially around stigmatized topics like eating disorders, tobacco and drug use, as well as more common topics like contraception, acne, and exercise habits (Leary, Tchividijian, & Kraxberger, 1994).

Impression management also plays a role in whether people will make lifestyle changes. For example, people who see themselves as overweight, flabby, or not fit are often embarrassed to be seen working out, putting on a swimsuit, or lifting weights that look light to others at a gym. Termed "physique anxiety," this can be paralyzing but not something people readily admit. A study of overweight women's reactions to exercise programs found the "most powerful influences seemed to be the social circumstances of the exercise setting, especially concerns about visibility, embarrassment, and judgment by others" (Bain, Wilson, & Chaikind, 1989).

Technology can help mediate face-to-face power dynamics. It can address and normalize unspoken patient concerns. It can also facilitate better relationships, create new lines of patient-clinician communication, improve understanding, and empower patents to engage.

SOLUTIONS AND RECOMMENDATIONS

Technology was once thought of as cold and impersonal. Today we know technology and the online world can be deeply engaging. Something as simple as a text message or emoticon can generate experiences of connection and care. A survey of people age 19 to 29 indicated they are so attached to these devices they sleep with their smartphone or tablet in their bed (Schocker, 2013). These devices connect us to the larger world, allowing us to interact with friends, family, and colleagues. They connect us to others with similar interests, health conditions, political views, and help us find everything from romance to employment.

When technological tools and information are designed in partnership with both patients and clinicians, they can become powerful ways to engage patients, and to share understandable, reliable information. This formative research helps ensure this information resonates with their current pain, problems, and even embarrassing concerns.

For decades, patients have been sent home with brochures, booklets, printouts, and discharged with binders full of instructions. These tomes make good doorstops, but reading them feels like a task. They can be an intimidating format even for educated and highly motivated patients. And for those with literacy and reading challenges, they are inaccessible.

People often sit down to read print materials or screens of static online text with a sigh, mustering the energy to begin. Reading takes effort, and stressful clinical information multiplies that burden. So when stressed, scared, ill, and weary patients go home with information critical for them to understand, narrated multimedia or video provides a more approachable format that reduces cognitive load and requires less mental effort. These formats can demonstrate procedural steps and can animate information in an unintimidating and diagrammatic way that anyone can understand. In fact, simplified medical information is preferred regardless of education level (Davis, Crouch, Wills, Miller, & Abdehou, 1990).

Prescribed, Web-Based Multimedia Programs

Multimedia combines voiceover, illustrations, animation, text, and interactions. Consistent with Mayer and Moreno's findings (2003) in the development of cognitive theory of multimedia learning, this type of orchestrated content creates a low-effort experience and enables patients to quickly view a lot of information in an easy-to-understand format.

Multimedia programs can connect with patients in language they understand, at a time when they are ready to learn, and on the devices they already own. This consumer-friendly technology helps patients engage in more productive conversations with their healthcare team and to take action around healthcare events or conditions.

Multimedia can help patients understand newly diagnosed health conditions, how and why to use a device like a nebulizer or CPAP device, or educate people about new skills and behaviors like injecting insulin or breastfeeding. It can help people understand their treatment options and consider their goals, values and preferences. Programs developed in these formats can also help people understand an upcoming test or procedure while augmenting and helping to document more thorough and authentic informed consent.

Multimedia programs can also be part of a technology platform so that clinicians can prescribe the programs to patients. Other times, multimedia programs can be placed on a patient portal. However, when a clinician or a member of the care team, hospital, or health plan recommends and prescribes programs, and each patient receives a personalized and unique access code, this confers a level of importance. This creates a sense of intention and feeling cared for and both patients know they are getting exactly the information their physician wants them to see. The recommendation of the clinicians helps patients recognize the information is essential, helpful, worth their time. Clinicians also know the information the patient views is up to date and relevant; as opposed to the variable information people may come across when doing an online search.

An individualized prescription (often delivered via email as web link) for information that is relevant to that individual can be delivered to a patient before, after, or between clinical encounters.

For example, if a patient is being scheduled for a surgical procedure, a multimedia or video program can be ordered, the patient is notified, they can view the program on any web-enabled device, and the experience can also be tracked. A program can be prescribed when a patient is scheduled for their procedure. It can also be prescribed or automated through an electronic medical record (EMR).

Patients can opt to receive their personalized access code however it is most convenient for them: by email, phone, text message, or a print out. Patients can view programs on any web-enabled device (tablet, desktop computer, laptop, or smartphone) when it is convenient for them. This type of choice autonomy gives people freedom to absorb information in the comfort of their home, where the stress and distraction of the clinical environment and patient-physician power dynamic do not interfere. People are truly "at home" as a person instead of as a "diabetic" or a patient. People can pause, go back, and re-play sections or watch the program as many times as they like. They are in control and can review the information as needed.

This type of web-based information also makes it easy to share it with other family members who often cannot be present to hear the clinician's explanation or instructions. It can also help families coordinate care; if an adult child lives half way across the country, without much effort, they can log on, watch, and understand their parent's procedure, recovery, why it is being done, and what the risks and alternatives are, and better plan a visit to help with the recovery.

These types of programs can also be tracked. This way patients can be reminded to start or finish watching a program if they forget. And questions patients type in captured for them in their patient portal or in personalized print summary. On some platforms, any questions the patient has can be typed in, tracked/captured for the clinician, who can then review the patient's questions and better prepare for their next conversation. This type of tracking can also help document best practices, such as providing education for topics like breastfeeding or counseling for smoking cessation.

A personal access code also creates a secure way for patients and clinicians to communicate with each other — a problem so often hindered by privacy concerns, and, in the United States, by compliance with the federal Health Insurance Portability and Accountability Act (HIPAA) of 1996 that protects the confidentiality and security of healthcare information.

Engaging Patients in Meaningful Informed Consent

Helping patients truly understand their procedures and the associated risks and alternatives is the true spirit of informed consent. Multimedia programs can provide more robust informed consent. It can give patients more realistic expectations and give them the knowledge they need to make truly informed decisions, and helps confirm whether a procedure will treat their symptoms and condition.

This helps address the culture of defensive medicine. In the United States, malpractice insurers like Beazley recognize the benefits this more robust patient education and engagement, and provide a reduced premium for hospitals that use this type of engagement technology.

Narrated Animation: Improved Understanding

Most patients have only a very basic understanding of physiology. Without much existing knowledge to build on, clinicians often struggle to help patients understand unfamiliar anatomy, health conditions, and procedures. Without strong visuals, these explanations frequently leave patients lost and confused.

However, when animation is coupled with narration patients can watch and understand key physiology (like how blood moves through the heart), or it can help them grasp more complex information (like ejection fraction). These challenging concepts are often essential to patients understanding their conditions or making decisions about procedures.

Other times, patients need to learn a new skill (like putting on compression stockings, or how to use a device (like a nebulizer). Multimedia demonstrations can provide a significant improvement over a series of static images that can leave out key information and make the reader or viewer do more interpretative work to understand the progression.

Research done by Meppelink, van Weert, Haven and Smit (2015) found that when animation is combined with narration, people with limited health literacy have better recall of the information. Interestingly, narrated information also creates better attitudes to the information. When narration was used to inform people about colon cancer screening, it resulted in better attitudes towards the message itself, which positively influenced screening attitudes. These positive attitudes resulted in stronger intentions to get screened. This is supported by previous research showing multimedia learning leads to increased motivation because of the autonomy, self pacing, and review opportunities (Schunk, Pintrich, & Meece, 2008). Better motivation and attitudes have also been associated with multimedia education. Abdoolatiff and Narod (2009) found students who completed a computer-based science lab performed significantly better on a test measuring understanding of the lab and reported increased motivation and enthusiasm for the material.

In the study done by Meppelink et al. (2015), researchers concluded that voice narration paired with animations "is the best way to communicate complex health information to people with low health literacy." This is essential for reaching the most vulnerable and underserved patients.

The Ease of Listening to a Conversation

Reading demands a high level of effort and concentration. Pain, discomfort, worry about a diagnosis, or the shock of being diagnosed with a serious condition puts people in a state of flight or flight and creates "attentional narrowing," where the brain can only focus on the most frightening statements (Kessels, 2003). These diagnoses can have a profound effect on a patient's emotional state. One study of over 1000 women found 23% of women diagnosed with breast cancer experienced post-traumatic stress disorder (PTSD), with 16.5% still experiencing PTSD two to three months later (Vin-Raviv et al., 2013). The physical and emotional stress makes it challenging for patients to focus, absorb, and remember information or thoughtfully consider treatment options.

With narration, the viewer can listen instead of read. Words are processed in the verbal channel instead of visually. This helps offload the cognitive load placed on the brain to process and understand information. With narration "the processing demands on the visual channel are thereby reduced, so the learner is better able to select important aspects of animation for further processing" (Mayer & Moreno, 2003).

And when narration is friendly, conversational, and empathic, viewers report they can listen to information they otherwise find too overwhelming to read. The voiceover seems to replace or temper patients' own more anxious internal voice that tends to take over when they read.

Conversational narration creates the experience of a well-informed friend is sitting next to people and walking them through the information. Casual conversation is our most familiar and comfortable mode of language and communication. As linguists like John McWhorter (2012, 2013) explain, "pragmatic particles" (also called "discourse particles") such as "well" and "you know" are a common way to indicate empathy. These colloquial moments "help establish a warm shared frame of reference".

According to Clark and Mayer (2011), multiple studies found conversational narration helps learners identify with the content and understand it better than more formal language (pp. 184-185). Casual speech also has a way of reaching out, whereas the technical and clinical language of medicine excludes people and reminds them they are not "in the know," even though the experience of their illness or procedure is often deeply personal.

Understanding Patient Concerns, Reducing Anxiety, and Improving Outcomes

When multimedia content is developed with both patients and clinicians providing input and feedback, the programs can then anticipate common patient questions and concerns. For example, acute back pain can be frightening and seem debilitating, and it is rife with misconceptions. When patients schedule appointments to see their physician for low back pain, at the same time a multimedia program about that topic can be prescribed so they can view it before their appointment. With this pre-appointment education, patients learn back pain usually is *not* serious, imaging is *not* usually needed, and findings like a herniated disc are common and are *not* necessarily the cause of their pain. With these assumptions and worries addressed, the patient is much less likely to arrive in a nervous state, catastrophizing their pain and asking for imaging, which is often unnecessary and counterproductive. Instead, they arrive with their worst fears already allayed.

For a procedure like colonoscopy, there is a lot of procedure-related anxiety because it sounds uncomfortable, unfamiliar, and embarrassing. Patients often cancel or do not show up for scheduled procedures. Patients often worry about something they are too embarrassed to ask about, like an existing hemorrhoid, thinking it may cause serious pain during a colonoscopy. Working with patients when creating this content can help anticipate these types of questions so they can be addressed and normalized. Patients realize that even though the topic felt embarrassing, it must be common enough to address it in a general program.

Of course, the answers to these questions are not always good. In those instances, the conversational narration can level with people, creating a moment of candor. Knowing and feeling like they were told the truth is still less stressful than the anxiety of the unknown.

When topics like hemorrhoids, sex, gas, and bowel movements are addressed, it also makes people feel comfortable to ask other questions.

Content designed with patients have also been shown to reduce patient anxiety and lead to better outcomes. In a study at the University of Chicago Medical Center, the gastroenterology department prescribed a multimedia colonoscopy program to patients when they scheduled them for their procedure. Most of the patients who viewed the program (89%) showed up for their colonoscopy, compared with only 68% of patients who did not watch it (Thomas, Kedia, & Cohen, 2007).

Multimedia programs have also been shown to reduce anxiety and improve outcomes. In a randomized controlled study at Dartmouth-Hitchcock Medical Center, 51 patients were given a standard printed pre-procedural packet. A second group of 52 patients received both the print packet and were also prescribed the multimedia colonoscopy program. Patients' perception of their anxiety level was measured with a state trait anxiety inventory before and after patients reviewed the print packet or the packet plus the multimedia program. Of the patients who viewed the multimedia program, 58% reported reduced anxiety (Parker, Zipurksy, Ma, & Siegel, 2013).

In addition, those who viewed the multimedia colonoscopy program were 11% more knowledgeable. And even though the physicians performing the colonoscopies did not know which patients had watched the multimedia program, analysis found patients who viewed it also required 18% less sedation medication and their procedure times were 14% shorter (Parker et al., 2013). This was further confirmation that those patients were less anxious.

Normalizing the Patient Experience

Helping patients feel comfortable so they will ask the questions weighing on their minds and disclose personal information is key to engagement. Patients often get home and realize they do not understand instructions, what a medication or treatment is meant to do, or when to call about problems or side effects, etc. The onus is then on them to find out, and to admit they do not remember or understand.

Virtual interactions with multimedia and interactive voice response (IVR) phone calls help create a sense of privacy and safety. Research shows people are more likely to honestly self-reveal personal information in a virtual setting (Lucas, Gratch, King, & Morency, 2014). Once another human is no longer present, impression management is diminished. People have a "sense of invulnerability to criticism... and an impression their responses 'disappear' into the computer" (Weisband & Kiesler, 1996, p. 3).

Taking this a step further, multimedia can enable patients to ask questions virtually. The program can even prompt and encourage people to ask questions. This can help patients feel it is safe and acceptable to ask questions, and that it is even something they are invited and expected to do.

For example, it is always difficult to broach the topic of smoking. Clinicians do not like bringing it up, and patients feel ashamed and judged. Even though most people want to quit, it usually takes about seven attempts to quit permanently. And before that final, successful quit attempt, people feel like failures. However, when information about quitting is presented in a virtual environment, when another human is not present, patient viewers are less likely to feel pressured, shamed, or lectured.

Likewise, when it comes to the risks of a procedure, patients and families are often hesitant to ask questions. They may fear it will be interpreted as litigious or as questioning the physician's skill or experience. Multimedia programs can walk patients through risk information at home. Interface design and narration can invite patients to flag risks in virtual setting, which helps them feel safe and normalizes it. The technology can also enable the physician's office to receive any flagged risk in advance so they have time to prepare for the conversation with the patient before their next meeting.

Creating a Safe, Honest Environment

As discussed above, virtual interactions have been shown to make people feel safe and they are more likely to honestly disclose information. Personalized, interactive voice response (IVR) phone calls can also be used to reach out and provide small doses of information to help keep patients and family members on point with daily tasks and to collect information like outstanding patient questions, new symptoms or side effects.

Research shows patients are comfortable engaging with IVR calls across a variety of health conditions. In a study done by Piette et al. (2013), patients completed 83% of attempted IVR assessments. Participation rates for heart failure and cancer were 90%, 81% for the diabetes, and 71% among patients with depression. That same study found that "older patients had higher call completion rates, even among patients > 75 years of age."

For example, a single IVR call can be used to reach patients to find out if they had a diabetes eye exam. If they have, this information can be reported back to their physician for documentation. If they have not, the IVR call can help patients understand why this is important and a "warm-transfer" can be done so the patient can immediately speak with an office to schedule their exam. This takes advantage of the patient's intention to act, but does not leave it to the patient's motivation or memory to make a separate call to schedule it during business hours.

Other times, a series of IVR calls can be used with our without multimedia programs to help patients engage and more successfully transition from hospital to home. For example, when a patient with heart failure is discharged to home, they and members of their family (both local and remote) can be signed up to receive regular IVR calls for a number of weeks or even months. An automated IVR call series can deliver and reinforce necessary instructions, like making sure they schedule and have transportation to their follow-up appointment. IVR calls can also collect data on patients' status to ensure recovery is progressing. Patients can be asked if they have any questions about taking their medications, or if they have any new symptoms or side effects. In this virtual setting, patients feel safe honestly disclosing personal information like their weight, or admitting they are still confused about the changes to their medications.

In the case of heart failure, patients can be asked if they have a scale to weigh themselves, the call can explain why getting a daily weight is important, ask if they weighed themselves, and how much they weigh each day. The hospital can then get a daily report, and an algorithm can be used to identify if any patients have gained weight over the course of a week (as this is usually an early warning sign of trouble). If they have, this can be noted as a red flag. The hospital staff can then use their human resources more intelligently and efficiently to reach out to those patients to engage them.

In a small study of 20 patents with heart failure most participants 95% said receiving IVR calls helped them feel more connected to their health care team and more confident in performing care plan activities. 90% also felt better prepared to start discussions about their health with their doctor (Zan et al., 2015).

Engaging Patients in Shared Decision Making

Often, there is no single best treatment option for something like low-risks prostate cancer, and patients are ideally invited to take part in shared decision making (SDM). SDM is a process where the provider helps the patient understand the decision, its consequences, and then helps them apply their values and preferences in order to make the best decision for that individual. This can be very challenging. And decision aids are tools that can be used during or between clinical encounters to help walk patients through this information in a more understandable and unbiased way.

The benefit of decision aids generally is well documented. In its review of the impact of decision aids, the Cochrane Collaboration reviewed 115 randomized controlled studies. When decision aids were compared to usual care, patients who used decision aids were more knowledgeable and had much more realistic expectations. 74% of people had more realistic expectations, 31% were less passive in decisions, with fewer people left undecided (Stacey et al., 2014).

Unfortunately, clinicians often view patients as unwilling or unable to engage in SDM. For example, a survey of 106 gastroenterologists found that 34% were enthusiastic about SDM and 47% were actually skeptical of it, with only 12% stating they have a "systemic, consistent, and formally documented approach to SDM" (Siegel et al., 2015). In contrast, a survey of 460 patients with a serious digestive disease, namely ulcerative colitis (UC), across a wide age range (19 to 81) found that most patients (87%) wanted to share treatment decision-making with their doctors. In fact, the majority (98%) also wanted more than just a basic understanding of UC (Thompson et al., 2016). A systematic review of patient preferences for shared decisions found that 71% of patients want to be involved in decisions (Chewning et al., 2012).

Meeting Patients Where They Are

Patients are often very interested to understand their condition or options. Many people are simply overwhelmed and have no idea where to begin asking questions or discussing their preferences. They lack the orientation and understanding to participate in a clinical conversation. As one mother explained, "When we were told my four year old son had Crohn's, our world flipped upside down. The attending doc… saw the mom-panic in my eyes, sat down, put his feet up on my son's bed and settled in for a nice long chat. However, I didn't have any idea what to ask." (personal communication, Sept 11, 2014). This sense of feeling both panicked and adrift is common. Yet we expect patients to settle in for a conversation when they are neither oriented nor calm. What is often interpreted as unwillingness or inability of patients to participate may be the healthcare system's failure to give people the understanding and support they need to engage.

Anxiety about a condition or treatment options can continue to exist even when patients have been living with a condition for many years. Helping people consider all the treatment options for a condition like ulcerative colitis (UC) is challenging. UC impacts patients' quality of life and increases their risk of colon cancer. Despite having serious problems for many years, people with UC are often afraid to learn about surgical treatment, which usually involves getting a temporary or permanent ostomy (where a bag is placed over an opening on their abdomen to collect feces). People tend to underestimate their emotional resilience and ability to adapt and bounce back from things that seem unimaginable, like an ostomy or learning to self-inject a medication.

This is a known challenge in SDM that social psychologists have termed: "immune neglect," because people think it will take longer and be harder for their so-called psychological immune system to cope and adapt. People often refer to an ostomy bag it as a "poop bag" and cannot imagine living with it, let alone that it could provide a better quality of life. In fact, research shows that not only do people with colostomies report the same moods and similar levels of life satisfaction as those who do not have them, but "overall life satisfaction and quality of life increased with time for patients with permanent, but not temporary, ostomies" (Smith, Lowenstein, Rozin, Sherriff, & Ubel, 2007).

Unfortunately, this leads people to make poor decisions. A UK study found increased UC-related mortality when treating UC with colectomy [ostomy] surgery was only considered as a last resort (Roberts, Williams, Yeates, & Goldacre, 2007). Delaying surgery for UC to the point of last resort also increases post-op complications (Randall et al., 2010). Therefore, it is essential to help UC patients consider treatments they fear and put off. Unfortunately, fear of UC surgery tends to persist even when others who have gotten an ostomy say how it much better their life is now — even that they wished they had done it years earlier. People are often too scared to read about it online or research surgery on their own.

This was borne out by a study done by Thompson et al. (2016) of 460 UC patients, which found that patients' second biggest concern after the risk of developing colon cancer was surgery to remove their colon, resulting in a temporary or permanent ostomy. In fact, 78% of the patients said they would consider surgery only as a last resort. The article discussion concludes that, "De-mystification of colectomy, and in particular of ileostomy-related and colorectal cancer-related concerns, can dramatically change patient perception of colectomy by directly addressing their 'fear of the unknown'." The same study found that most UC patients (85%) indicated they would find it most helpful to view a web-based decision aid prior to meeting with their doctor to discuss their treatment options.

One benefit of multimedia programs that play like a video or movie is that it is effortlessness to allow the program to play on. Even when the program reaches a stressful topic, the program continues to convey information and does not rely on the viewer's volition to keep moving through it. The format reverses the equation, so that instead of making an effort to keep reading, the patient-viewer needs to make an effort to stop or pause the program – essentially creating a "default effect."

As per self-determination theory, because this type of program is usually viewed at home, there is also time and opportunity to support autonomy by acknowledging emotions that accompany new diagnoses or treatment decision, providing rationale in a way that the patient does not feel judged and minimizes pressure (Deci & Flaste, 1996, p. 101). For example, since most UC patients are resistant to hearing about surgery, a multimedia program can validate and normalize their anxiety and aversion to surgery. The program can acknowledge that for most people surgery to remove the colon is a daunting topic and something that is often thought of as a last resort – creating a moment of empathy.

A multimedia program can provide context, in this case as to why surgery can be a good option at some point and why people should talk with their doctor about when it would be a viable option for them. The animations of the different surgical options (ileostomy or "J-pouch"; see example in Figure 1) demonstrate the procedures in a format that demystifies them and is more understandable than still drawings and less frightening than real video footage.

Pressure is minimized and patient autonomy is created when a program provides opportunities to decide whether they want more in-depth information about topics such as the risks of ileostomy or J-pouch surgery, and what life is like afterward. Participants do not feel like information about surgery is being forced on them and are then interested to hear more in-depth information.

While clinicians may often ask patients if they would like more information about a treatment, the interpersonal dynamic may intrude. Patients may feel they would be asking for too much of a clinician's time, or they may feel too overwhelmed to

Figure 1. Example from explanation of J-pouch surgery
© 2014 Emmi Solutions, LLC. Treatment Options for Ulcerative Colitis program

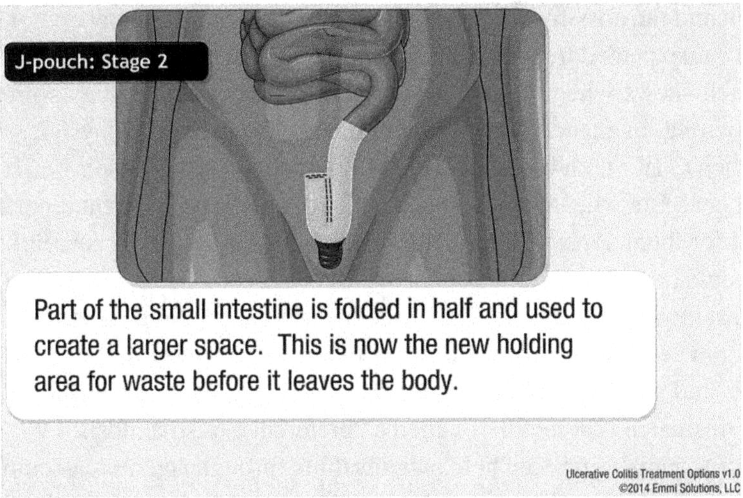

try and absorb it in the office setting. In other cases, they may feel pressured or like they are being a "bad patient" if they decline to hear more information.

Research shows most patients hold back showing emotions like sadness in front of providers. But in a virtual setting people are more likely to display more intense emotions (Lucas et al., 2014). Being able to review an online program at home gives patients the latitude to view it when distractions are minimal, and in a private setting where they are not regulating or suppressing emotions.

In this private setting, multimedia can also take the time to walk patients through thought exercises. For example, this can walk women through various scenarios to help them think about how they would feel wearing a prosthetic under a party dress or bathing suit, how they would feel changing in a gym locker room, how it would impact activities like swimming, and each woman's relationship with her partner.. This is a more emotionally engaging experience that moves beyond the facts of treatment pros, cons, and tradeoffs to help women think about what the reality of day-to-day life would be like. These preferences are uniquely personal and not typically elicited as part of a standard clinical assessment. Research shows that patients who use decision aids that include these types of explicit values clarification exercises are more likely to choose an option congruent with their values (Stacey et al., 2014).

If the patient's doctor is not aware of how she feels about these matters, a treatment might be selected based on criteria that are less important to her. If the doctor assumed a woman wanted to preserve her breast, whereas the patient just wanted to deal with the problem once and for all and avoid the inconvenience of radiation therapy, the doctor might recommend a lumpectomy when a mastectomy might be a better fit. Clinicians cannot predict each patient's unique preferences. Every patient is different and the possible reasons patients and their families may opt for counter-intuitive or unexpected treatment decisions are impossible to predict.

Research shows when clinicians assume they know what patients prefer, they are often wrong. In a study done by Montgomery et al. (2007), physicians thought most women (71%) with breast cancer would rank conserving their breast as a top treatment goal. But when women were surveyed, only seven percent reported it was a top goal for them. And while no physicians in this study (zero percent) believed women would be very concerned about avoiding a prosthetic breast, 33% of patients placed great importance on this. This disconnect between clinician assumptions and reality would send many women down a treatment pathway that does not reflect their goals and would potentially leave them with a greatly diminished quality of life. This mismatch is sometimes called a "preference misdiagnosis."

Interactive capabilities can help patients think through and more document their concerns, goals, and preferences at home where they feel comfortable disclosing what is often very sensitive information (see Figure 2). This creates a better starting point for the conversation with their treatment team.

Decision science continues to investigate virtual interactions to help patients understand not just their preferences, but also the trade-offs of treatment options. Interactive, dynamic slider bars may help people grasp trade-offs to make treatment

Figure 2. Example of patient values clarification interaction
© 2012 Emmi Solutions, LLC. Early-stage Invasive Breast Cancer: Considering Your Treatment Options program

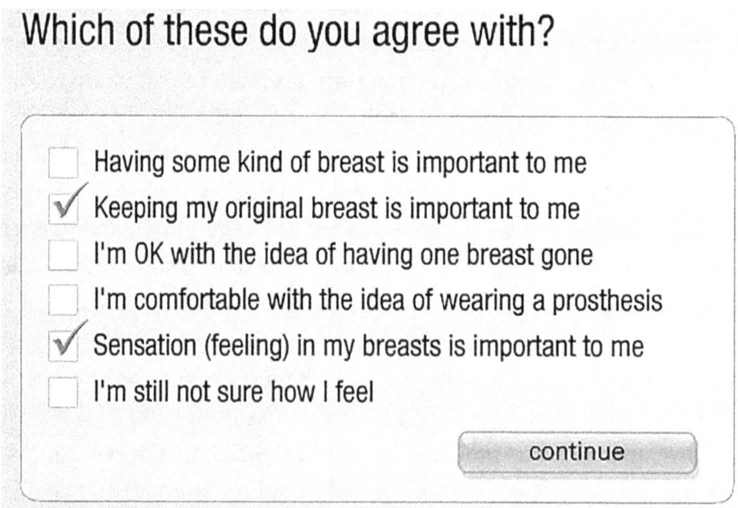

choices more in line with their values. Instead of asking people what matters to them or having them check or rank it, sliders that adjust based on each other's position as people pull them out or push them back help people understand what is important to them and how this then maps to their treatment options. In work done by Witteman et al. (2012), this kind of interactive exercise reduced the number of patients who experienced discordance between their choices and their stated values from 23% down to 14%.

FUTURE RESEARCH DIRECTIONS

The research and patient feedback on virtual interactions with IVR calls and multimedia program are encouraging. While some outcomes have already been measured, such as patient attendance at procedures and shorter procedure times for colonoscopy, the opportunity to measure numerous other outcomes after patients interact with virtual tools is fertile ground. For example, many patients who view decision aids for chronic hip, knee, and low back pain indicate they are now leaning away from surgery and toward less aggressive treatment like physical therapy. But finding out what treatment patients actually receive is key to understanding to the full impact of these tools and to understanding what kind of training clinicians need so they do not deter or mitigate their impact.

Anecdotally, clinicians often report better experiences when patients use these tools as well. In an era of clinician burnout, it is essential physicians feel they have tools and resources to improve their conversations and help them with the challenges engaging patients in processes that informed consent and shared decision making pose. A growing body of evidence indicates patients who receive this type of multimedia program arrive with a better base understanding of the physiology, their condition, what it means, and what the treatment or procedure entails. Instead of feeling lost, they have better questions rooted in information their provider knows is reliable. There is also opportunity to assess to what degree these tools can improve patient and physician satisfaction, and whether it creates more efficient visits.

Dr. Corey Siegel, Director of the IBD Center at Dartmouth-Hitchcock Medical Center describes his encounters with patients to discuss treatment options for Crohn's disease after they view a multimedia decision aid: "They understand the stakes and are more comfortable being involved in decisions since they have a better grasp of the issues. People are also more comfortable asking me questions" (personal communication, July 19, 2013). It would be valuable to study how and to what degree multimedia tools improve the quality of patient-physician conversations and whether it affects clinicians' perceptions of patients' understanding and their willingness to engage in SDM.

CONCLUSION

Multimedia programs and IVR can help break down patient-clinician communication barriers, reduce patient anxiety, and improve competence, understanding, relational dynamics and autonomy, to create more productive and empowered patients. These tools can create better and more engaging experience for patients, providers, and caregivers. Once patients get information in a way they can understand, review, and share outside of the clinical setting, this gives them the orientation, foundation, privacy, and confidence they need to engage more fully in their care and are empowered to ask the questions that matter to them; and this engagement is an essential for a meaningful and valuable healthcare experience.

REFERENCES

Abdoolatiff, S., & Narod, F. B. (2009). Investigating the effectiveness of computer simulations in the teaching of "atomic structure and bonding". In *Chemistry Education in the ICT Age* (pp. 85-100).

Bain, L. L., Wilson, T., & Chaikind, E. (1989). Participant perceptions of exercise programs for overweight women. *Research Quarterly for Exercise and Sport*, *60*(2), 134–143. doi:10.1080/02701367.1989.10607428 PMID:2489834

Chewning, B., Bylund, C., Shah, B., Arora, N. K., Gueguen, J. A., & Makoul, G. (2012). Patient preferences for shared decisions: A systematic review. *Patient Education and Counseling*, *86*(1), 9–18. doi:10.1016/j.pec.2011.02.004 PMID:21474265

Clark, R., & Mayer, R. (2011). *E-Learning and the Science of Instruction: Proven Guidelines for Consumers and Designers of Multimedia Learning*. New York: Pfeiffer. doi:10.1002/9781118255971

Davis, T. C., Crouch, M. A., Wills, G., Miller, S., & Abdehou, D. M. (1990).. . *The Journal of Family Practice*, *31*(5), 533–538. PMID:2230677

Deci, E. L., & Flaste, R. (1996). *Why We Do What We Do: Understanding Self-Motivation*. New York: Penguin Books.

Fang, M. C., Panguluri, P., Machtinger, E. L., & Schillinger, D. (2009). Language, literacy, and characterization of stroke among patients taking warfarin for stroke prevention: Implications for health communication. *Patient Education and Counseling*, *75*(3), 403–410. Retrieved from http://www.ajmc.com/journals/supplement/2014/a465_ma14_transitions/a465_mar14_owen_s81t91/P-3#shash.SfblJhR1.dpuf doi:10.1016/j.pec.2008.12.009 PMID:19171448

Gerr, R., Saulsberry, K., Clark, M., & Kerns, C. (2014). *The Shared Accountability Care Model: Keeping Patients Activated, In-Network, and Brand Loyal*. The Advisory Board Company.

Harper, D. (2001). *Online Etymology Dictionary*. Retrieved from http://www.etymonline.com/index.php?term=patience&allowed_in_frame=0

Health Insurance Portability and Accountability Act. (1996). *CMS.gov*. Retrieved from https://www.cms.gov/Regulations-and-Guidance/HIPAA-Administrative-Simplification/HIPAAGenInfo/downloads/hipaalaw.pdf

Himmelstein, D. U., Warren, E., Thorne, D., & Woolhandler, S. (2005, February). MarketWatch: Illness And Injury As Contributors To Bankruptcy. *Health Affairs*. Retrieved from:http://content.healthaffairs.org/content/early/2005/02/02/hlthaff.w5.63/suppl/DC1

Katz, M. G., Jacobson, T. A., Veldar, E., & Kripalani, S. (2007). Patient Literacy and Question-asking Behavior During the Medical Encounter: A Mixed-metholds Analysis. *Journal of General Internal Medicine*, *22*(6), 782–786. doi:10.1007/s11606-007-0184-6 PMID:17431697

Kessels, R. P. (2003). Patients' Memory for Medical Information. *Journal of the Royal Society of Medicine*, *96*(5), 219–222. doi:10.1258/jrsm.96.5.219 PMID:12724430

Leary, M. R., & Kowalski, R. M. (1990). Impression management: A literature review and two-component model. *Psychological Bulletin*, *107*(1), 34–47. doi:10.1037/0033-2909.107.1.34

Leary, M. R., Tchividijian, L. R., & Kraxberger, B. E. (1994). Self-presentation can be hazardous to your health: Impression management and health risk. *Health Psychology*, *13*(6), 461–470. doi:10.1037/0278-6133.13.6.461 PMID:7889900

Lucas, G. M., Gratch, J., King, A., & Morency, L. (2014). It's only a computer: Virtual humans increase willingness to disclose. *Computers in Human Behavior*, *37*, 94–100. doi:10.1016/j.chb.2014.04.043

Mayer, R., & Moreno, R. (2003). Nine Ways to Reduce Cognitive Load in Multimedia Learning. *Educational Psychologist*, *38*(1), 43–52. doi:10.1207/S15326985EP3801_6

McWhorter, J. (2012). Gosh, Golly, Gee. *New Republic*. Retrieved from htttp://www.newrepublic.com/article/politics/magazine/103945/romney-language-mcwhorter

McWhorter, J. (2013, February). Txting is killing language. JK!!! *TED2013*. Retrieved from http://www.ted.com/talks/john_mcwhorter_txtng_is_killing_language_jk#t-126831

Meppelink, C., van Weert, J., Haven, C. J., & Smit, E. G. (2015). The Effectiveness of Health Animations in Audiences with Different Health Literacy Levels: An Experimental Study. *Journal of Medical Internet Research, 17*(1), e11. doi:10.2196/jmir.3979 PMID:25586711

Montgomery, A. A., Emmett, C. L., Fahey, T., Jones, C., Ricketts, I., Patel, R. R., & Murphy, D. J. et al. (2007). Two decision aids for mode of delivery among women with previous caesarean section: Randomised controlled trial. *BMJ (Clinical Research Ed.), 334*(7607), 1305. doi:10.1136/bmj.39217.671019.55 PMID:17540908

Parker, S., Zipurksy, J., Ma, H., & Siegel, C. (2013, October). Randomized controlled trial demonstrates a web-based multimedia program used prior to first-time colonoscopy decreased patient anxiety, sedation requirement and procedure time while increasing knowledge. Dartmouth-Hitchcock Medical Center, Geisel School of Medicine at Dartmouth. *Poster presented at theMeeting of the American College of Gastroenterology*, San Diego, CA.

Piette, J., Rosland, A., Marinec, N., Striplin, D., Bernstein, S., & Silveira, M. (2013). Engagement With Automated Patient Monitoring and Self-Management Support Calls. *Medical Care, 51*(3), 216–223. doi:10.1097/MLR.0b013e318277ebf8 PMID:23222527

Randall, J., Singh, B., Warren, B., Travis, S., Mortensen, N., & George, B. (2010). Delayed surgery for acute severe colitis is associated with increased risk of post-operative complications. *British Journal of Surgery, 97*(3), 404–409. doi:10.1002/bjs.6874 PMID:20101648

Roberts, S., Williams, J., Yeates, D., & Goldacre, M. (2007). Mortality in patients with and without colectomy admitted to hospital for ulcerative colitis and Crohn's disease: Record linkage studies. *British Medical Journal, 17*(7628), 1033–3. doi:10.1136/bmj.39345.714039.55 PMID:17977817

Safran, C. (2004). *United States House Ways and Means Health Subcommittee testimony*. Washington, D.C.

Schocker, L. (2013). Young People Are Sleeping With Their Phones. Their Parents Are Sleeping With People. Retrieved from http://www.huffingtonpost.com/2013/09/16/sleep-phone-tablet-bed_n_3924161.html

Schunk, D. H., Pintrich, P. R., & Meece, J. L. (2008). *Motivation in education: Theory, research, and applications*. Upper Saddle River, New Jersey: Pearson/Merrill Prentice Hall.

Siegel, C., Lofland, J., Naim, A., Gollins, J., Walls, D., Rudder, L., & Reynolds, C. (2015). Gastroenterologists' Views of Shared Decision Making for Patients with Inflammatory Bowel Disease. *Digestive Diseases and Sciences*, *60*(9), 2636–2645. doi:10.1007/s10620-015-3675-z PMID:25939543

Smith, D. M., Lowenstein, G., Rozin, P., Sherriff, R. L., & Ubel, P. A. (2007). Sensitivity to disgust, stigma, and adjustment to life with a colostomy. *Journal of Research in Personality*, *41*(4), 787–803. doi:10.1016/j.jrp.2006.09.006 PMID:17940585

Stacey, D., Légaré, F., Col, N. F., Bennett, C. L., Barry, M. J., Eden, K. B., & Wu, J. H. C. et al. (2014). Decision aids for people facing health treatment or screening decisions. *Cochrane Database of Systematic Reviews*, *January*. doi:10.1002/14651858.CD001431.pub4 PMID:24470076

Thomas T., Kedia, P. & Cohen, R. D. (2007). Impact of an Internet-based educational program on colonoscopy attendance and quality (abstract). *American Journal of Gastroenterology* Supplement S454.

Thompson, K. D., Connor, S. J., Walls, D., Gollins, J., Stewart, S. K., Bewtra, M., … & Siegel, C. A. (2016). Patients with ulcerative colitis are more concerned about complications of their disease than side effects of medications. *Inflamm. Bowel Dis.*, 22(4), 940-947.

Vin-Raviv, N., Hillyer, G. C., Hershman, D. L., Galea, S., Leoce, N., Bovbjerg, D. H., & Neugut, A. I. et al. (2013). Racial Disparities in Posttraumatic Stress After Diagnosis of Localized Breast Cancer: The BQUAL Study. *Journal of the National Cancer Institute*, *107*(7). doi:10.1093/jnci/djt024 PMID:23434900

Weisband, S., & Kiesler, S. (1996, April). Self disclosure on computer forms: Meta-analysis and implications. Proceedings of the SIGCHI conference on human factors in computing systems (pp. 3-10). ACM.

Witteman, H. O., Scherer, L. D., Angott, A. M., Ubel, P. A., Dickson, M., Holtzman, L. G., . . . Zikmund-Fisher, B. J. (2012). Hold My Hand: Explicitly Showing Tradeoffs and Fit Between Values and Options Helps People Make Choices Concordant With Their Stated Values. Proceedings of 34th. Chicago: Annual Meeting of The Society for Medical Decision Making. Retrieved from https://smdm.confex.com/smdm/2012az/webprogram/Paper7417.html

Zan, S., Agboola, S., Moore, S. A., Parks, K. A., Kvedar, J. C., & Jethwani, K. (2015). Patient Engagement With a Mobile Web-Based Telemonitoring System for Heart Failure Self Management: A Pilot Study. *Journal of Medical Internet Research*, *3*(2), e33. doi:10.2196/mhealth.3789 PMID:25842282

KEY TERMS AND DEFINITIONS

Attentional Narrowing: The brain tends to focus on the most frightening statements. This focus draws all or most of an individual's attention, and it becomes difficult for him or her to listen to and absorb any other information.

Cognitive Load: The amount of mental effort and resources the brain's limited short-term memory needs to process and understand information.

Default Effect: A phenomenon where people leave an existing choice, setting, or state (such as a media program continuing to play) in place because changing it requires an active decision and effort (such as clicking "pause").

Immune Neglect: Also called "immune bias." People tend to underestimate their own ability to cope and adapt to challenging or negative events. This bias leads to poor decision-making.

Impression Management (Self Presentation): Whether consciously or unconsciously, patients may not respond honestly or withhold information because they want to be viewed positively and create a good impression on the clinician or healthcare worker.

Information Therapy: When clinicians or healthcare teams prescribe patient-friendly, trusted information to people that is relevant to their condition, medical decision, or procedure at that point in time.

Interactive Voice Response (IVR) Phone Calls: Scheduled, automated phone calls that use speech recognition and keypad responses to understand their responses and dynamically interact with them. Information can also be collected with this type of system.

Preference Misdiagnosis: When a clinician assumes they know what a patient would prefer regarding their treatment, does not ask the patient about their preferences, and the clinician's assumption is often wrong. Also referred to as a "silent misdiagnosis."

Progressive Disclosure: A design technique to prevent users from getting overwhelmed by information, where the information is sequenced across multiple screens and becomes more detailed as the user moves through it.

Shared Decision Making: A process where the provider helps the patient understand the decision, its consequences, and then helps them apply their values and preferences in order to make a decision.

Chapter 7
Using the Communication AssessmenT Checklist in Health to Assess the Communication Quality of Web Based Resources for Prostate Cancer

Juliana Genova
University of Ottawa, Canada

Curtis A. Olson
Geisel School of Medicine at Dartmouth, USA

Jackie Bender
University Health Network, Canada

ABSTRACT

Introduction: The communication quality of web resources for patients is unknown. The purpose of this study was to assess prostate cancer websites using the Communication AssessmenT Checklist in Health (CATCH). Methods: CATCH is a theory-based tool consisting of 50 elements nested in 12 concepts. Two raters independently applied it to 35 HON certified websites containing information on prostate cancer treatment. Results: Websites contained a mean 24.1 (SD= 3.6) CATCH items. The concepts Language, Readability, Layout, Typography and Appearance were present in over

DOI: 10.4018/978-1-5225-0663-8.ch007

80% of sites. Content, Risk Communication, Usefulness, and Scientific Value were present in 50% or less. Discussion: The prostate cancer websites evaluated in this study did not present treatment information in a useful, informative or credible way for patients. The communication quality of these resources could be improved with a clear strategic intent focused on decision-making, using CATCH as a guiding framework.

INTRODUCTION

There is a growing emphasis on shared decision-making (Makoul & Clayman, 2006; Wong et al., 2000) as a means to enhance patient care. Partnerships with patients can improve the planning and carrying out of therapies (Brett et al., 2014; Brown, Brown, & Sharma, 2000), facilitate adaptation of new knowledge to specific patient communities (Brett et al., 2014; Collier, 2011; Fagerlin, Zikmund-Fisher, & Ubel (2011); Frank, Basch, & Selby, 2014) and make information more accessible to patients by making it more user-friendly (Brett et al., 2014).

There is, however, a gap in our understanding of the process that occurs between the creation of knowledge and its use (Bero et al., 1998; Dopson, Locock, Gabbay, Ferlie, & Fitzgerald, 2003; Lang, Wyer, & Haynes, 2007). In fact, academic researchers have often studied knowledge dissemination and implementation as a two-step process, the first step of which is distilling and packaging the evidence (Cohen et al., 2008; Grimshaw et al., 2006), and the second step is studying the adoption of evidence, taking into consideration behaviour-change factors (Ajzen & Albarracen, 2007; Ajzen, Czasch, & Flood, 2009; Michie, Johnston, Abraham, & Walker, 2005; Michie, van Stralen, & West, 2011). Those steps overlap and are well documented. But the factors affecting the effectiveness of the resources used to communicate new health knowledge and influence behaviour remains largely unexplored.

There are several instruments designed to help streamline health information, filter it and make it more usable. Four instruments evaluate the implementability of clinical guidelines and incorporate a communication dimension. The Guideline Implementability Appraisal tool (GLIA) (Shiffman et al., 2005) proposes a "Presentation and Formatting" dimension comprising two items, while ADAPTE (T. A. Collaboration, 2009) highlights the importance of Context of Use", "Strength of Evidence" and " Risks and Benefits". Two others– Appraisal of Guidelines for Research & Evaluation (AGREE) (Brouwers et al., 2010; A. Collaboration, 2001; Klazinga, 2003) and GRADE (Guyatt et al., 2011; Guyatt et al., 2012; Oxman & GRADE Working Group, 2004) assess the scientific value of the evidence, its scope and purpose, rigor of development, clarity and presentation. Another set of instruments analyses the quality of information provided in web resources for prostate cancer. LIDA (Borgmann et al., 2015; Soobrah & Clark, 2012) and DISCERN (Charnock, Shepperd, Needham, & Gann, 1999) measure the accessibility, usability and reliability of the information; the Information Comprehensiveness Tool (Warren, Footman, Tinelli, McKee, & Knai, 2014) assesses its comprehensiveness; and a framework developed by Ferreira, Carreira, Silva and Lunet (2013) evaluates its relevance.

The first instrument to address the overall suitability of materials for patients, is Suitability Assessment of Materials (SAM), developed by Doak, Doak and Root (1994). Although SAM was developed for use with print materials, it has also been used to assess video- and audio-taped instructions to patients.

However, the existing tools give little or no attention to the communication characteristics of the resource and the message it contains. To the best of our knowledge, there is no instrument for evaluating the communication qualities of online health-related materials and the concepts that could trigger behaviour change and to ensure that patients have accurate, spin-free information.

In this chapter, we present a version of CATCH (Communication AssessmenT Checklist in Health), a new instrument based on communication theories for assessing health messages. We modified the original CATCH tool for application to web-based resources. We will demonstrate its use by applying it to web-based resources for prostate cancer patients. Our aim is to show how the modified CATCH tool can be used to identify the communication concepts exemplified on prostate cancer treatment websites designed for patients and suggest ways to further tailor those online messages to make them more effective.

BACKGROUND

Prostate cancer is the most common cancer among men in Canada (Society, Records, & Registries, 1987), and the fourth most common cancer worldwide, after lung, breast and bowel cancer (Collin et al., 2008). In Canada, every year 23,600 men are diagnosed with prostate cancer (Carter, Miller, Murphy, Payne, & Bryant-Lukosius, 2014). Prostate cancer is also one of the more difficult cancers for patients to comprehend because of the variety of treatment options available (Clark, Wray, & Ashton, 2001; Stamey, McNeal, Yemoto, Sigal, & Johnstone, 1999) including: watchful-waiting, active surveillance, surgery, external beam radiation, brachytherapy, hormone therapy, cryotherapy, chemotherapy and high frequency ultrasound therapy (Loblaw et al., 2007). Each option has its pros and cons, which vary according to the patient's age, genetics and overall health.

It is important that prostate cancer patients educate themselves on the treatment options available to them, because treatment options are numerous, decisions are largely patient driven and the side effects can be distressing, and in some cases, long term.

Nowadays the most popular source for health information is the Internet. It may have the greatest potential for health related behaviour change and decision-making (Chua et al., 2011). Data from the World Bank (2015) indicates that at least 85.6% of people in Canada and 84.2% in US use the Internet. According to the Pew Internet and American Life Project Health Fact Sheet (2012), 72% of adults in the US use the Internet to obtain health information.

Not surprisingly, the Internet is a popular source for prostate cancer information for patients. A 2014 multi-province, population-based survey of Canadian men with prostate cancer found that 79% reported using the Internet and 68% reported using the Internet for information on prostate cancer treatment during the diagnosis and treatment period (Wong et al., 2000).

There are, however, significant challenges, the first of which is the low eHealth literacy of much of the population (Jacobs, Lou, Ownby, & Caballero, 2014; Sullivan, 2011; Tennant et al., 2015). eHealth literacy is defined as "the ability to seek, find, understand, and appraise health information from electronic sources and apply the knowledge gained to addressing or solving a health problem" (Norman & Skinner, 2006a; Norman & Skinner, 2006b). 50% of Canadian men with prostate cancer reported not knowing how to judge the quality of information on the Internet and whether it was personally applicable, and 25 to 30% reported poor search skills and difficulty finding information that they could understand (Norman & Skinner, 2006a; Norman & Skinner, 2006b). As evidence suggests, low levels of eHealth literacy are associated with inferior health outcomes, increased hospitalization and morbidity (Van der Vaart et al., 2011). One approach to address the issue is to tailor online messages to individuals' needs, preferences and circumstances and make them easy to understand, acceptable, easily deployed, accessible and cost-effective (Chua et al., 2011), (Aakhus, Granlund, Oxman, & Flottorp, 2015; Davison, Szafron, Gutwin, & Visvanathan, 2014; Falk et al., 2014; Salonen, Ryhänen, & Leino-Kilpi, 2014). Tailored interventions, consistently proven to be more effective in inducing behavior change (Hoffman et al., 2013; Norman & Skinner, 2006), can help consumers find and evaluate information, monitoring their health status, and understand financial constraints (Kobayashi, Wardle, & von Wagner, 2014; Smith et al., 2015)

Numerous studies have assessed the quality of prostate cancer information on the Internet (Black & Penson, 2006; Pruthi, Belsante, Kurpad, Nielsen, & Wallen, 2011; Routh, Gong, Cannon, & Nelson, 2011) (Hellawell, Turner, Le Monnier, & Brewster, 2000). When systematically reviewed by Black and Penson (2006), websites containing information on prostate cancer were found to be of sufficient quality to aid in decision making but lacked currency, attribution, balance of evidence and comprehensiveness. Prostate cancer websites have also been assessed for readability – the ease with which information is read and understood. Using Flesch Kindcaid Grade Level and Flesch Reading Ease Level tools, Ellimoottil, Polcari, Kadlec and Gupta (2012) analysed 62 eligible websites containing information on prostate cancer treatment options and only found 3 that were written below a high school reading level. Concerning findings given that one third of the US population reads below a high school reading level (Ellimoottil et al., 2012). To our knowledge, the communication quality of prostate cancer websites has not been studied.

The CATCH Instrument

CATCH (Table 1), whose development and preliminary validation is described in a prior publication, (Genova et al., 2014) is based on SAM (Doak et al., 1994), fundamental communication concepts from the theories of risk communication (Fischhoff, Brewer, & Downs, 2011), Tarde's theory of social values (Tarde, 1890; Tarde, 1902a; Tarde, 1902b), and concepts related to user-centred design (Neuhauser, 2011; Nielsen, 2004). The original CATCH is composed of 55 elements nested in 12 concepts ranging from appearance, form and content to fundamental communication concepts such as numeracy, objectivity, credibility, effectiveness, scientific value and usefulness. CATCH was initially applied to a set of PEMs with proven effectiveness (Giguière et al., 2012) distributed to clinicians and demonstrated good ability to discriminate between resources that are different based on the quality of communication concepts, suggesting good construct validity (Genova et al., 2014). As a theory-based instrument, CATCH can, in our view, be applied to print or online content, using different medias and targeting different audiences.

Because we modified CATCH specifically for web-based resources for prostate-cancer patients, its validity and reliability must be re-assessed. The present study is a pilot designed to show how CATCH can be applied to online resources; further studies are needed to formally assess its performance.

Tailoring of CATCH for Web Resources

The concepts underlying CATCH (Table 1) for patients and CATCH for physicians are the same. Both versions contain the same 12 concepts, but the CATCH for patients contains 5 fewer elements. Table 1 presents each concept and element.

The concepts of Layout, Typography, and Clarity of Content (elements 2 to 11) which relate to information design, as well as the elements of risk communication (elements 20 to 30) were appropriate for PEMs and for web resources, as well as for physicians and patients.

We adjusted the concepts "Source Credibility" and "Usefulness" from Tarde's Theory of Social Value (Katz, 1999; Lazzarato, 2002; Tarde, 1890; Tarde, 1902).

Table 1. Concepts and elements for the Communication AssessmenT Checklist in Health (CATCH)

Concept	Element: description
Appearance	
	1. Pictures, special fonts and colors
	2. Length: the material is no more than a page long.
Layout and typography	
	3. Clear layout: the text and graphics attract the reader's attention and create a visual path.
	4. Short to-the-point paragraphs: the resource uses short sentences of no more than 12 words, paragraphs of no more than 10 sentences with a single idea, and short and simple words.
	5. Subtitles: subtitles or subheadings are used to clearly group the information.
	6. Font size: the text is easy to read because the font size is not excessively small or large, at least 12 point, serif.
	7. Text clearly laid out and delimited by spaces: the text is well organized and easy to follow.
	8. Italics and capitals are used appropriately for references and subtitles or to enhance the layout.
Content	
	9. Purpose of the text is clearly stated in the title, illustration, or introduction.
	10. Limited scope: the scope of the resource is relevant to the stated purpose and is limited to defining the problem and the rationale, and providing a solution.
	11. Summary: the resource provides a summary or a review that reiterates and explains the central information.
	12. Information limited to key messages: the resource covers only a few key messages, ideally no more than three or four.
	13. Desired behaviours explained or modeled: best practices or recommended therapy procedures are clearly described.
Language and readability	
	14. Active voice: Sentences are written in the active voice whenever possible.
	15. Context given first: the situation is explained to the reader at the beginning of the message.
	16. Organizers (sometimes called "road signs") such as headers, captions, or transition words or statements briefly inform the reader of what is coming next.
Graphics	
	17. Graphics to facilitate understanding: the graphics are self-explanatory and facilitate understanding of the text.
	18. Relevance of graphics: graphics match and enhance the content; they should be simple in their meaning, without additional details that distract the reader. Moreover, they depict the recommended behaviour.
	19. Captions: captions and/or legends are used for each figure, list, table, or other display supporting the text.

continued on following page

Table 1. Continued

Concept	Element: description
Risk communication	
	20. Risk clarity: the risk is clearly presented and defined. There is no ambiguity.
	21. Likelihood of the event: there is a greater than 50% likelihood that the event described in the message will happen.
	22. Risks presented in order of priority: risks are presented starting with the most important, to clarify all the issues at stake at each level of risk.
	23. Objective presentation of both harms and benefits: the resource provides complete information on harms and benefits. For example, reporting survival rates for 1 year is incomplete compared to 5 years.
	24. Standardized presentation of harms and benefits: for all the outcomes, harms are defined the same way and use the same variable as benefits.
	25. Absolute risk difference used
	26. Consistent denominators and whole numbers: the resource uses the same denominators to present harms and benefits to ensure consistency, as well as whole numbers, which are easier to understand than fractions or decimals.
	27. Consistent time frames for harms and benefits: the resource expresses harms and benefits in the same temporal patterns.
	28. Clear difference between the risks at baseline and the risks at follow-up: Risks at baseline and following treatment are clearly presented so that the reader can evaluate the degree of change between the two time periods.
	29. Use of positive and negative frames: the message highlights not only the harms, but also the benefits of the recommended action, and uses positive framing that is more productive than negative framing (e.g., survival versus mortality).
	30. Symbols (numbers, graphs, statistics, etc.): symbols are used to clearly convey the meaning of the probabilities presented.
Scientific value	
	31. Effectiveness of the recommendations: it is stated in the resources that adherence to the recommendations yields concrete and specific results.
	32. Robustness of the evidence: it is stated in the resource that the message is supported by sufficient, high quality data. It is convincing for professionals.
Emotional appeal	
	33. Communication of urgency: the message raises concerns that should be answered immediately to reduce the morbidity or mortality of patients.
	34. Timeliness and visibility of the topic: the resource addresses a topic covered by popular media because of a public debate, a scientific controversy, or because it features a celebrity with a disease.
	35. Vibrancy or intensity: a fast pace and the choice of words show that the author is invested in the subject or driven by the urgency to convey something. The resource, through its appearance and language, conveys a sense of urgency.
	36. Threat of the event: the message depicts a serious threat that cannot be ignored.
	37. Newness of the message: the document provides a new perspective or represents an innovation.

continued on following page

Table 1. Continued

Concept	Element: description
	38. Highlighting of danger: the message highlights a potential threat or danger relative to the topic presented.
Relevance	
	39. Consistency with experience, logic, and language of reader: the message's language, format, and structure correspond to the reader's level of education, language, and/or professional background.
	40. Cultural match: the resource is adapted to the culture of readers and takes into account their background, customs, beliefs, and expectations.
	41. Narrative included: contains personal testimonies or real life-examples to drive the message home.
Social value/Source credibility	
	42. Endorsement by renowned individuals or organizations: the document is "validated" by renowned clinicians, research scientists, professional organizations, or the government.
	43. Background of the author: the resource clearly states that its author has relevant experience.
	44. Disclaimer of conflict of interests: an official statement attests to the absence of any conflict of interest.
Social value/Usefulness for the patient	
	45. Time saving the resource states that the recommended behaviour saves time.
	46. Money saving: the resource states that the recommended behaviour helps save money.
	47. Non-threatening: the message does not highlight deficiencies or lack of training in the medical staff or the health system.
	48. Building of self-efficacy: the resource describes a technology or innovation that will give more self-confidence to the clinician and allow them to make an informed decision or trust his or her own judgment.
	49. Increased ease: the resource offers an easier and better way to do things.
	50. Better quality of life: the resource states that adherence to the targeted behaviour will facilitate healthcare processes and improve organization of the environment.

The adjustment was simple: we removed all elements pertaining to usefulness for the physician or the health system. The rest (elements 42 to 50) remain the same.

Also, we did not include the element of Increased Ease, as it related to the ease of operation for the physician, or the elements Incentive and Promotion of Health, because they seemed irrelevant for patients as written.

THEORETICAL FRAMEWORK FOR CATCH

CATCH is a new evaluation framework based on several theories.

Risk Communication

The first theory is risk communication, and one of its most important dimensions is objectivity. We operationalized objectivity and included the elements numeracy, standard definitions, constant denominators and timeframes. If risks and benefits are in numerical expressions, they are easier to use and more comprehensible for patients in distress with a decreased ability to process information (Fagerlin et al., 2011). In decision-making, patients with better numeracy skills rely more on abstract information, such as numbers and graphs, while less numerated patients use emotion-based information, such as narratives (Salmon & Atkin, 2003), and whole numbers (e.g., 1 in 10,000) (Peters, 2012b; Sheridan et al., 2011).

Objectivity is better conveyed with standard definitions, constant denominators and timeframes about risks, costs and benefits, especially if they are enumerated in order of importance (Fischhoff, 2012; Fischhoff et al., 2011; Fischhoff, Watson, & Hope, 1984; Peters, 2012b). While enumerating choices, less is more: research shows that less cognitive effort results in better decision quality choices for patients (Peters, Dieckmann, Dixon, Hibbard, & Mertz, 2007) - less messages and fewer options for patients have bigger impact (Zikmund-Fisher, Windschitl, Exe, & Ubel, 2011).

Novelty, urgency and visibility of the danger are three elements that are usually intertwined. Novelty and urgency increase the perception of risk (Bandura, 2001) and this has more impact on arguments (Ajzen, 1971) and opinion change (Murphy et al., 1998). The relationship between stronger fear-arousing conditions and greater message acceptance is a linear one (Berkowitz & Cottingham, 1960; Sutton & Eiser, 1984). Witte and Allen (2000) conclude in their meta-analysis of over hundred fear appeal articles "the stronger the fear aroused by a fear appeal, the more persuasive it is" (p. 601). Visibility increases the impact of those elements.

There is also a subjective dimension to risk communication. A patient with high self-efficacy (Witte & Allen, 2000) is more likely to perform the recommended action. Michie and Abraham (2008) and Woolf, Grol, Hutchinson, Eccles and Grimshaw (1999) define self-efficacy as control of material and social environment, perceived behavioural control, self-esteem and self-confidence. Also, Ruiter and Kok (2011) show that people are more likely to act if the response will lead to a quick, sure and efficient change (Witte & Allen, 2000). The effectiveness of the recommended response may lead to behaviour change.

The message has to be relevant to the public. People relate to a message that is consistent with their experience, logic and language and they are more likely to adopt it. Patients tend to make sense of their environment through narrative, they think with stories (Morris, 2001) and are influenced by their own history and memories. Cultural match, as the expression " on-going negotiation within societal groups and conflicts of cultures" (Harter, Japp, & Beck, 2005), allows them to identify with the information and ultimately, to adopt it.

Conveying risks and benefits depend also on the formulation of the message. Effective messages highlight the positive outcomes of a treatment or behaviour (gain frames), especially when the outcome is clear (Ruiter & Kok, 2011; Salmon & Atkin, 2003). When the tone of the message is vibrant, commanding or intense, the conviction of the author is perceived by people and they use better the information (Peters, 2012a).

Tarde's Theory of Social Value

Gabriel Tarde based his theory on societal change on innovation and imitation, both triggered by value-credit (Tarde, 1902). Value-credit is composed of value-usefulness, value-beauty and value-truth. We operationalized value-truth, related to credibility of the source (Atkin, 1994), as endorsement by experts and disclaimer of interests. Value-usefulness is operationalized as time-saving, money-saving (Brownson, Fielding, & Maylahn, 2009) and non-threatening for the patient. Value-beauty is operationalized as "healthy environment" that promotes healing, or a treatment that avoids unnecessary surgical interventions or undesirable side effects.

Plain Language, Graphics and Content

CATCH incorporates also some elements of SAM (Doak et al., 1994) and comprises notions related to the plain language, such as active voice, use of short sentences and words which break the information into easier-to-process words (US Federal Plain Language Guidelines, 2010) and clean layout that facilitates reading (US Department of Health and Human Services, 2010) and creates a visual path (Doak, Doak, & Root, 1996) (Neuhauser, 2011). As for graphics, they should be culturally appropriate (Doak et al., 1996; Potomac & Doak, 2002), simple (Wright, 2001) and show only the behaviours to be encouraged (US Federal Plain Language Guidelines, 2010).

METHODS

Conceptualization and Operationalization

CATCH was created based on a literature review of commonly accepted communication theories. We defined some concepts that could be applied to evidence-based material, operationalized them and applied them, using a mapping approach, first to PEMs and then to web-based resources for prostate-cancer patients.

Sample of Web-Based Resources for Prostate-Cancer Patients

We conducted a search using the HON code search engine and the key words "prostate cancer treatment'. The Health on the Net Code (HON Code) is the oldest and most common quality standard for health related online information (Health On the Net Foundation, 2014). To achieve the HON code seal of approval, websites must conform to a number principles: have authoritative, reliable and accessible information, support patient-physician relation and confidentiality, and mention funding sources (Health On the Net Foundation, 2014) We hypothesized that the HON code certification guarantees, at least to some degree, the credibility of health information or the fact that it is reviewed by medical professionals. In addition, the results from the HON code search engine correspond well with the top ten web sites obtained using Google. More than 75% of patients begin their search with one of these three search engines (Pew Internet and American Life Project Health Fact Sheet, 2012), and visit only the top 10 web sites listed in the results [16]. To assess a diverse sample of content, we included the first four search results from each organization that pointed to different content, and selected the first 35 search results.

Application of CATCH

A conceptual mapping approach was used to apply CATCH to the selected sample of web pages. Two raters (JB, JG) independently applied the 50 elements of the CATCH instrument to each web-based resources for prostate-cancer patients.

Each web resource was rated along each CATCH element using a dichotomous scale indicating the presence/absence of the element. We wanted to find the presence or absence of each CATCH element and to compute the total occurrences. Once all the elements computed, this would give a comprehensive picture of the strategies used, their advantages and also disadvantages.

Analysis and Scoring

We used Excel and SPSS Version 21 to calculate the sum and sum percentage for each CATCH item and the total summary score for each web resource. We computed the scores for CATCH concepts by calculating the mean value of the items pertaining to each concept.

Rating Procedure

The raters compared their ratings and resolved any disagreements through discussion, which in some cases resulted in rewording of an element. Most disagreements among raters resulted from an unclear description of the elements or misunderstandings as to the degree of specificity required when coding for the presence or absence of an element.

RESULTS

Frequent Concepts

Table 2 and Figure 1 show that the most commonly addressed CATCH concepts. In order of frequency, they were Language and Readability, Layout & Typography, and Appearance. These elements were present in 80% to 93% of the web resources. As shown in Figure 2, the majority of the web resources evaluated contained less than 50% of the CATCH items. The mean CATCH summary score of the web- resources was 24.1 (SD= 3.6). The scores ranged from 15 to 33, out of a possible 50.

Table 2. Summary scores for CATCH concepts and elements (N=35)

CATCH Concepts and Items		Summary Score Sub-scale: X, SD (%) Item: n (%)
Appearance		28, 7.1 (80)
	1. Pictures, special fonts and colours	33 (94)
	2. Length: the material is no more than a page long.	23 (66)
Layout and Typography		31.3, 1.6 (86)
	3. Clear layout	31 (89)
	4. Short to-the-point paragraphs	30 (86)
	5. Subtitles	33 (94)
	6. Font size	29 (83)
	7. Text clearly laid out and delimited by space	32 (91)
	8. Italics and capitals	33 (94)
Content		19, 11.7, (54)
	9. Purpose of the text	27 (77)
	10. Limited scope	32 (91)
	11. Summary	4 (11)
	12. Information limited to key messages	10 (29)
	13. Desired behaviours explained or modelled	22 (63)

continued on following page

Table 2. Continued

CATCH Concepts and Items		Summary Score Sub-scale: X, SD (%) Item: n (%)
Language and Readability		32.7, 2.1 (93)
	14. Active voice	32 (91)
	15. Context given first	35 (100)
	16. Organizers	31 (89)
Graphics		13, 1.7 (37)
	17. Graphics to facilitate understanding	14 (40)
	18. Relevance of graphics.	14 (40)
	19. Captions	11 (31)
Risk Communication		11.6, 12.2 (33)
	20. Risk clarity	27 (77)
	21. Likelihood of the event	33 (94)
	22. Risks presented in order of priority	15 (43)
	23. Objective presentation of both harms and benefits	7 (20)
	24. Standardized presentation of harms and benefits	1 (3)
	25. Absolute risk difference used	0 (0)
	26. Consistent denominators and whole numbers	0 (0)
	27. Consistent time frames for harms and benefits	0 (0)
	28. Clear difference between the risks at baseline and the risks at follow-up	2 (6)
	29. Use of positive and negative frames	20 (57)
	30. Symbols (numbers, graphs, statistics, etc.)	0 (0)
	Scientific Value	16, 7.1 (51)
	31. Effectiveness of the recommendations	23 (66)
	32. Robustness of the evidence	13 (37)
Emotional Appeal		19.2, 11.8 (55)
	33. Communication of urgency	7 (20)
	34. Timeliness and visibility of the topic	34 (97)
	35. Vibrancy or intensity	7 (20)
	36. Threat of the event	32 (91)
	37. Newness of the message	15 (43)
	38. Highlighting of danger	20 (57)
Relevance		12.7, 16.3 (36)
	39. Consistency with experience, logic, and language of reader	31 (89)
	40. Cultural match	7 (20)

continued on following page

Table 2. Continued

CATCH Concepts and Items		Summary Score Sub-scale: X, SD (%) Item: n (%)
	41. Narrative included	0 (0)
Social Value/ Source Credibility		8.0, 8.0 (23)
	42. Endorsement by renowned individuals or organizations	16 (46)
	43. Background of the author	8 (23)
	44. Disclaimer of conflict of interests	0 (0)
Social Value/Usefulness for the Patient		8.3, 11.8 (24)
	45. Time saving	1 (3)
	46. Money saving	2 (6)
	47. Non-threatening	31 (89)
	48. Building of self-efficacy	2 (6)
	49. Increased ease	12 (34)
	50. Better quality of life	2 (6)

Figure 1. CATCH element scores

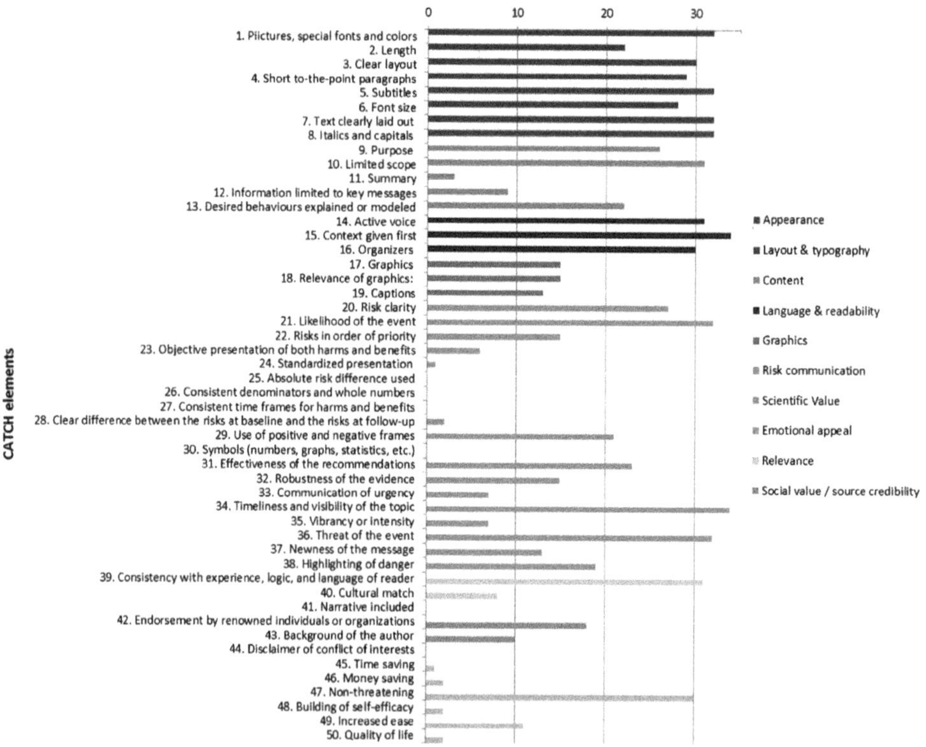

For a more accurate representation of this figure, please see the electronic version

Figure 2. CATCH instrument score

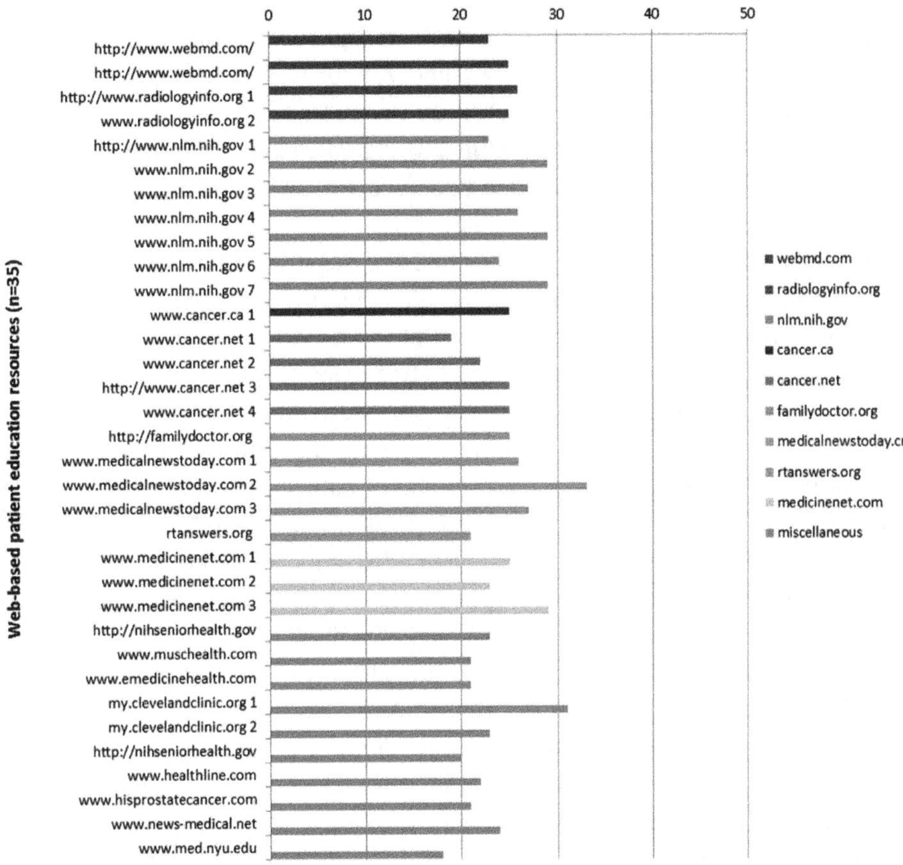

For a more accurate representation of this figure, please see the electronic version

Nearly all the web resources appropriately used italics and capitals, had clearly laid out text, sub-titles and easy to read fonts. Although Appearance came in a close second, only 66% of the resources were the appropriate length for the web, about a screen long, and while many had graphics, most graphics were a simple stock image of the prostate gland. A handful of web resources contained embedded videos. In most cases, these were relevant to and facilitated understanding of the text.

Poorly Represented Concepts

The concept Content was unequally distributed. Almost all of the resources had limited scope, clearly stated the context and were written in active voice. But only 4 had summaries and 29% contained key messages or recommended a particular behaviour or course of action. Web-based resources that did provide a recommendation, advised their readers to consult their physician.

Risk communication was poorly covered, beyond Risk Clarity and Likelihood of the Event, which were present in 94% and 77% of web resources respectively. Only 20% of resources contained a clear and objective presentation of the risks and benefits associated with each treatment option. Few web resources contained numeric presentation of the information, such as in a chart, graph or table, and none reported absolute risks or used consistent denominators or timeframes to describe the likelihood of harms and benefits. Positive and negative (gain and loss) frames, to invite patients to adopt a recommended behaviour, were not used.

The Scientific Value of the web resources for prostate-cancer patients was also poorly addressed. Two-thirds conveyed the effectiveness of the treatment options, but only 37% indicated that the message was supported by high quality evidence. This finding goes hand-in-hand with the results for the concept Credibility. Less than 50% of the web resources for prostate-cancer patients reported that they were reviewed by a medical professional or organisation, and only 23% reported the background of the author. We did not find any disclaimers of conflict of interests.

As for the concept Emotional Appeal, only two elements were consistently covered: Threat of the Event, Timeliness and Visibility. With regards to the concept Newness of the Message, less than half of the web resources provided a new perspective or reported an innovation in prostate cancer treatment, and only about 20% of web resources conveyed the concepts Vibrancy or Intensity, or Urgency.

The concept Usefulness for the patient was also poorly addressed, ranging from 6 to 34%, with the exception of the element Non-Threatening which was evident in 89% of web resources.

DISCUSSION

In this section we discuss the communication concepts exemplified on Web sites for prostate cancer patients. We will also highlight concepts and features that are missing or could be given more attention to improve the communication of the evidence.

CATCH was used to assess the Appearance, Layout and Typography, Content, Language and Readability, Graphics, Communication of Risks, Emotional Appeal, Scientific Value, Relevance, Usefulness for the patient and Source Credibility of HON certified sites for prostate cancer patients.

In general, only the concepts of Appearance, Layout and Typography and Language and Readability were well represented in the web resources on prostate cancer treatment options. This result can be explained with the fact that there are established user-centered design standards and guidelines to present content on websites (Nielsen, 1999, 2004; User-Centered Design Basics, 2015).

However, essential concepts were frequently missing. We found only 14 graphics, mostly similar stock images of the prostate gland. Pictures speak volumes, especially to an audience with lower literacy levels, like the general public (Ellimoottil et al., 2012). Similarly, Bender, Yue, To, Deacken and Jadad (2013) found that a significant proportion of smartphone apps for cancer (at least 30%) used basic and repetitive images. Genova et al. (2014) also found poor use of graphics in printed education materials for clinicians; the pictures were only remotely connected to the content and overly complicated.

As far as the concept of Content is concerned, the most revealing finding is that there was no explicit statement of the purpose of the web-based resources for prostate-cancer patients, except in the fact that the title of the page corresponded to the content. In that sense, these resources lacked a clear *strategic intent.* The purpose of the web resources for prostate cancer patients had to be inferred from the content and the organization of the materials. The purpose was not well defined and this ambiguity translated into poor communication of risks and incomplete information. If we suppose that patient education materials are supposed to inform and guide patient action, our evaluation shows these materials were not well-designed to achieve that purpose. In terms of guidance, only a few web resources took what might be called a minimalist approach to patient empowerment (e.g., recommending that patients ask their doctor about participation in a clinical trial).

This lack of strategic intent may in fact explain why many prostate cancer websites lack sufficient detail about treatment options (Ogah & Wassersug, 2013). It may also account for why risk factors were not presented objectively or consistently. We did not find any numerical representations of risks and advantages, such as charts, graphs, or numbers, aiming to facilitate decision-making and give them clear understanding of the situation. Timeframes, symbols and risk difference were not at all used. As for the organization of risks, most web materials did not present the serious side effects of prostate cancer treatments, the risks associated, and the eventual benefits. All those factors are important for informed shared decision making.

Also, the web resources did not use the strength of Emotional Appeal elements to encourage or empower patients: positive frames were barely used; the tone was neutral, without patient narratives or a mention of cultural match.

The lack of strategic intent of the web-based materials evaluated is further illustrated by the low summary scores for credibility and scientific value. The names, credentials and background of the authors or reviewers were rarely present, and none of the sites provided disclaimers of conflict of interests - results that are quite curious for medical web sites. This finding is consistent with studies of the quality or credibility of information on prostate cancer websites, which has been reported to be lacking in currency, attribution, balance of evidence and disclosure (Black & Penson, 2006).

Web resources are not ends in themselves but rather a means to an end. Evaluating web resources entails assessing the fit between the content and the intended purpose. If a health information material is designed with a strategy in mind - whether it is to inform, change perceptions or even attract visitors - it should be useful for the intended purpose. The prostate cancer websites in our sample did not score well in terms of Usefulness for patients - they did not adequately address the concerns that motivate patients to seek out this information: quality of life (except for impotency); reducing physical and emotional discomfort; saving time and money; or inconvenience. Warren et al. (2014) found that many prostate cancer websites do not adequately address topics identified as important to patients, particularly related to treatment, recovery and quality of life issues (Warren et al., 2014). To improve the usefulness of websites containing information on prostate cancer treatment options, Ogah and Wassersug (2013) advise website developers to: (1) present all evidence-based treatment options, (2) regularly update and time stamp information, (3) acknowledge that treatment recommendations may become out of date quickly, and (4) direct viewers to information on relevant, active clinical trials (Rot, Ogah, & Wassersug, 2012).

CONCLUSION

CATCH is a theoretically based framework that can be used to evaluate the quality of various materials, whether they are patient or physician oriented, print or web-based.

The present study reveals that frequently consulted websites for prostate-cancer patients are not optimally designed to present health information in a way that is useful, informative and credible for patients. If the strategic intent is what guides content developers to create meaningful and valuable resources, with attention to detail, this was not the case here.

Communicating risks can be improved with more objective presentations of risks and benefits, numerical presentation of facts and consistent timeframes. The purpose of the information on the web sites must be clearer. The information should be more credible and geared towards informed decision-making, not just gaining knowledge about diseases and treatments. The web resources did not show any innovative approach or new treatment, the danger was downplayed and the risks and benefits were organized just by gravity of the treatment. If the web resources are to change attitudes and behaviour and more effectively support patients' active involvement in decisions related to their own care, communication elements such as vibrant tone and empathy with patients should become more common features of Web-based patient resources.

REFERENCES

Aakhus, E., Granlund, I., Oxman, A., & Flottorp, S. (2015). Tailoring interventions to implement recommendations for the treatment of elderly patients with depression: a qualitative study. *International journal of mental health systems, 9*(1), 1-24.

Ajzen, I. (1971). Attitudinal vs. normative messages: An investigation of the differential effects of persuasive communications on behavior. *Sociometry, 34*(2), 263–280. doi:10.2307/2786416

Ajzen, I., & Albarracen, D. (2007). *Predicting and changing behavior: A reasoned action approach.* Mahwah, NJ: Lawrence Erlbaum Associates Publishers.

Ajzen, I., Czasch, C., & Flood, M. G. (2009). From Intentions to Behavior: Implementation Intention, Commitment, and Conscientiousness1. *Journal of Applied Social Psychology, 39*(6), 1356–1372. doi:10.1111/j.1559-1816.2009.00485.x

Atkin, C. (1994). Designing persuasive health messages. *Effective dissemination of clinical health information*, 95-0015.

Bandura, A. (2001). Social cognitive theory: An agentic perspective. *Annual Review of Psychology, 52*(1), 1–26. doi:10.1146/annurev.psych.52.1.1 PMID:11148297

Bender, J., Yue, R., To, M., Deacken, L., & Jadad, A. (2013). A lot of action, but not in the right direction: Systematic review and content analysis of smartphone applications for the prevention, detection, and management of cancer. *Journal of Medical Internet Research, 15*(12), e287. doi:10.2196/jmir.2661 PMID:24366061

Berkowitz, L., & Cottingham, D. R. (1960). The interest value and relevance of fear arousing communications. *Journal of Abnormal and Social Psychology, 60*(1), 37–43. doi:10.1037/h0045247 PMID:13799520

Bero, L. A., Grilli, R., Grimshaw, J. M., Harvey, E., Oxman, A. D., & Thomson, M. A. (1998). Closing the gap between research and practice: An overview of systematic reviews of interventions to promote the implementation of research findings. *BMJ (Clinical Research Ed.), 317*(7156), 465–468. doi:10.1136/bmj.317.7156.465 PMID:9703533

Black, P., & Penson, D. (2006). Prostate cancer on the Internet-information or misinformation? *The Journal of Urology*, *175*(5), 1836–1842. doi:10.1016/S0022-5347(05)00996-1 PMID:16600774

Borgmann, H., Wölm, J., Vallo, S., Mager, R., Huber, J., Breyer, J., & Tsaur, I. et al. (2015). Prostate Cancer on the Web-Expedient Tool for Patients' Decision-Making? *Journal of Cancer Education*. PMID:26234650

Brett, J., Staniszewska, S., Mockford, C., Herron-Marx, S., Hughes, J. R., Tysall, C., & Suleman, R. (2014). Mapping the impact of patient and public involvement on health and social care research: A systematic review. *Health Expectations*, *17*(5), 637–650. doi:10.1111/j.1369-7625.2012.00795.x PMID:22809132

Brouwers, M., Kho, M., Browman, G., Burgers, J., Cluzeau, F., Feder, G., & Hanna, S. et al. (2010). AGREE II: Advancing guideline development, reporting and evaluation in health care. *Canadian Medical Association Journal*, *182*(18), E839–E842. doi:10.1503/cmaj.090449 PMID:20603348

Brown, G., Brown, M., & Sharma, S. (2000). Health care in the 21st century: Evidence-based medicine, patient preference-based quality, and cost effectiveness. *Quality Management in Health Care*, *9*(1), 23–31. doi:10.1097/00019514-200009010-00004 PMID:11185879

Brownson, R. C., Fielding, J. E., & Maylahn, C. M. (2009). Evidence-based public health: A fundamental concept for public health practice. *Annual Review of Public Health*, *30*(1), 175–201. doi:10.1146/annurev.publhealth.031308.100134 PMID:19296775

Canadian Cancer Society, National Cancer Institute of Canada. Advisory Committee on Records, & Registries. (1987). Canadian cancer statistics. Canadian Cancer Society.

Carter, N., Miller, P., Murphy, B., Payne, V., & Bryant-Lukosius, D. (2014). Healthcare providers' perspectives of the supportive care needs of men with advanced prostate Cancer. *Paper presented at theOncology nursing forum*. doi:10.1188/14.ONF.421-430

Charnock, D., Shepperd, S., Needham, G., & Gann, R. (1999). DISCERN: An instrument for judging the quality of written consumer health information on treatment choices. *Journal of Epidemiology and Community Health*, *53*(2), 105–111. doi:10.1136/jech.53.2.105 PMID:10396471

Chua, H. F., Ho, S. S., Jasinska, A. J., Polk, T. A., Welsh, R. C., Liberzon, I., & Strecher, V. J. (2011). Self-related neural response to tailored smoking-cessation messages predicts quitting. *Nature*, *20*(1), 1. PMID:21358641

Clark, J., Wray, N., & Ashton, C. (2001). Living with treatment decisions: Regrets and quality of life among men treated for metastatic prostate cancer. *Journal of Clinical Oncology*, *19*(1), 72–80. PMID:11134197

Cohen, D. J., Crabtree, B. F., Etz, R. S., Balasubramanian, B. A., Donahue, K. E., Leviton, L. C., & Green, L. W. et al. (2008). Fidelity versus flexibility. *American Journal of Preventive Medicine*, *35*(5), 381–389. doi:10.1016/j.amepre.2008.08.005 PMID:18929985

Agree Collaboration. (2001). Appraisal of guidelines for research & evaluation (AGREE) instrument.

Collaboration, The ADAPTE. (2009). *The ADAPTE Process: Resource Toolkit for Guideline Adaptation. Version 2.0.* Retrieved from http://www.adapte.org

Collier, R. (2011). Federal government unveils patient-oriented research strategy. *Canadian Medical Association Journal*, *183*(13), E993–E994. doi:10.1503/cmaj.109-3978 PMID:21876023

Collin, S. M., Martin, R. M., Metcalfe, C., Gunnell, D., Albertsen, P. C., Neal, D., & Donovan, J. et al. (2008). Prostate-cancer mortality in the USA and UK in 1975-2004: An ecological study. *The Lancet Oncology*, *9*(5), 445–452. doi:10.1016/S1470-2045(08)70104-9 PMID:18424233

Davison, B., Szafron, M., Gutwin, C., & Visvanathan, K. (2014). Using a web-based decision support intervention to facilitate patient-physician communication at prostate cancer treatment discussions. *Revue canadienne de soins infirmiers en oncologie [Canadian Oncology Nursing Journal]*, 24(4), 241-247.

Doak, C. C., Doak, L. G., & Root, J. H. (1994). Suitability assessment of materials (SAM). *Paper presented at theAmerican Public Health Association Annual Meeting*, Washington, DC.

Doak, C. C., Doak, L. G., & Root, J. H. (1996). Teaching patients with low literacy skills. *AJN The American Journal of Nursing*, *96*(12), 16M. doi:10.1097/00000446-199612000-00022

Dopson, S., Locock, L., Gabbay, J., Ferlie, E., & Fitzgerald, L. (2003). Evidence-based medicine and the implementation gap. *Health*, *7*(3), 311–330. doi:10.1177/1363459303007003004

Ellimoottil, C., Polcari, A., Kadlec, A., & Gupta, G. (2012). Readability of websites containing information about prostate cancer treatment options. *The Journal of Urology*, *188*(6), 2171–2176. doi:10.1016/j.juro.2012.07.105 PMID:23083852

Fagerlin, A., Zikmund-Fisher, B. J., & Ubel, P. A. (2011). Helping patients decide: Ten steps to better risk communication. *Journal of the National Cancer Institute*, *103*(19), 1436–1443. doi:10.1093/jnci/djr318 PMID:21931068

Falk, E. B., O'Donnell, M. B., Tompson, S., Gonzales, R., Chin, S. D., Strecher, V., & An, L. (2014). *Neural systems associated with self-related processing predict population success of health messages*. Mass Commun Health.

Ferreira, D., Carreira, H., Silva, S., & Lunet, N. (2013). Assessment of the contents related to screening on Portuguese language websites providing information on breast and prostate cancer. *Cadernos de Saude Publica*, *29*(11), 2163–2176. doi:10.1590/0102-311x00150312 PMID:24233032

Fischhoff, B. (2012). *Communicating Risks and Benefits: An Evidence Based User's Guide*. Government Printing Office.

Fischhoff, B., Brewer, N. T., & Downs, J. S. (2011). *Communicating risks and benefits: an evidence-based user's guide*. Food and Drug Administration.

Fischhoff, B., Watson, S. R., & Hope, C. (1984). Defining risk. *Policy Sciences*, *17*(2), 123–139. doi:10.1007/BF00146924

Frank, L., Basch, E., & Selby, J. (2014). The PCORI Perspective on Patient-Centered Outcomes Research. *Journal of the American Medical Association*, *312*(15), 1513–1514. doi:10.1001/jama.2014.11100 PMID:25167382

Genova, J., Nahon-Serfaty, I., Dansokho, S. C., Gagnon, M. P., Renaud, J. S., & Giguère, A. (2014). The Communication AssessmenT Checklist in Health (CATCH): A Tool for Assessing the Quality of Printed Educational Materials for Clinicians. *The Journal of Continuing Education in the Health Professions*, *34*(4), 232–242. doi:10.1002/chp.21257 PMID:25530293

Giguière, A., Légaré, F., Grad, R., Pluye, R., Haynes, B., Cauchon, M., & Labrecque, M. et al. (2012). Decision boxes for clinicians to support evidence-based practice and shared decision making: The user experience. *Implementation Science; IS*, *7*(72). PMID:22862935

Grimshaw, J., Eccles, M., Thomas, R., MacLennan, G., Ramsay, C., Fraser, C., & Vale, L. (2006). Toward Evidence-based Quality Improvement. *Journal of General Internal Medicine*, *21*(Suppl. 2), S14–S20. PMID:16637955

Guyatt, G., Oxman, A., Akl, E., Kunz, R., Vist, G., Brozek, J., & deBeer, H. et al. (2011). GRADE guidelines: 1. Introduction-GRADE evidence profiles and summary of findings tables. *Journal of Clinical Epidemiology*, *64*(4), 383–394. doi:10.1016/j.jclinepi.2010.04.026 PMID:21195583

Guyatt, G., Oxman, A. D., Sultan, S., Brozek, J., Glasziou, P., Alonso-Coello, P., ... & Jaeschke, R. (2012). GRADE guidelines: 11. Making an overall rating of confidence in effect estimates for a single outcome and for all outcomes. *Journal of clinical epidemiology*.

Harter, L. M., Japp, P. M., & Beck, C. S. (2005). *Narratives, health, and healing: Communication theory, research, and practice*. Mahwah, NJ: Lawrence Erlbaum.

Health On the Net Foundation. (2014). Retrieved from http://www.healthonnet.org/HONcode/Conduct.html

Hellawell, G., Turner, K., Le Monnier, K., & Brewster, S. (2000). Urology and the Internet: An evaluation of Internet use by urology patients and of information available on urological topics. *BJU International*, *86*(3), 191–194. doi:10.1046/j.1464-410x.2000.00831.x PMID:10930912

Hoffman, A., Volk, R., Saarimaki, A., Stirling, C., Li, L., Härter, M., & Llewellyn-Thomas, H. et al. (2013). Delivering patient decision aids on the Internet: Definitions, theories, current evidence, and emerging research areas. *BMC Medical Informatics and Decision Making*, *13*(Suppl. 2), S13. doi:10.1186/1472-6947-13-S2-S13 PMID:24625064

Jacobs, R., Lou, J., Ownby, R., & Caballero, J. (2014). A systematic review of eHealth interventions to improve health literacy. *Health Informatics Journal*. PMID:24916567

Katz, E. (1999). Theorizing diffusion: Tarde and Sorokin revisited. *The Annals of the American Academy of Political and Social Science*, *566*(1), 144–155. doi:10.1177/000271629956600112

Klazinga, N. (2003). Development and validation of an international appraisal instrument for assessing the quality of clinical practice guidelines: The AGREE project. *Quality & Safety in Health Care*, *12*(1), 18–23. doi:10.1136/qhc.12.1.18 PMID:12571340

Kobayashi, L. C., Wardle, J., & von Wagner, C. (2014). Limited health literacy is a barrier to colorectal cancer screening in England: Evidence from the English Longitudinal Study of Ageing. *Preventive Medicine*, *61*, 100–105. doi:10.1016/j.ypmed.2013.11.012 PMID:24287122

Lang, E., Wyer, P., & Haynes, R. (2007). Knowledge translation: Closing the evidence-to-practice gap. *Annals of Emergency Medicine, 49*(3), 355–363. doi:10.1016/j.annemergmed.2006.08.022 PMID:17084943

Lazzarato, M. (2002). *Puissances de l'invention: la psychologie Économique de Gabriel Tarde contre l'Économie politique.* Paris: Empêcheurs de penser en rond.

Loblaw, D., Virgo, K., Nam, R., Somerfield, M., Ben-Josef, E., Mendelson, D., & Talcott, J. et al. (2007). Initial hormonal management of androgen-sensitive metastatic, recurrent, or progressive prostate cancer: 2007 update of an American Society of Clinical Oncology practice guideline. *Journal of Clinical Oncology, 25*(12), 1596–1605. doi:10.1200/JCO.2006.10.1949 PMID:17404365

Makoul, G., & Clayman, M. L. (2006). An integrative model of shared decision making in medical encounters. *Patient Education and Counseling, 60*(3), 301–312. doi:10.1016/j.pec.2005.06.010 PMID:16051459

Michie, S., & Abraham, C. (2008). Advancing the science of behaviour change: A plea for scientific reporting. *Addiction (Abingdon, England), 103*(9), 1409–1410. doi:10.1111/j.1360-0443.2008.02291.x PMID:18783495

Michie, S., Johnston, M., Abraham, C., & Walker, A. (2005). Making psychological theory useful for implementing evidence based practice: A consensus approach. *Quality & Safety in Health Care, 14*(1), 26–33. doi:10.1136/qshc.2004.011155 PMID:15692000

Michie, S., van Stralen, M. M., & West, R. (2011). The behaviour change wheel: A new method for characterising and designing behaviour change interventions. *Implementation Science; IS, 6*(1), 42. doi:10.1186/1748-5908-6-42 PMID:21513547

Morris, D. B. (2001). Narrative, ethics, and pain: Thinking with stories. *Narrative*, 55-77.

Murphy, M., Black, N., Lamping, D., McKee, C., Sanderson, C., Askham, J., & Marteau, T. (1998). Consensus development methods, and their use in clinical guideline development. *Health Technology Assessment (Winchester, England), 2*(3), i. PMID:9561895

Neuhauser, L. (2011). Readability, Comprehension and Usability. In B. Fischhoff, N. Brewer, & J. S. Downs (Eds.), *Communicating Risks and Benefits: An Evidence-Based User's Guide. US Department of Health and Human Services Food and Drug Administration. Risk Communication Advisory Committee and consultants.*

Nielsen, J. (1999). *Designing web usability: The practice of simplicity*. New Riders Publishing.

Nielsen, J. (2004). *Designing web usability*. Pearson Deutschland GmbH.

Norman, C. D., & Skinner, H. A. (2006a). eHEALS: The eHealth literacy scale. *Journal of Medical Internet Research*, *8*(4), e27. doi:10.2196/jmir.8.4.e27 PMID:17213046

Norman, C. D., & Skinner, H. A. (2006b). eHealth literacy: Essential skills for consumer health in a networked world. *Journal of Medical Internet Research*, *8*(2), e9. doi:10.2196/jmir.8.2.e9 PMID:16867972

Ogah, I., & Wassersug, R. (2013). How reliable are "reputable sources" for medical information on the Internet? The case of hormonal therapy to treat prostate cancer. *Paper presented at the Urologic Oncology: Seminars and Original Investigations*.

Oxman, A.GRADE Working Group. (2004). Grading quality of evidence and strength of recommendations. *BMJ (Clinical Research Ed.)*, *328*(19), 1490–1494. PMID:15205295

Peters, E. (2012a). Affect and emotion. Communicating Risks and Benefits: An Evidence Based User's Guide, 89.

Peters, E. (2012b). Quantitative information. In B. B Fischhoff, N. Brewer, & J. S. Downs (Ed.), Communicating Risks and Benefits: An Evidence Based User's Guide: An Evidence Based User's Guide (pp. 53). US Department of Health and Human Services Food and Drug Administration. Risk Communication Advisory Committee and consultants.

Peters, E., Dieckmann, N., Dixon, A., Hibbard, J. H., & Mertz, C. K. (2007). Less is more in presenting quality information to consumers. *Medical Care Research and Review*, *64*(2), 169–190. doi:10.1177/1077558707064002030l PMID:17406019

Pew Internet and American Life Project Health Fact Sheet. (2012). *Pew Internet*. Retrieved from http://www.pewinternet.org/fact-sheets/health-fact-sheet/

Potomac, M., & Doak, C. C. (2002). Pfizer Principles for Clear Health Communication.

Pruthi, R., Belsante, J., Kurpad, R., Nielsen, M., & Wallen, E. (2011). Robotic cystectomy and the Internet: Separating fact from fiction. *Paper presented at the Urologic Oncology: Seminars and Original Investigations*. doi:10.1016/j.urolonc.2009.04.010

Rot, I., Ogah, I., & Wassersug, R. (2012). The language of prostate cancer treatments and implications for informed decision making by patients. *European Journal of Cancer Care*, *21*(6), 766–775. doi:10.1111/j.1365-2354.2012.01359.x PMID:22574619

Routh, J. C., Gong, E. M., Cannon, G. M. Jr, & Nelson, C. P. (2011). Does a controversial topic affect the quality of urologic information on the Internet? *Urology, 78*(5), 1051–1056. doi:10.1016/j.urology.2011.06.050 PMID:21945281

Ruiter, R. A. C., & Kok, G. (2011). Planning to frighten people? Think again! In *Writing Health Communication: An Evidence-Based Guide for professionals.*

Salmon, C. T., & Atkin, C. (2003). Using media campaigns for health promotion. Handbook of health communication, 285-313.

Salonen, A., Ryhänen, A., & Leino-Kilpi, H. (2014). Educational benefits of Internet and computer-based programmes for prostate cancer patients: A systematic review. *Patient Education and Counseling, 94*(1), 10–19. PMID:24021418

Sheridan, S. L., Draeger, L. B., Pignone, M. P., Keyserling, T. C., Simpson, R. J., Rimer, B., & Gizlice, Z. et al. (2011). A randomized trial of an intervention to improve use and adherence to effective coronary heart disease prevention strategies. *BMC Health Services Research, 11*(1), 331. doi:10.1186/1472-6963-11-331 PMID:22141447

Shiffman, R., Dixon, J., Brandt, C., Essalhi, A., Hsiao, A., Michel, G., & O'Connell, R. (2005). The GuideLine Implementability Appraisal (GLIA): Development of an instrument to identify obstacles to guideline implementation. *BMC Medical Informatics and Decision Making, 5*(23). doi:10.1186/1472-6947-5-23 PMID:16048653

Smith, S. C., O'Conor, R., Curtis, L., Waite, K., Deary, I., Paasche-Orlow, M., & Wolf, M. S. (2015). Low health literacy predicts decline in physical function among older adults: findings from the LitCog cohort study. *Journal of epidemiology and community health*, jech-2014-204915.

Soobrah, R., & Clark, S. K. (2012). Your patient information website: How good is it? *Colorectal Disease, 14*(3), e90–e94. doi:10.1111/j.1463-1318.2011.02792.x PMID:21883807

Stamey, T. A., McNeal, J. E., Yemoto, C. M., Sigal, B. M., & Johnstone, I. M. (1999). Biological determinants of cancer progression in men with prostate cancer. *Journal of the American Medical Association, 281*(15), 1395–1400. doi:10.1001/jama.281.15.1395 PMID:10217055

Sullivan, G. M. (2011). A primer on the validity of assessment instruments. *Journal of graduate medical education, 3*(2), 119-120.

Sutton, S. R., & Eiser, J. R. (1984). The effect of fear-arousing communications on cigarette smoking: An expectancy-value approach. *Journal of Behavioral Medicine*, *7*(1), 13–33. doi:10.1007/BF00845345 PMID:6716470

Tarde, G. (1890). *Les lois de l'imitation*. Paris: Kimé éditeur.

Tarde, G. (1902). *Pstchologie économique. Tome second.* Paris.

Tarde, G. (1902). *Psychologie économique. Tome premier.* Paris.

Tennant, B., Stellefson, M., Dodd, V., Chaney, B., Chaney, D., Paige, S., & Alber, J. (2015). eHealth Literacy and Web 2.0 Health Information Seeking Behaviors Among Baby Boomers and Older Adults. *Journal of Medical Internet Research*, *17*(3), e70. doi:10.2196/jmir.3992 PMID:25783036

The World Bank Group. (2015). Retrieved from http://Worldbank.org

US Department of Health and Human Services. (2010). *CfMMS*. Toolkit for Making Written Material Clear and Effective.

US Federal Plain Language Guidelines. (2010). Retrieved from http://www.plainlanguage.gov/howto/guidelines/bigdoc/fullbigdoc.pdf

User-Centered Design Basics. (2015). Retrieved from http://www.usability.gov/what-and-why/user-centered-design.html

Van der Vaart, R., van Deursen, A., Drossaert, C., Taal, E., van Dijk, J., & van de Laar, M. (2011). Does the eHealth Literacy Scale (eHEALS) measure what it intends to measure? Validation of a Dutch version of the eHEALS in two adult populations. *Journal of Medical Internet Research*, *13*(4), e86. doi:10.2196/jmir.1840 PMID:22071338

Warren, E., Footman, K., Tinelli, M., McKee, M., & Knai, C. (2014). Do cancer-specific websites meet patient's information needs? *Patient Education and Counseling*, *95*(1), 126–136. doi:10.1016/j.pec.2013.12.013 PMID:24447523

Witte, K., & Allen, M. (2000). A meta-analysis of fear appeals: Implications for effective public health campaigns. *Health Education & Behavior*, *27*(5), 591–615. doi:10.1177/109019810002700506 PMID:11009129

Wong, F., Stewart, D., Dancey, J., Meana, M., McAndrews, M., Bunston, T., & Cheung, A. (2000). Men with prostate cancer: Influence of psychological factors on informational needs and decision making. *Journal of Psychosomatic Research*, *49*(1), 13–19. doi:10.1016/S0022-3999(99)00109-9 PMID:11053599

Woolf, S. H., Grol, R., Hutchinson, A., Eccles, M., & Grimshaw, J. (1999). Clinical guidelines: Potential benefits, limitations, and harms of clinical guidelines. *BMJ: British Medical Journal, 318*(7182), 527–530. doi:10.1136/bmj.318.7182.527 PMID:10024268

Wright, S. M. (2001). Contribution of a lecturer-practitioner in implementing evidence-based health care. *Clinical Effectiveness in Nursing, 5*(1), 30–34. doi:10.1054/cein.2000.0170 PMID:11761876

Zikmund-Fisher, B. J., Windschitl, P. D., Exe, N., & Ubel, P. A. (2011). 'I'll do what they did": Social norm information and cancer treatment decisions. *Patient Education and Counseling, 85*(2), 225–229. doi:10.1016/j.pec.2011.01.031 PMID:21367557

KEY TERMS AND DEFINITIONS

Better Quality of Life or Better Organization of the Environment: In some cases, treating the disease requires a full reorganization of the patient environment, daily routine or practices (e.g. cases of depression). Better quality of life refers also to a treatment that is not intrusive and respects the person – for instance, a breast cancer operation may be life-saving, but is very invasive for the patient and does not enhance her quality of life.

Effectiveness of the Recommended Response: The recommended response (in evidence-based practice) will be efficient and quick, promoting the user to adopt it.

Narrative: Quite often, diseases are personified and different social groups color the description of the disease. Cancer is a typical example – patients describe it as "a silent killer" and they often see themselves as "warriors", a narrative that will appeal to readers who are cancer patients.

Negative Frame: The message is negative, p.ex. "If you smoke, you will die a painful death."

Objective Presentation of Harms and Benefits: Evidence-based practice aims to provide complete information on risks and advantages for the patient, based on standardized presentation of harms and benefits, outcomes, dosages and periods of evaluation, and using consistent denominators and whole numbers. The difference between the risks at baseline and the risks at follow-up should be clearly explained. Risks are presented in order of priority.

Positive Frame: The message is expressed in positive terms, p.ex. "If you stop smoking, you will see your grandchildren grow".

Purpose of the Text: The main messages of the text are clearly stated in the title, the illustration are relevant and the introduction and conclusion sum up clearly the content. The content is limited in scope and relevant – it defines the problem, the rationale and suggests a solution.

Risk Clarity: The risk is clearly presented and defined. There is no ambiguity. Presenting the risks. Absolute risk reduction is more objective than relative risk reduction.

Self-Efficacy: Feeling of confidence in one's abilities. Self-confidence is considered a game changer when it comes to behavior-change and adoption of new practices.

Urgency, Vibrancy or Intensity of the Tone: The reader can feel, in the tone of the message, in the choice of words, active voice and dynamic verbs, that the author is sincere and communicates his or her emotions on the topic. This feeling is usually communicated to the reader and it has a bigger impact.

Chapter 8
A Stepped Care mHealth-Based Approach for Promoting Patient Engagement in Chronic Care Management of Obesity with Type 2 Diabetes

Gianluca Castelnuovo
Catholic University of the Sacred Heart, Italy

Giada Pietrabissa
Catholic University of the Sacred Heart, Italy

Gian Mauro Manzoni
Catholic University of the Sacred Heart, Italy

Stefania Corti
Istituto Auxologico Italiano IRCCS, Italy

Margherita Novelli
Istituto Auxologico Italiano IRCCS, Italy

Maria Borrello
University of Bergamo, Italy

Emanuele Maria Giusti
Catholic University of the Sacred Heart, Italy

Francesco Borgia
Istituto Auxologico Italiano IRCCS, Italy

Enrico Molinari
Catholic University of the Sacred Heart, Italy

Nicole Ann Middleton
University of South Australia, Australia

Roberto Cattivelli
Istituto Auxologico Italiano IRCCS, Italy

Susan Simpson
University of South Australia, Australia

DOI: 10.4018/978-1-5225-0663-8.ch008

ABSTRACT

Diabesity could be defined as a new global epidemic of obesity and being overweight with many complications and chronic conditions. The financial direct and indirect burden of diabesity is a real challenge in many Western health-care systems. Even if multidisciplinary protocols have been implemented, significant limitations in the chronic care management of obesity with type 2 diabetes concern costs and long-term adherence and efficacy. mHealth approach could overcome limitations linked with the traditional, restricted and highly expensive in-patient treatment of diabesity. The mHealth approach could help clinicians by motivating patients in remote settings to develop healthier lifestyles and could be implemented in the Chronic Care Model. A practical stepped-care model for diabesity, including mhealth approach and psychological treatments with different intensity, is discussed.

FACING DIABESITY WITH A CHRONIC CARE MANAGEMENT APPROACH: REDUCING COSTS AND IMPROVING LONG-TERM ADHERENCE AND EFFICACY

Francine Kaufman coined the term "diabesity" (diabetes + obesity) to describe the dangerous combination of obesity, insulin resistance, metabolic syndrome and type 2 diabetes (Jones, 2006; Kresser, 2014a, 2014b; Leiter et al., 2013).

Diabesity could be defined as a new global epidemic of obesity and being overweight with many complications and chronic conditions. Such conditions include not only type 2 diabetes, but also cardiovascular diseases, hypertension, dyslipidemia, hypercholesterolemia, cancer, and various psychosocial and psychopathological disorders (Byrne, Cooper, & Fairburn, 2004; Castelnuovo et al., 2014; Flegal, Graubard, Williamson, & Gail, 2005; Wadden, Brownell, & Foster, 2002; Whitlock et al., 2009).

The etiology of diabesity is universally recognized as multifactorial with a complex interaction between genetic, individual, and environmental factors (Marcus & Wildes, 2009). Genetics plays an important role, but behavioral factors, such as a dysfunctional diet and low physical activity, are among the main modifiable and proximal causes strictly connected to obesity and obesity-related complications (Dombrowski et al., 2012).

Diabetes is emerging as a relevant chronic disease in the USA, particularly among children. The financial direct and indirect burden (considering also the clinical resources involved and the loss of productivity) is a real challenge in many Western health-care systems (Malvey & Slovensky, 2014). The total costs of diagnosed diabetes grew from US$ 174 billion in 2007 to US$ 245 billion in 2012 with an increasing of 41 (American Diabetes Association [ADA], 2013).

With respect to the significant health care costs associated with treating obesity and type 2 diabetes, recently the Lancet journal defined diabetes as a 21st-century challenge: "the economic effect of diabetes is enormous. In 2010, global health expenditure attributable to diabetes was estimated to be US$376 billion—that is, 12% of all global health expenditure. In the USA in 2012, the direct medical cost of diabetes was $176 billion" (McCormick & Stone, 2007, p. 60; Zimmet, Magliano, Herman, & Shaw, 2014).

About obesity, different opportunities for prevention and treatment approaches targeting a part of or the entire population have been studied and are well described in (Rothberg, Peeters, & Herman, 2014): "Obesity may be viewed as a continuum with at least three opportunities for intervention... Primary prevention targets the entire population. Indeed, almost everyone in the population is at risk for obesity... Delaying the onset of obesity or limiting its severity may reduce its comorbidities and complications. Interventions for primary prevention focus on decreasing energy intake, increasing energy expenditure, or both. They may include health-care, community, or environmental measures to encourage people to eat less, be more active, and maintain a healthy weight.

Secondary interventions target people with obesity at high risk for complications, such as those with glucose intolerance at risk for type 2 diabetes or those with hypertension or dyslipidemia at risk for cardiovascular disease. Targeted lifestyle interventions and medications may produce and maintain weight loss, improve risk factors, and delay or prevent complications.

Tertiary interventions target people with severe obesity and its attendant complications, such as type 2 diabetes and coronary artery disease. For such individuals, bariatric surgery can induce weight loss and delay or prevent the development of additional complications including diabetic microvascular and neuropathic complications, myocardial infarction, and death. All interventions have the potential to delay comorbidities and complications, reduce costs, and improve quality of life and survival" (pp. 453-454).

In order to promote patient engagement and compliance in diabesity treatment while reducing costs, evidence-based interventions to improve weight-loss, maintain a healthy weight, and reduce related comorbidities combine different treatment approaches: dietetic, nutritional, physical, behavioral, psychological, and, in some situations, pharmacological and surgical. Moreover new technologies can provide useful solutions in this multidisciplinary approach.

Even if multidisciplinary protocols have been implemented, significant limitations in the chronic care management of obesity with type 2 diabetes concern costs and long-term adherence and efficacy.

Another limitation is the difficulty associated with maintaining long-term compliance and adherence in order to ensure clinical efficacy. "In fact, most overweight and obese individuals regain about one third of the weight lost with treatment within one year and they will typically come back to baseline in three to five years" (Pietrabissa et al., 2012, p. 317). Specifically in relation to diabetes, "Lifestyle intervention has been effective in several countries, but its success depends on uptake of intervention programmes and on compliance ... An urgent priority is to identify ways to effectively engage people at risk of diabetes. Long-term sustainability is also a concern" (Zimmet et al., 2014, pp. 61-62).

THE KEY ROLE OF PSYCHOLOGICAL INTERVENTIONS TO IMPROVE MOTIVATION, COMPLIANCE AND ENGAGEMENT IN DIABESITY TREATMENT

Assessment of patients' motivation, compliance, and engagement is a key factor of treatment for obesity with type 2 diabetes (Barello, Graffigna, & Vegni, 2012; Waller, Stringer, & Meyer, 2012).

Psychological therapies with diet and exercise plans could better help patients in achieving weight loss outcomes, both inside hospitals and clinical centers and during out-patient follow-up sessions (Swencionis & Rendell, 2012; Wing, 2002).

Some psychological skills should be implemented for functional chronic care management of obesity and its complications. Such skills include determining the client's ability to self-monitor (e.g., using diaries), assistance with stimulus control through restricting quantities of food, and behavioral modification strategies (e.g., chewing slowly, taking time to enjoy food, and increasing awareness of the pleasure associated with taste and food) (Foster, Makris, & Bailer, 2005; Swencionis & Rendell, 2012; Wing, 2002). Specific psychological actions are also required in order to maintain goals that have initially been achieved, manage possible relapses, and learn strategies to cope with critical situations (Capodaglio et al., 2013; Dombrowski, Avenell, & Sniehott, 2011; Dombrowski et al., 2012; Manzoni et al., 2010; Manzoni et al., 2011b).

In the management of chronic diseases clinical psychology plays a key role (Castelnuovo, 2010a, 2010b), due to the need of working on psychological conditions of patients, their families and their caregivers (de Ridder, Geenen, Kuijer, & van Middendorp, 2008; Levy, Nocerini, & Grazier, 2007; Pagnini et al., 2012; Pagnini et al., 2011; Pagnini et al., 2010), particularly with cardiovascular diseases where psychological variables (anxiety, stress, depression, etc.) have a significant impact in the organic worsening and demanding caregiving with developed case management skills is requested, even if relatives and caregivers are not well trained in accomplishing healthcare tasks (Hemingway & Marmot, 1999a, 1999b; Manzoni, Castelnuovo, & Proietti, 2011; Rozanski, Blumenthal, & Kaplan, 1999). About chronic disease management programs focused on containing costs and improve health outcomes (Villagra, 2004; Villagra & Ahmed, 2004), Mercer noted that "What emerged from these early programs was an understanding that quality improvement and cost reductions could be achieved through enhancing disease process understanding and attending to the psychological aspects of health and illness (Levy et al., 2007; Schneiderman, Antoni, Saab, & Ironson, 2001)" (Mercer, 2011, p. 151).

THE MHEALTH OPPORTUNITY

eHealth could be traditionally defined as a growing field of health services provided through the Internet and other new technologies (Eysenbach, 2001). mHealth (also m-health, mhealth, or mobile health) could be considered an evolution of eHealth and could be defined as the practice of medicine and public health supported by mobile communication devices, such as mobile phones, tablet computers, and PDAs, for health services and information (Castelnuovo et al., 2014; Cipresso et al., 2012; Eysenbach, 2011; Fiordelli, Diviani, & Schulz, 2013; Riper et al., 2010; Whittaker, 2012). Another interesting definition of mHealth, provided in an engineering field, defines it as "the practice of eHealth supported by mobile devices and smartphones, which are used to capture, analyze, store, and transmit health-related information from various sources including personal inputs, sensors, and other biomedical acquisition systems" (Adibi, 2015, p. 2).

mHealth approach could overcome limitations linked with the traditional, restricted and highly expensive in-patient treatment of many chronic pathologies: one of the best up-to-date application is the management of obesity with type 2 diabetes, where mHealth solutions can provide remote opportunities for enhancing weight reduction and reducing complications from clinical, organizational and economic perspectives (Castelnuovo et al., 2015b; Khaylis, Yiaslas, Bergstrom, & Gore-Felton, 2010; Manzoni, Castelnuovo, & Molinari, 2008; Manzoni, Pagnini, Corti, Molinari, & Castelnuovo, 2011a; Rao et al., 2011). Specifically for diabetes management Chomutare, Fernandez-Luque, Arsand and Hartvigsen (2011) reported more than 260 different diabetes applications (for Nokia Symbian, BlackBerry, Apple iPhone and Google Android), able to manage many features of the diabetes management, self-monitoring, blood glucose, weight, physical activity, diet, insulin and medication, blood pressure, education, disease-related alerts and reminders, integration of social media functions (Santoro, 2013; Santoro, Caldarola, & Villella, 2011; Santoro & Quintaliani, 2013), disease-related data export and communication, synchronization with personal health record (PHR) systems, and patient portals (Chomutare et al., 2011).

Programs with mHealth, defined as the practice of medicine and public health supported by mobile communication devices (Castelnuovo et al., 2014; Cipresso et al., 2012; Eysenbach, 2001, 2011; Fiordelli et al., 2013; Riper et al., 2010; Whittaker, 2012), could overcome limitations connected to the traditional in-patient chronic care management of obesity with type 2 diabetes by providing promising opportunities for enhancing weight reduction and reducing complications in terms of long-term efficacy and effectiveness across clinical, organizational, and economic perspectives (Khaylis et al., 2010; Manzoni et al., 2011a; Rao et al., 2011). These technology-based strategies provided in out-patient settings are based on a collaborative approach derived from central planning and grounded in chronic care logic (Rao et al., 2011).

Applications have also been shown to increase participation, compliance, and engagement (Graffigna, Barello, & Riva, 2013; Graffigna, Barello, Wiederhold, Bosio, & Riva, 2013).

Khaylis et al. (2010) underlined five psychological components (Self-monitoring, Counselor feedback and communication, Social support, Structured program, Individually-tailored program) necessary for functional necessary for functional mHealth-based chronic case management in order to facilitate weight loss and a reduction of comorbidities such as type 2 diabetes.

There is a critical need for scientific research to evaluate the specific outcomes of collaborative approaches for weight management that utilize the Internet and mobile-based tools (Turner-McGrievy et al., 2013).

The mHealth approach could help clinicians by motivating patients in remote settings to develop healthier lifestyles (Castelnuovo, 2010a; Pietrabissa et al., 2012), to accept more intrusive medical treatments, and to cope with chronic conditions by reducing complications (such as type 2 diabetes, hypertension, and cardiovascular disease) (Nguyen & Lau, 2012). In order to deal with lifestyle diseases and to prevent chronic medical conditions, mobile applications are able to measure the physical activity of a patient or user, also in a free-living monitoring environment (Torres-Huitzil & Alvarez-Landero, 2015).

The mHealth approach could be implemented in the Chronic Care Model, developed by Wagner (Glasgow, Orleans, & Wagner, 2001; Wagner et al., 2001a; Wagner et al., 2001b), that is based on the collaboration between a well coordinated team of clinicians-providers and an activated-engaged patient, promoting self-management skills, tracking and sharing information about patient health status and treatment programs, focusing on the family, social and community networks (O'Donnell, 2011).

mHealth provides the possibility to monitor oneself or for a clinician to monitor a patient through a mobile platform or device accessing to important information in real time. The smartphone applications can also deliver "education about diet, exercises, health reminders, community resources, and local healthcare providers"

(Moss Richins, 2015, p. 24). These opportunities are very important above all for seniors and for people living alone and dealing with diabetes (Javitt, 2014), encouraging the elderly to carry on a healthy lifestyle.

Different clinical applications have been developed about the utility of mobile phones in promoting weight loss behaviors, healthy lifestyle and comorbidities reduction (Bacigalupo et al., 2013; Burke et al., 2012; Cafazzo, Casselman, Hamming, Katzman, & Palmert, 2012; Castelnuovo et al., 2010; Chomutare et al., 2011; Fiordelli et al., 2013; Hebden et al., 2013; Manzoni et al., 2011a; Martinez-Perez, de la Torre-Diez, & Lopez-Coronado, 2013; Park & Kim, 2012; Pellegrini et al., 2012; Rao et al., 2011; Rodrigues, Lopes, Silva, & Torre Ide, 2013; Schiel, Kaps, & Bieber, 2012; Schoffman, Turner-McGrievy, Jones, & Wilcox, 2013; Sharifi et al., 2013; Shaw et al., 2013; Simpson & Slowey, 2011; Turner-McGrievy et al., 2013)

Even if 1 million mobile device applications have been developed (Chouffani, 2013), up to date diabesity monitoring methods do not satisfy patients' requirements and are not so effective in helping people control the disease. As noted by (Shaheen, Mohammed, & Grbic, 2015), results performed for e-health in Finland (Ekroos & Jalonen, 2007) expressed the potential to provide interactive devices useful to engage diabetic patients in the self-management and to improve communications between patients and healthcare providers, but mobile services and biosensors are lacking in encouraging physical activities for diabetic patients in community settings for achieving a better lifestyle. "What is needed is an effective self-management wireless solution that collects, stores, and transmits these important parameters in real time to the health professionals and receives a feedback correspondingly" (Shaheen et al., 2015, p. 52).

THE STEPPED-CARE OPPORTUNITY

In the pioneering book *Stepped Care and e-Health Practical Applications to Behavioral Disorders*, O'Donohue and Draper (2011b, pp. 5-6) proposed a practical stepped-care model for many pathologies, including chronic conditions. A list of the health care "steps" is indicated below:

1. **Assessment and Triage:** This information can be used to determine which step is the best step for an individual in beginning treatment... also consider*ing* how there can be a stepped-care model within the assessment process. For example... consider*ing* more and less intense screening and assessment modules and those that can be used with and without a trained therapist or varying degrees of using therapist time.

2. **Watchful Waiting:** This information can be used to determine which disorders may show a natural return to baseline and disappear without specific intervention... *considering* the idea that immediate treatment after the incident may actually be iatrogenic and... when an individual may want to seek the next level of care.
3. **Psychoeducation:** This type of low-intensity intervention includes several modalities of providing simple information about disorders, treatment for disorders, or other expectations. This can be delivered via web sites, books, pamphlets, groups and classes, or any other mode of information delivery.
4. **Bibliotherapy:** Bibliotherapy, or self-help, is broadly the use of text to implement behavior change or to see movement on a given disorder. The most widely used form of bibliotherapy is self-help books, but *there are also* non interactive web sites and occasionally even videos. Bibliotherapy generally provides consumers with an active intervention including homework (usually in the form of workbooks).
5. **E-Health:** E-health is a broad term, which in this text refers to the use of technology to provide tailored or interactive modules in addition to the treatment that may be used in bibliotherapy. This includes both computer-based interventions (CBIs), in which there is little or no therapist contact, and computer-assisted interventions (CAIs), in which a therapist plays a role in the treatment, although the treatment is delivered largely via computer and may also include adjuncts including the use of electronics such as palm devices or text messaging to enhance other modalities of treatment.
6. **Group Therapy:** This form of therapy may vary greatly in where it falls in the stepped-care model, depending on the structure and purpose of the group. Groups can range from support groups led by non therapists to psychoeducational groups delivered between one or several meetings, to treatments similar to individual treatments, but minimizing therapist time by providing the same information and intervention for multiple people at once.
7. **Individual Therapy:** This step is what we usually would refer to as simply "therapy" and is the portion in the model that has received by far the most research. This step is commonly among the first step for most people who seek treatment (along with medication), and many practitioners accept this and do not triage to lower levels when indicated... This norm is not necessarily the most practical and does not necessarily provide better outcomes.
8. **Medical and Medication:** This step is, for some disorders, often found to be the first line of treatment even when this is counter-indicated by current research. In the treatment of many disorders, this may actually be considered among the last steps of a fail-forward attempt, generally due to side effects and often showing higher cost in the long-term.

9. **Inpatient Treatment:** This step is widely seen as the highest step in the treatment of any disorder and is often only indicated in the event of failures of previous steps.

New technologies play an important role in this model (point 5), even if mHealth does not express all its potentiality in the O'Donohue and Draper model (2011b).

Working out the previous Von Korff and Tiemens's proposal (Von Korff & Tiemans, 2000), a strong model of stepped care based on mhealth is proposed by O'Donnell (2011, p. 265): "The stepped care model is based on the acknowledgement that (1) different patients require different levels of care; (2) the most appropriate level of care is based on closely monitoring outcomes; and (3) moving from lower to more intensive levels of care based on patient response can increase the effectiveness of care while lowering overall costs". Stepped care is "potentially much more consistent with the ethical imperative of choosing the least intrusive intervention for one's patient" (O'Donohue & Draper, 2011a, p. 3). Using this approach, many efforts in the research field have to be focused not only on the development of new clinical protocols or therapies, but in the validation of new health-care delivery model, measuring its reliability, affordability, safety, efficiency and user satisfaction (where users are patients, professionals, stakeholders, etc.) and demonstrating that this model can improve the quality of care and reduce costs (Mercer, 2011; Neumeyer-Gromen, Lampert, Stark, & Kallischnigg, 2004; O'Donohue & Draper, 2011a; Ofman et al., 2004; Weingarten et al., 2002).

According to Bower and Gilbody (2005), psychological treatments with different intensity are necessary in a stepped care approach and they can offer less intensive treatments, such as brief therapies, group approaches, self-help opportunities (bibliotherapy, pc-based treatments). Moreover the stepped care framework could provide significant benefits: minimal interventions can ensure health gains equivalent or similar to that of traditional psychotherapies, reduce costs optimizing healthcare resources in an efficient way, be recognized and considered acceptable for both patients and clinicians.

About a possible economic evaluation of stepped care models in diabesity management, unfortunately empirical data from long term randomized controlled clinical trials are lacking, above all in providing few years of follow-up (less than 4 years and 1 or 2 years of reliable empirical data (Rothberg et al., 2014).

A deep and interesting economic analysis for the US situation is reported by Rothberg et al. (2014, p. 468): "Although lifestyle, pharmacologic, and surgical interventions to prevent and treat obesity appear to be cost-effective, they may have very different cost implications to a health system or society. To understand the cost of an intervention, one must consider the size of the target population and the cost of the intervention... The normal weight and overweight population (66% of U.S.

adults ≥20 years of age) is large compared to the population with obesity (28% of U.S. adults) and those populations are large compared to the population with severe obesity (6% of U.S. adults). Conversely, the per person cost of a mass media campaign, a new tax, or a regulatory policy, or even a healthy lifestyle intervention for the general population, is low compared to that of a targeted intensive lifestyle intervention, pharmacotherapy, or bariatric surgery. The total costs of an intervention are the product of the number of people in the target population and the per person cost of the intervention. An inexpensive intervention applied to many people may incur total costs as large as those of an expensive intervention applied to a few people. For this reason, even inexpensive interventions applied to large populations may have a substantial cost burden, while very expensive interventions, targeted to small subsets of people, may have smaller cost burdens. At the same time, a less effective intervention broadly applied may result in a greater improvement in the health of the population than a very effective (and expensive) intervention applied to a few people. It is likely that a combination of effective and cost-effective approaches will be needed to address the epidemic of obesity. A range of cost-effective interventions appropriate for each stage of prevention and treatment, from childhood to adulthood, should be implemented".

A STEPPED CARE MHEALTH-BASED APPROACH AS A PERSPECTIVE IN CHRONIC CARE MANAGEMENT OF OBESITY WITH TYPE 2 DIABETES

This section will discuss the feasibility of a stepped care mHealth-based approach as a perspective in chronic care management of obesity with type 2 diabetes. One promising future direction could be treating obesity, considered as a chronic multifactorial disease, using a stepped-care approach (Castelnuovo et al., 2015b; Organization, 2011) as well described in Castelnuovo et al. (2015a):

- The lower level of treatment could be simply a *mhealth or traditional based lifestyle psychoeducational and nutritional approach* to weight management. This step could be also considered as a prevention phase at the population level.
- The following step, useful in moderate conditions, could be represented by the inclusion in *health professionals-driven multidisciplinary protocols* tailored for each patient. The mhealth approach could be useful for providing many parts of the clinical program reducing costs and limiting hospitalizations.
- Another step of care, useful in severe conditions, could be the *inpatient approach with the inclusion of drug therapies and other multidisciplinary treat-*

ments if necessary. The mhealth contribution could be useful for monitoring and motivating patients after the inpatient phase and for reducing costs above all in the follow-up steps.

- Another step, in more severe conditions, needs the solution of *bariatric surgery* and with this option the mhealth approach could be useful for monitoring eating attitudes, motivating patients in changing dysfunctional behaviors and for reducing costs above all in the follow-up steps.

In the chronic care management of globesity mhealth solutions cannot substitute traditional approaches, but they can supplement some steps in obesity prevention and weight loss management, above all in the follow-up phase where the mobile technology can ensure a continuity of care saving costs and avoiding long term lack of connections between patients-citizens and the health care team. (Castelnuovo et al., 2015b, p. 4).

A similar scenario will be possible, from a technological point of view, with the growing development of biomedical devices, sensors and smartphone applications, as well described in (Torres-Huitzil & Alvarez-Landero, 2015): "Micro electro-mechanical systems (MEMS) sensors have already enable smartphones to provide services that deeply affect the user style of life. For instance, through embedded inertial sensors, smartphones are able to respond to hand gestures, support virtual reality applications, or provide information about physical activities that a user performs and infer knowledge about health status. Currently smartphones are able to hear, see, touch, feel and smell and truly act as sensor hubs and their derived services increasingly rely on how well they know the user and user context. Such smartphone perceptual capabilities are possible thanks to the seamless integration of sensors, at hardware level, into the smartphone complex software stack... In spite of the continuous advance of mobile multicore processors, the resources demands and bandwidths of new and future sensors will become so significant that current mobile operating systems, such as Android, for sensor-streams handling will not be enough. Sensors with high bandwidth demands will require additional processing power that can only be provided by additional hardware working closely to the sensor chip... Thus, developing industry standards for sensor integration in smartphone platforms coupled with the almost unlimited computing capabilities from the cloud is required so as to meet the sensor-processing demand of future cognitive smartphones. With the advance of sensing technology for gathering data about human health and the environment integrated in smartphones it is possible to envisage a great impact in mHealth for the next years" (pp. 165-166).

If the technological component is ready to sustain a stepped care mhealth-based approach, the ideal management and organization of stepped care is not so clear (Bower & Gilbody, 2005). "Although there is some supportive evidence for the use of stepped care, rigorous evaluations of the underlying assumptions are scarce, and a significant research agenda remains. Modelling may be a useful research method in the shorter term" (Bower & Gilbody, 2005, p. 15).

HOW A MHEALTH-BASED APPROACH CAN ENHANCE THE PATIENT ENGAGEMENT IN OBESITY WITH TYPE 2 DIABETES

According to Rodriguez (2013), patients with obesity and diabetes could have different abilities and engaging motivations about the necessary self-management behaviors: these differences are due to several intrinsic and extrinsic factors, such as health beliefs, self-efficacy, level of diabetes knowledge and technical skills, functional health literacy and medication adherence.

About health beliefs, patients with diabesity usually think that a good parameter to evaluate their health status could be the presence/absence of symptoms, whereas obesity with diabetes is a silent condition "until hypoglycemia occurs or the development of a complication arises" (Rodriguez, 2013, p. 172). So engaging patients using the long term risk of complications is not successful. The most motivating approach is to show short-term gains working on day-to-day challenges patients face in managing their diabetes. Mobile health solutions can foster the achievement of these results providing progressive feedbacks where and when necessary, even in everyday life situations.

About self-efficacy mhealth can improve the self-perceived coping skills of each patient in keeping on diabetes self-management activities. Providing real-time and on-line feedbacks about patients' actions, mhealth solutions can foster the active participation of clients (and caregivers) in their own care.

About knowledge-technical skills and functional health literacy, new technologies could create useful solutions in providing up-to-date reliable clinical knowledge in real time that can enhance functional self-management approaches. Moreover mhealth-based clinical records and social media could improve documentation sharing and communication between patients, parents, caregivers, health care professionals, researchers, and stakeholders (Santoro, 2015; Santoro, Castelnuovo, Zoppis, Mauri, & Sicurello, 2015).

CONCLUSION

In diabesity, a key role for a successful chronic care management is to engage patients in healthy behaviors, such as a diet and physical exercise. mhealth approach can provide good solutions such as smartphone-based apps that can create or receive from a server a daily list of things to do, a system to track patients' exercises and reminders to take their medications (Brimmer, 2014; Moss Richins, 2015).

REFERENCES

Adibi, S. (2015). Introduction. In S. Adibi (Ed.), *mHealth Multidisciplinary Verticals* (pp. 1–10). London: CRC Press, Taylor & Francis Group.

American Diabetes Association. (2013). American Diabetes Association releases new research estimating annual cost of diabetes at $ 245 billion. Retrieved from http://www.diabetes.org/for-media/2013/annual-costs-of-diabetes-2013.html?loc=cost-of-diabetes

Bacigalupo, R., Cudd, P., Littlewood, C., Bissell, P., Hawley, M. S., & Buckley Woods, H. (2013). Interventions employing mobile technology for overweight and obesity: An early systematic review of randomized controlled trials. *Obesity Reviews*, *14*(4), 279–291. doi:10.1111/obr.12006 PMID:23167478

Barello, S., Graffigna, G., & Vegni, E. (2012). Patient engagement as an emerging challenge for healthcare services: Mapping the literature. *Nursing Research and Practice*, *2012*, 905934. doi:10.1155/2012/905934 PMID:23213497

Bower, P., & Gilbody, S. (2005). Stepped care in psychological therapies: Access, effectiveness and efficiency. Narrative literature review. *The British Journal of Psychiatry*, *186*(1), 11–17. doi:10.1192/bjp.186.1.11 PMID:15630118

Brimmer, K. (2014, June 2). New technologies, hospital strategies promote patient engagement. *Healthcare Finance News*.

Burke, L. E., Styn, M. A., Sereika, S. M., Conroy, M. B., Ye, L., Glanz, K., & Ewing, L. J. et al. (2012). Using mHealth technology to enhance self-monitoring for weight loss: A randomized trial. *American Journal of Preventive Medicine*, *43*(1), 20–26. doi:10.1016/j.amepre.2012.03.016 PMID:22704741

Byrne, S. M., Cooper, Z., & Fairburn, C. G. (2004). Psychological predictors of weight regain in obesity. *Behaviour Research and Therapy*, *42*(11), 1341–1356. doi:10.1016/j.brat.2003.09.004 PMID:15381442

Cafazzo, J. A., Casselman, M., Hamming, N., Katzman, D. K., & Palmert, M. R. (2012). Design of an mHealth app for the self-management of adolescent type 1 diabetes: A pilot study. *Journal of Medical Internet Research*, *14*(3), e70. doi:10.2196/jmir.2058 PMID:22564332

Capodaglio, P., Lafortuna, C., Petroni, M. L., Salvadori, A., Gondoni, L., Castelnuovo, G., & Brunani, A. (2013). Rationale for hospital-based rehabilitation in obesity with comorbidities. *European Journal of Physical and Rehabilitation Medicine*, *49*(3), 399–417. PMID:23736902

Castelnuovo, G. (2010a). Empirically supported treatments in psychotherapy: Towards an evidence-based or evidence-biased psychology in clinical settings? *Frontiers in Psychology*, *1*, 27. PMID:21833197

Castelnuovo, G. (2010b). No medicine without psychology: The key role of psychological contribution in clinical settings. *Frontiers in Psychology*, *1*, 4. doi:10.3389/fpsyg.2010.00004 PMID:21833187

Castelnuovo, G., Manzoni, G. M., Cuzziol, P., Cesa, G. L., Tuzzi, C., Villa, V., & Molinari, E. et al. (2010). TECNOB: Study design of a randomized controlled trial of a multidisciplinary telecare intervention for obese patients with type-2 diabetes. *BMC Public Health*, *10*(1), 204. doi:10.1186/1471-2458-10-204 PMID:20416042

Castelnuovo, G., Manzoni, G. M., Pietrabissa, G., Corti, S., Giusti, E. M., Molinari, E., & Simpson, S. (2014). Obesity and outpatient rehabilitation using mobile technologies: The potential mHealth approach. *Frontiers in Psychology*, *5*, 559. doi:10.3389/fpsyg.2014.00559 PMID:24959157

Castelnuovo, G., Pietrabissa, G., Manzoni, G. M., Corti, S., Ceccarini, M., Borrello, M., & Molinari, E. et al. (2015a). Chronic care management of globesity: Promoting healthier lifestyles in traditional and mHealth based settings. *Frontiers in Psychology*, October. PMID:26528215

Castelnuovo, G., Zoppis, I., Santoro, E., Ceccarini, M., Pietrabissa, G., Manzoni, G. M., & Sicurello, F. et al. (2015b). Managing chronic pathologies with a stepped mHealth-based approach in clinical psychology and medicine. *Frontiers in Psychology*, *6*, 407. doi:10.3389/fpsyg.2015.00407 PMID:25926801

Chomutare, T., Fernandez-Luque, L., Arsand, E., & Hartvigsen, G. (2011). Features of mobile diabetes applications: Review of the literature and analysis of current applications compared against evidence-based guidelines. *Journal of Medical Internet Research*, *13*(3), e65. doi:10.2196/jmir.1874 PMID:21979293

Chouffani, R. (2013). mHealth clinical apps impacting care, not just with consumers. *TechTarget*. Retrieved from http://searchhealthit.techtarget.com/opinion/MHealth-clinical-apps-impacting-care-not-just-with-consumers?asrc=EM_ERU_27369471&utm_medium=EM&utm_source=ERU&utm_campaign=20140320_ERU%20Transmission%20for%2003/20/2014%20(UserUniverse:%20732731)_myka-reports@techtarget.com&src=5223540

Cipresso, P., Serino, S., Villani, D., Repetto, C., Selitti, L., Albani, G., & Riva, G. et al. (2012). Is your phone so smart to affect your states? An exploratory study based on psychophysiological measures. *Neurocomputing*, *84*, 23–30. doi:10.1016/j.neucom.2011.12.027

de Ridder, D., Geenen, R., Kuijer, R., & van Middendorp, H. (2008). Psychological adjustment to chronic disease. *Lancet*, *372*(9634), 246–255. doi:10.1016/S0140-6736(08)61078-8 PMID:18640461

Dombrowski, S. U., Avenell, A., & Sniehott, F. F. (2011). Behavioural interventions for obese adults with additional risk factors for morbidity: Systematic review of effects on behaviour, weight and disease risk factors. *Obes Facts*, *3*(6), 377–396. doi:10.1159/000323076 PMID:21196792

Dombrowski, S. U., Sniehotta, F. F., Avenell, A., Johnston, M., MacLennan, G., & Ara, Ã. (2012). Identifying active ingredients in complex behavioural interventions for obese adults with obesity-related co-morbidities or additional risk factors for co-morbidities: A systematic review. *Health Psychology Review*, *6*(1), 7–32. doi:10.1080/17437199.2010.513298

Ekroos, N., & Jalonen, K. (2007). E-Health and diabetes care. *Journal of Telemedicine and Telecare*, *13*(1), 22–23. doi:10.1258/135763307781645013

Eysenbach, G. (2001). What is e-health? *Journal of Medical Internet Research*, *3*(2), e20. doi:10.2196/jmir.3.2.e20 PMID:11720962

Eysenbach, G. (2011). Can tweets predict citations? Metrics of social impact based on Twitter and correlation with traditional metrics of scientific impact. *Journal of Medical Internet Research*, *13*(4), e123. doi:10.2196/jmir.2012 PMID:22173204

Fiordelli, M., Diviani, N., & Schulz, P. J. (2013). Mapping mHealth research: A decade of evolution. *Journal of Medical Internet Research*, *15*(5), e95. doi:10.2196/jmir.2430 PMID:23697600

Flegal, K. M., Graubard, B. I., Williamson, D. F., & Gail, M. H. (2005). Excess deaths associated with underweight, overweight, and obesity. *Journal of the American Medical Association*, *293*(15), 1861–1867. doi:10.1001/jama.293.15.1861 PMID:15840860

Foster, G. D., Makris, A. P., & Bailer, B. A. (2005). Behavioral treatment of obesity. *The American Journal of Clinical Nutrition*, *82*(Suppl. 1), 230S–235S. PMID:16002827

Glasgow, R. E., Orleans, C. T., & Wagner, E. H. (2001). Does the chronic care model serve also as a template for improving prevention? *The Milbank Quarterly*, *79*(4), 579–612. doi:10.1111/1468-0009.00222 PMID:11789118

Graffigna, G., Barello, S., & Riva, G. (2013). Technologies for patient engagement. *Health Affairs (Project Hope)*, *32*(6), 1172. doi:10.1377/hlthaff.2013.0279 PMID:23733998

Graffigna, G., Barello, S., Wiederhold, B. K., Bosio, A. C., & Riva, G. (2013). Positive technology as a driver for health engagement. *Studies in Health Technology and Informatics*, *191*, 9–17. PMID:23792833

Hebden, L., Balestracci, K., McGeechan, K., Denney-Wilson, E., Harris, M., Bauman, A., & Allman-Farinelli, M. (2013). 'TXT2BFiT' a mobile phone-based healthy lifestyle program for preventing unhealthy weight gain in young adults: Study protocol for a randomized controlled trial. *Trials*, *14*(1), 75. doi:10.1186/1745-6215-14-75 PMID:23506013

Hemingway, H., & Marmot, M. (1999a). Clinical Evidence: Psychosocial factors in the etiology and prognosis of coronary heart disease: systematic review of prospective cohort studies. *The Western Journal of Medicine*, *171*(5-6), 342–350. PMID:18751201

Hemingway, H., & Marmot, M. (1999b). Evidence based cardiology: Psychosocial factors in the aetiology and prognosis of coronary heart disease. Systematic review of prospective cohort studies. *BMJ (Clinical Research Ed.)*, *318*(7196), 1460–1467. doi:10.1136/bmj.318.7196.1460 PMID:10346775

Javitt, J. (2014). Case study: Using mHealth to manage diabetes. *mHealth News*. Retrieved from http://www.mhealthnews.com/print/24916

Jones, V. (2006). The "Diabesity" Epidemic: Let's Rehabilitate America. *Medscape General Medicine*, *8*(2), 34–34. PMID:16926773

Khaylis, A., Yiaslas, T., Bergstrom, J., & Gore-Felton, C. (2010). A review of efficacious technology-based weight-loss interventions: Five key components. *Telemedicine Journal and e-Health*, *16*(9), 931–938. doi:10.1089/tmj.2010.0065 PMID:21091286

Kresser, C. (2014a). Diabesity Retrieved from http://chriskresser.com/diabesity#

Kresser, C. (2014b). Diabesity: the #1 cause of death and disease? Retrieved from http://chriskresser.com/diabesity-the-1-cause-of-death-and-disease

Leiter, E. H., Strobel, M., O'Neill, A., Schultz, D., Schile, A., & Reifsnyder, P. C. (2013). Comparison of Two New Mouse Models of Polygenic Type 2 Diabetes at the Jackson Laboratory, NONcNZO10Lt/J and TALLYHO/JngJ. *J Diabetes Res*, *2013*, 165327. doi:10.1155/2013/165327 PMID:23671854

Levy, P., Nocerini, R., & Grazier, K. (2007). Paying for disease management. *Disease Management*, *10*(4), 235–244. doi:10.1089/dis.2007.104646 PMID:17718662

Malvey, D., & Slovensky, D. J. (2014). mHealth. Transforming Healthcare. New York: Springer.

Manzoni, G. M., Castelnuovo, G., & Molinari, E. (2008). Weight loss with a low-carbohydrate, Mediterranean, or low-fat diet. *The New England Journal of Medicine*, *359*(20), 2170, author reply 2171–2172. PMID:19009669

Manzoni, G. M., Castelnuovo, G., & Proietti, R. (2011). Assessment of psychosocial risk factors is missing in the 2010 ACCF/AHA guideline for assessment of cardiovascular risk in asymptomatic adults. *Journal of the American College of Cardiology*, *57*(14), 1569–1570. doi:10.1016/j.jacc.2010.12.015 PMID:21453841

Manzoni, G. M., Cribbie, R. A., Villa, V., Arpin-Cribbie, C. A., Gondoni, L., & Castelnuovo, G. (2010). Psychological well-being in obese inpatients with ischemic heart disease at entry and at discharge from a four-week cardiac rehabilitation program. *Frontiers in Psychology*, *1*, 38. PMID:21833207

Manzoni, G. M., Pagnini, F., Corti, S., Molinari, E., & Castelnuovo, G. (2011a). Internet-based behavioral interventions for obesity: An updated systematic review. *Clinical Practice and Epidemiology in Mental Health*, *7*(1), 19–28. doi:10.2174/1745017901107010019 PMID:21552423

Manzoni, G. M., Villa, V., Compare, A., Castelnuovo, G., Nibbio, F., Titon, A. M., & Gondoni, L. A. et al. (2011b). Short-term effects of a multi-disciplinary cardiac rehabilitation programme on psychological well-being, exercise capacity and weight in a sample of obese in-patients with coronary heart disease: A practice-level study. *Psychology Health and Medicine*, *16*(2), 178–189. doi:10.1080/13548506.2010.542167 PMID:21328146

Marcus, M. D., & Wildes, J. E. (2009). Obesity: Is it a mental disorder? *International Journal of Eating Disorders*, *42*(8), 739–753. doi:10.1002/eat.20725 PMID:19610015

Martinez-Perez, B., de la Torre-Diez, I., & Lopez-Coronado, M. (2013). Mobile health applications for the most prevalent conditions by the World Health Organization: Review and analysis. *Journal of Medical Internet Research*, *15*(6), e120. doi:10.2196/jmir.2600 PMID:23770578

McCormick, B., & Stone, I. (2007). Economic costs of obesity and the case for government intervention. *Obesity Reviews*, *8*(Suppl. 1), 161–164. doi:10.1111/j.1467-789X.2007.00337.x PMID:17316321

Mercer, V. (2011). Chronic Disease Management. In W. T. O'Donohue & C. Draper (Eds.), *Stepped Care and e-Health: Practical Applications to Behavioral Disorders* (pp. 151–179). New York: Springer. doi:10.1007/978-1-4419-6510-3_9

Moss Richins, S. (2015). *Emerging Technologies in Healthcare*. London: CRC Press, Taylor & Francis Group. doi:10.1201/b18431

Neumeyer-Gromen, A., Lampert, T., Stark, K., & Kallischnigg, G. (2004). Disease management programs for depression: A systematic review and meta-analysis of randomized controlled trials. *Medical Care*, *42*(12), 1211–1221. doi:10.1097/00005650-200412000-00008 PMID:15550801

Nguyen, T., & Lau, D. C. (2012). The obesity epidemic and its impact on hypertension. *The Canadian Journal of Cardiology*, *28*(3), 326–333. doi:10.1016/j.cjca.2012.01.001 PMID:22595448

O'Donnell, R. R. (2011). Stepped Care and E-Health in Behavioral Managed Care. In W. T. O'Donohue & C. Draper (Eds.), *Stepped Care and e-Health: Practical Applications to Behavioral Disorders* (pp. 263–282). New York: Springer. doi:10.1007/978-1-4419-6510-3_14

O'Donohue, W. T., & Draper, C. (2011a). The Case for Evidence-Based Stepped Care as Part of a Reformed Delivery System. In W. T. O'Donohue & C. Draper (Eds.), *Stepped Care and e-Health: Practical Applications to Behavioral Disorders* (pp. 1–16). New York: Springer. doi:10.1007/978-1-4419-6510-3_1

O'Donohue, W. T., & Draper, C. (Eds.). (2011b). *Stepped Care and e-Health: Practical Applications to Behavioral Disorders*. New York: Springer.

Ofman, J. J., Badamgarav, E., Henning, J. M., Knight, K., Gano, A. D. Jr, Levan, R. K., & Weingarten, S. R. et al. (2004). Does disease management improve clinical and economic outcomes in patients with chronic diseases? A systematic review. *The American Journal of Medicine*, *117*(3), 182–192. doi:10.1016/j.amjmed.2004.03.018 PMID:15300966

Organization, W. H. (2011). mHealth: New horizons for health through mobile technologies: Second global survey on eHealth. Global observatory for eHealth series (Vol. 3). Retrieved from http://www.who.int/goe/publications/goe_mhealth_web.pdf

Pagnini, F., Banfi, P., Lunetta, C., Rossi, G., Castelnuovo, G., Marconi, A., & Molinari, E. et al. (2012). Respiratory function of people with amyotrophic lateral sclerosis and caregiver distress level: A correlational study. *BioPsychoSocial Medicine*, *6*(1), 14. doi:10.1186/1751-0759-6-14 PMID:22721255

Pagnini, F., Lunetta, C., Rossi, G., Banfi, P., Gorni, K., Cellotto, N., & Corbo, M. et al. (2011). Existential well-being and spirituality of individuals with amyotrophic lateral sclerosis is related to psychological well-being of their caregivers. *Amyotrophic Lateral Sclerosis; Official Publication of the World Federation of Neurology Research Group on Motor Neuron Diseases*, *12*(2), 105–108. doi:10.3109/17482968.2010.502941 PMID:20653520

Pagnini, F., Rossi, G., Lunetta, C., Banfi, P., Castelnuovo, G., Corbo, M., & Molinari, E. (2010). Burden, depression, and anxiety in caregivers of people with amyotrophic lateral sclerosis. *Psychology Health and Medicine*, *15*(6), 685–693. doi:10.1080/13548506.2010.507773 PMID:21154021

Park, M. J., & Kim, H. S. (2012). Evaluation of mobile phone and Internet intervention on waist circumference and blood pressure in post-menopausal women with abdominal obesity. *International Journal of Medical Informatics*, *81*(6), 388–394. doi:10.1016/j.ijmedinf.2011.12.011 PMID:22265810

Pellegrini, C. A., Duncan, J. M., Moller, A. C., Buscemi, J., Sularz, A., DeMott, A., & Spring, B. et al. (2012). A smartphone-supported weight loss program: Design of the ENGAGED randomized controlled trial. *BMC Public Health*, *12*, 1041. PMID:23194256

Pietrabissa, G., Manzoni, G. M., Corti, S., Vegliante, N., Molinari, E., & Castelnuovo, G. (2012). Addressing motivation in globesity treatment: A new challenge for clinical psychology. *Frontiers in Psychology*, *3*, 317. doi:10.3389/fpsyg.2012.00317 PMID:22969744

Rao, G., Burke, L. E., Spring, B. J., Ewing, L. J., Turk, M., Lichtenstein, A. H., & Coons, M. et al. (2011). New and emerging weight management strategies for busy ambulatory settings: A scientific statement from the American Heart Association endorsed by the Society of Behavioral Medicine. *Circulation*, *124*(10), 1182–1203. doi:10.1161/CIR.0b013e31822b9543 PMID:21824925

Riper, H., Andersson, G., Christensen, H., Cuijpers, P., Lange, A., & Eysenbach, G. (2010). Theme issue on e-mental health: A growing field in internet research. *Journal of Medical Internet Research*, *12*(5), e74. doi:10.2196/jmir.1713 PMID:21169177

Rodrigues, J. J., Lopes, I. M., Silva, B. M., & Torre Ide, L. (2013). A new mobile ubiquitous computing application to control obesity: SapoFit. *Informatics for Health & Social Care*, *38*(1), 37–53. doi:10.3109/17538157.2012.674586 PMID:22657250

Rodriguez, K. M. (2013). Intrinsic and extrinsic factors affecting patient engagement in diabetes self-management: Perspectives of a certified diabetes educator. *Clinical Therapeutics*, *35*(2), 170–178. doi:10.1016/j.clinthera.2013.01.002 PMID:23411000

Rothberg, A. E., Peeters, A., & Herman, W. H. (2014). Cost-Effectiveness of Obesity Prevention and Treatment. In A. G. Bray & C. Bouchard (Eds.), *Handbook of Obesity. Clinical Applications* (pp. 453–470). London: CRC Press, Taylor & Francis Group.

Rozanski, A., Blumenthal, J. A., & Kaplan, J. (1999). Impact of psychological factors on the pathogenesis of cardiovascular disease and implications for therapy. *Circulation*, *99*(16), 2192–2217. doi:10.1161/01.CIR.99.16.2192 PMID:10217662

Santoro, E. (2013). [Social media and medical apps: how they can change health communication, education and care]. *Recenti Progressi in Medicina*, *104*(5), 179–180. PMID:23748682

Santoro, E. (2015). [Social media and health communication: do we need rules?]. *Recenti Progressi in Medicina*, *106*(1), 15–16. PMID:25621774

Santoro, E., Caldarola, P., & Villella, A. (2011). [Using Web 2.0 technologies and social media for the cardiologist's education and update]. *Giornale Italiano di Cardiologia*, *12*(3), 174–181. PMID:21560473

Santoro, E., Castelnuovo, G., Zoppis, I., Mauri, G., & Sicurello, F. (2015). Social media and mobile applications in chronic disease prevention and management. *Frontiers in Psychology*, *6*, 567. doi:10.3389/fpsyg.2015.00567 PMID:25999884

Santoro, E., & Quintaliani, G. (2013). [Using web 2.0 technologies and social media for the nephrologist]. *Giornale Italiano di Nefrologia*, *30*(1). PMID:23832442

Schiel, R., Kaps, A., & Bieber, G. (2012). Electronic health technology for the assessment of physical activity and eating habits in children and adolescents with overweight and obesity IDA. *Appetite*, *58*(2), 432–437. doi:10.1016/j.appet.2011.11.021 PMID:22155072

Schneiderman, N., Antoni, M. H., Saab, P. G., & Ironson, G. (2001). Health psychology: Psychosocial and biobehavioral aspects of chronic disease management. *Annual Review of Psychology*, *52*(1), 555–580. doi:10.1146/annurev.psych.52.1.555 PMID:11148317

Schoffman, D. E., Turner-McGrievy, G., Jones, S. J., & Wilcox, S. (2013). Mobile apps for pediatric obesity prevention and treatment, healthy eating, and physical activity promotion: Just fun and games? *Translational Behavioral Medicine*, *3*(3), 320–325. doi:10.1007/s13142-013-0206-3 PMID:24073184

Shaheen, S., Mohammed, A., & Grbic, N. (2015). Mobile Services for Diabetic Patients' Sustainable Lifestyle. In S. Adibi (Ed.), *mHealth Multidisciplinary Verticals* (pp. 51–61). London: CRC Press, Taylor & Francis Group.

Sharifi, M., Dryden, E. M., Horan, C. M., Price, S., Marshall, R., Hacker, K., & Taveras, E. M. et al. (2013). Leveraging text messaging and mobile technology to support pediatric obesity-related behavior change: A qualitative study using parent focus groups and interviews. *Journal of Medical Internet Research*, *15*(12), e272. doi:10.2196/jmir.2780 PMID:24317406

Shaw, R. J., Bosworth, H. B., Silva, S. S., Lipkus, I. M., Davis, L. L., Sha, R. S., & Johnson, C. M. (2013). Mobile health messages help sustain recent weight loss. *The American Journal of Medicine*, *126*(11), 1002–1009. doi:10.1016/j.amjmed.2013.07.001 PMID:24050486

Simpson, S. G., & Slowey, L. (2011). Video therapy for atypical eating disorder and obesity: A case study. *Clinical Practice and Epidemiology in Mental Health*, *7*(1), 38–43. doi:10.2174/1745017901107010038 PMID:21559235

Swencionis, C., & Rendell, S. L. (2012). The psychology of obesity. *Abdominal Imaging*, *37*(5), 733–737. doi:10.1007/s00261-012-9863-9 PMID:22392131

Torres-Huitzil, C., & Alvarez-Landero, A. (2015). Accelerometer-Based Human Activity Recognition in Smartphones for Healthcare Services. In S. Adibi (Ed.), *Mobile Health: A Technology Road Map* (pp. 147–170). Berlin: Springer. doi:10.1007/978-3-319-12817-7_7

Turner-McGrievy, G. M., Beets, M. W., Moore, J. B., Kaczynski, A. T., Barr-Anderson, D. J., & Tate, D. F. (2013). Comparison of traditional versus mobile app self-monitoring of physical activity and dietary intake among overweight adults participating in an mHealth weight loss program. *Journal of the American Medical Informatics Association*, *20*(3), 513–518. doi:10.1136/amiajnl-2012-001510 PMID:23429637

Villagra, V. G. (2004). Integrating disease management into the outpatient delivery system during and after managed care. *Health Affairs (Project Hope)*, (Suppl. Web Exclusives), W4-281–283. PMID:15451998

Villagra, V. G., & Ahmed, T. (2004). Effectiveness of a disease management program for patients with diabetes. *Health Affairs (Project Hope)*, *23*(4), 255–266. doi:10.1377/hlthaff.23.4.255 PMID:15318587

Von Korff, M., & Tiemans, B. (2000). Individualized stepped care of chronic illness. *The Western Journal of Medicine*, *172*(2), 133–137. doi:10.1136/ewjm.172.2.133 PMID:10693379

Wadden, T. A., Brownell, K. D., & Foster, G. D. (2002). Obesity: Responding to the global epidemic. *Journal of Consulting and Clinical Psychology*, *70*(3), 510–525. doi:10.1037/0022-006X.70.3.510 PMID:12090366

Wagner, E. H., Austin, B. T., Davis, C., Hindmarsh, M., Schaefer, J., & Bonomi, A. (2001a). Improving chronic illness care: Translating evidence into action. *Health Affairs (Project Hope)*, *20*(6), 64–78. doi:10.1377/hlthaff.20.6.64 PMID:11816692

Wagner, E. H., Glasgow, R. E., Davis, C., Bonomi, A. E., Provost, L., McCulloch, D., & Sixta, C. et al. (2001b). Quality improvement in chronic illness care: A collaborative approach. *The Joint Commission Journal on Quality Improvement*, *27*(2), 63–80. PMID:11221012

Waller, G., Stringer, H., & Meyer, C. (2012). What cognitive behavioral techniques do therapists report using when delivering cognitive behavioral therapy for the eating disorders? *Journal of Consulting and Clinical Psychology*, *80*(1), 171–175. doi:10.1037/a0026559 PMID:22141595

Weingarten, S. R., Henning, J. M., Badamgarav, E., Knight, K., Hasselblad, V., Gano, A. Jr, & Ofman, J. J. (2002). Interventions used in disease management programmes for patients with chronic illness-which ones work? Meta-analysis of published reports. *BMJ (Clinical Research Ed.)*, *325*(7370), 925. doi:10.1136/bmj.325.7370.925 PMID:12399340

Whitlock, G., Lewington, S., Sherliker, P., Clarke, R., Emberson, J., Halsey, J., & Peto, R. et al.Prospective Studies Collaboration. (2009). Body-mass index and cause-specific mortality in 900 000 adults: Collaborative analyses of 57 prospective studies. *Lancet*, *373*(9669), 1083–1096. doi:10.1016/S0140-6736(09)60318-4 PMID:19299006

Whittaker, R. (2012). Issues in mHealth: Findings from key informant interviews. *Journal of Medical Internet Research*, *14*(5), e129. doi:10.2196/jmir.1989 PMID:23032424

Wing, R. R. (2002). Behavioral weight control. In T. A. Wadden & A. J. Stunkard (Eds.), *Handbook of obesity treatment* (pp. 301–316). New York: Guilford Press.

Zimmet, P. Z., Magliano, D. J., Herman, W. H., & Shaw, J. E. (2014). Diabetes: A 21st century challenge. *The Lancet Diabetes & Endocrinology*, *2*(1), 56–64. doi:10.1016/S2213-8587(13)70112-8 PMID:24622669

KEY TERMS AND DEFINITIONS

Bariatric Surgery: Surgery on the stomach and-or intestines to help patients with extreme obesity lose weight (traditionally it is an option for people who have a body mass index-BMI above 40).

Chronic Care Management: The comprehensive activities of education, prevention, monitoring and treatment conducted by health care professionals to help patients with chronic diseases and health conditions motivating patients to persist in necessary interventions to protect achieve a reasonable quality of life.

eHealth: A growing field of health services provided through the Internet and other new technologies.

mHealth: The practice of medicine and public health supported by mobile communication devices, such as mobile phones, tablet computers, and PDAs, for health services and information (it is an evolution of eHealth).

Obesity: A condition with a BMI (Body Mass Index, a person's weight in kilograms-kg divided by their height in meters-m squared) of 30 and above.

Social Media: Advanced forms of electronic communication through which users create online communities to share information, ideas, personal messages, and other content (as videos).

Stepped Care: Treatment that follows a predetermined sequence with a care approach adjusted in steps according to the failure or lack of effect of lower intensity interventions. The simplest and most affordable treatment regimen is used first: if that fails, other options are employed one after another until an endpoint is reached.

Type 2 Diabetes: A form of diabetes mellitus that is present especially in obese subjects with a condition of hyperglycemia resulting from impaired insulin utilization and with the body's inability to compensate with increased insulin production.

Chapter 9
Why, What and When in-Home Physiotherapy?

Gabriela Postolache
Universidade de Lisboa, Portugal

Isabel Moreira
Universidade do Porto, Portugal

Raul Oliveira
Universidade de Lisboa, Portugal

Octavian Postolache
Instituto de Telecomunicações, ISCTE-IUL, Portugal

ABSTRACT

In the last decade, rehabilitation process has shifted from medical management to issues that enhance quality of life, community participation, treatment and cost effectiveness. In this context physiotherapists design and implement new and/or tailored interventions that enhance physical and functional abilities, restore, maintain, and promote optimal physical function, wellness, fitness and quality of life. The aim of this review was to assess the extent, content, and outcomes of in-home physiotherapy interventions. A search was conducted in Medline, PEDro, and Cochrane Library and IEEE Xplore. RE-AIM and GRADE guidelines were used to report this review. The findings suggest that in-home physiotherapy tailored specifically to the people needs, functioning and disability has positive results, including patients' engagement in their healthcare. Integration of information and communication technology in-home physiotherapy has great potential to increase accessibility, quality and effectiveness of various interventions provided by physiotherapists.

DOI: 10.4018/978-1-5225-0663-8.ch009

INTRODUCTION

In-home physiotherapy is rapidly growing, in line with the current shift in emphasis toward: i) patient- centered healthcare, compliant with 4P medicine (personalized, preventive, predictive, participatory medicine) (see Hood & Galas, 2008); ii) self-management for people with long-term and/or chronic conditions, in which greater use of community settings and individual autonomy are being encouraged (see Lommi, Matarese, Alvaro, Piredda, & De Marinis, 2015); iii) healthcare delivery closer to patients' homes - aiming for increasing access to healthcare services, cost-effectiveness, and sustainability of healthcare system (see Coulter, 2005). With advances in information and communication technologies (ICT), dramatic changes are produced in health care provision. There is increasing evidence suggesting great potential of ICT (see list of definitions) to meet healthcare aspirations of patients and citizens (see Coulter, 2005) as: fast access to reliable information about illness and treatment options; attention to physical and environmental needs; participation in health care decision and service developments, etc. ICT through contribution to patient engagement (see Triberti & Riva, 2014a), particularly on patient engagement in physical rehabilitation process (see Triberti et al., 2014) lead to more appropriate health care, tailored treatment, better health outcome and cost effective use of health services (Graffigna & Barello, 2015; Triberti et al., 2014). Home health technologies are now emerging as a distinct segment within the larger ICT market, forecasting the increase of consumers using home health technologies from 14.3 million worldwide in 2014 to 78.5 million by 2020 (Tractica, 2015). This is produced by: rapidly advances in ICT; increased access to Internet - 82,1% of European and 60% American population has now Internet access at home; development of mobile technologies; and increased access to mobile technologies – approximately 80% of Europeans and Americans have active mobile broadband subscriptions (ITU, 2015).

The interest on model, determinants, and technologies for in-home health care has led to a rise in the number of studies addressing the same, or very similar research questions, with a concurrent increase in discordant findings in terms of direction and magnitude of in-home physiotherapy interventions. Differences in scope, methods, and results in studies realized by health care professionals, engineers or information technology specialists cause great confusion, and make it difficult for decision makers to analyze the level of evidence towards finding solutions to improve practice and identify areas where new research is needed.

We investigated the extent (demographic, health, functioning/disability characteristics of patients, level of evidence, amplitude of practice implementation and adoption), content (what type of physiotherapy intervention, in which clinical condition, what technique or technology is used) and outcomes (e.g. balance, posture, coordination) of in-home physiotherapy. The aim of this chapter is characterization of the level of evidence of in-home physiotherapy in various clinical conditions, and on technology use for in-home physiotherapy. We present the framework for the analysis of the level of evidence related with in-home physiotherapy (Study Design and Methodology section) and the results (Main Evidence section) on what and when in-home physiotherapy, emphasizing why in-home physiotherapy may contribute to patient engagement in health care. Ongoing research and trends in technology for in-home physiotherapy are presented in Future Researches section.

BACKGROUND: WHY IN-HOME PHYSIOTHERAPY

In-home health care provided by governmental healthcare services are rapidly growing in industrialized countries, as a result of: i) increase in elderly population, ii) general increase of population with non-communicable, chronic diseases, and iii) epidemiological transition triggered by medical innovation in disease or sickness therapy and treatment (see Omran, 2005). In Europe, all countries are experiencing an ageing of their populations, a trend that is projected to continue until at least the middle of the twenty-first century (Rechel, Doyle, Grundy, & McKee, 2009). Nowadays, in Portugal, elderly population is already around 20%. This adds significant cost to the healthcare system. One study performed in eight countries from Organisation for Economic Co-operation and Development (OECD) found that between one third and one half of total health expenditure was spent on health care for older people (Anderson & Hussey, 2001). In industrialized countries larger proportions of people increased life expectancy, but also larger proportions of patients in these countries live with more than one disease. The monthly costs per patient of co-morbidity increase exponentially, and rise more with mental disorders (Naylor et al., 2012). Most of the subject receiving physiotherapy - elderly population, people with chronic diseases or people with disabilities - often receive a mix of health and social care provided by several formal and informal workers. In this context, to achieve the intent and sustainability of meaningful use of health care services, and to balance rising cost pressure in healthcare system, focus on prevention and prediction became a priority of many health services, particularly in physiotherapy services.

Patient-centered models of health care services were implemented worldwide, in order: to look actively and systematically for conditions in their early stages; to identify factors that are known to be health risk; and to provide tailored, efficient care. Services for continuing care, or long term care are provided in assisted living or nursing home but also at patient home. The Alliance for Home Health Quality & Innovation organization (2014), from U.S.A., that is comprised of home health care providers and organizations committed to advancing research and initiatives on the value of home health care, underlines that '*the value of health care delivery at home will grow because it is a patient-preferred, cost-effective means of delivery high quality care*'.

An important contribution to quality and efficiency of home health care has been the integration of ICT in healthcare services. For instance, various mobile technologies are currently used in-home setting in a broad range of interventions. Most commonly, health professionals use mobile technology for collecting health data; tele-monitoring; management of practice (e.g. schedule of appointments, register of clinical summary of the patient during and after each visit); messaging between health professionals and patients; patient specific health education; better communication with patients (e.g. through interactive communication – video sharing, video games, augmented reality, virtual reality, etc.). Recent studies suggest that mobile technologies present promising opportunities to improve the range, quality and cost-effectiveness of services provided by health professionals (see Nhavoto & Gronlundt, 2014; Berratarrechea et al., 2014). However, demographic, socio-economic and clinical heterogeneity of the patients requiring home health care, in addition to lack of standardization of in-home health services, lack of strong evidence on the optimal model for providing home health care services and optimal model of payment and reimbursement for these services, create a confusing picture regarding in-home healthcare. In-home physiotherapy (also known as domiciliary physiotherapy) as part of home health care services is more challenging, as more uncertainty exists in physiotherapists status and complexity of interventions provided by physiotherapists - some overlapping with other therapies or in-home health services (see Figure 1).

Physiotherapy, also known as physical therapy or kinesitherapy, has different definition worldwide (see Jull, 2013) despite being recognized as the assessment, prevention and treatment of movement disorders as a core of expertise, practice, education and research in physiotherapy. Physiotherapists are often associated with spine and sports injuries treatment although they promote and prescribe physical activity programmes in the area of prevention and maintenance, promotion and treatment across lifespan. They are involved in a large variety of healthcare services (e.g. care for the premature babies; care for the children with impaired motor functionalities; rehabilitation of cardiac and respiratory system; therapy for musculo-skeletal disorders; programs for preventions of functional decline in older adults). Physiotherapists can prescribe aerobic and resistance exercise (e.g. for

Figure 1. Physiotherapy practice and relationships with other health care services

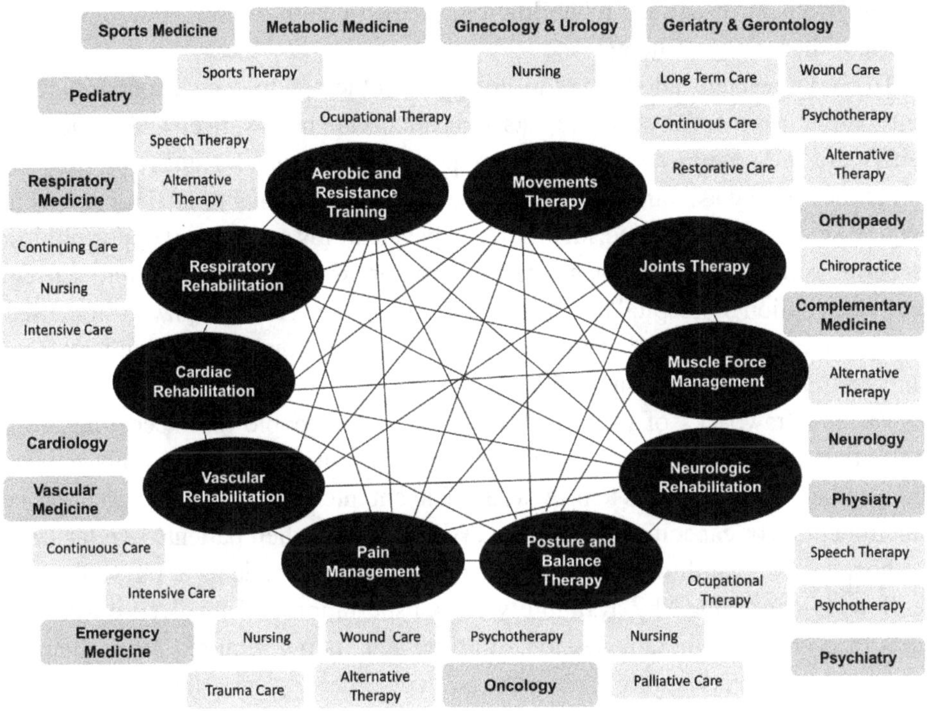

athletes, or people with metabolic diseases like obesity or diabetes), movement therapy (e.g. in upper or lower limbs rehabilitation), joints therapy (e.g. rehabilitation after knee arthroplasty, shoulder dislocation), muscle force management (e.g. strength training, muscle spasticity and rigidity treatment), exercises for neurologic or neuro-motor rehabilitation (e.g. mobility and stability exercises, sensory-motor training, posture and balance training for people with cerebral palsy), therapy for pain reduction (e.g. for rheumatoid arthritis), therapy for vascular rehabilitation (e.g. for therapy for venous or lymphatic edema, physical exercises for people with abdominal aneurism), physical exercises for cardiac rehabilitation (e.g. after cardiac surgery), or respiratory rehabilitation (e.g. after pulmonary surgery), etc. In most countries, patients must have a prescription or referral from a licensed medical doctor before physiotherapy. Some competencies, skills and knowledge of physiotherapists are overlapping with those of others health professionals (e.g. wound care, alternative therapy, occupational therapy) but there are always several differences in the approach and interventions. Physiotherapists can practice either alone or in different teams (see Figure 1) in hospital, primary health centers, private clinics, and community centers. They can be specialized in respiratory physiotherapy, cardiac rehabilitation, woman health, family and community health, in-home physiotherapy, etc.

To our knowledge, adoption of in-home physiotherapy in many countries is currently limited as most physiotherapists and patients are not aware on techniques and benefits of in-home physiotherapy. They perceive various advantages on hospital and clinics setting as: various equipment and multidisciplinary staffing; access to 'expert' support and guideline; facilitation of peer learning and support opportunities; 'economies of scale' when physiotherapy program is delivered in a group setting; safety perception of hospital or clinics environment, and risk of injury in-home setting (although few adverse events were reported until now) (see Gunn, Cattaneo, Finlayson, Freeman, & Sosnoff, 2014).

Various drawbacks of these services, mainly for people that need long term physiotherapy (months, years) were reported: i) programs away from home are unlikely to be frequent enough to provide a sufficient intensity of exercises to improve functionalities or capacities; ii) less accessibility (e.g. when patients live far from the hospital or rehabilitation centers and participation of patients at physiotherapy sessions is constrained by availability of transportation and involved costs); iii) costs of each physiotherapy session; iv) time and energy required for regular attendance, adding an additional burden on people dealing with the challenges of ongoing health conditions. Therefore, in-home physiotherapy may be a solution for the above-mentioned problems.

According to a systematic review based on the analysis of 23 randomized controlled trials and 3 controlled trials (Novak, 2011), strong and moderate evidence supporting in-home physiotherapy was published. Many systematic reviews on various interventions in which physiotherapists may be involved (e.g. stroke rehabilitation, cardiac rehabilitation) have supported that in-home setting physiotherapy have favorable outcomes (Outpatient Service Trialists, 2004; Jolly et al., 2007; Chien, Lee, Wu, Chen, & Wu, 2008; Thomas, Simpson, Riley, & Grant, 2010; Health Quality Ontario, 2013; Crocker et al., 2013; Coulter, Scarvell, Neeman, & Smith, 2013; Siemonsma et al., 2014; Anderson & Taylor, 2014, Chan et al., 2015). However, there are inconclusive data, and some studies showing no positive outcomes for several physiotherapy interventions, mainly when complications or the presence of co-morbidities are also considered in the study (Mehta & Roy, 2011; Al-Jundi, Madback, Beard, Nawaz, & Tew, 2013; Papalia et al., 2013; Valdes, Naughton, & Michlovitzl, 2014). Moreover, it is easy to understand that in-home physiotherapy is not appropriate for every patient. Some patients in need for therapy after hospital discharge may be able to obtain outpatient therapy in-home or clinic environment and adequately meet their needs. Other patients may only need to follow up with their in-home exercises. For some patients, in-home physiotherapy would not offer either quality or effectiveness of traditional physiotherapy. Taking into account the accumulating evidence from the last years, it should be noted that for many patients with multiple chronic conditions or with disabilities, in-home physiotherapy would be cost-effective and adequate care. It is required, therefore, description and comprehensive analysis of evidence related with interventions that are better suited for in-home setting. With rapidly growing of in-home physiotherapy practice as well as changes in health services produced nowadays by ICT integration, the analysis of evidence should be a dynamic process in which various dimensions (e.g. perspectives of patients and physiotherapists on various kind of ICT technologies, usability of new technologies for in-home physiotherapy, effectiveness, wellbeing or quality of life provision) should be integrated.

WHAT AND WHEN IN-HOME PHYSIOTHERAPY: A SYSTEMATIC REVIEW

Study Design and Methodology

Medline via PubMed, PEDro, Cohrane Central Register of Controlled Trials and IEEE/IET Electronic Library were searched from January 2013 up to December 2014 for review of the evidence on technologies and type of physiotherapy that can be applied in-home setting. Search was made by using the following terms: 'in-home physiotherapy', 'in-home rehabilitation', 'balance monitoring' 'Wii,' 'Kinect,' 'exergame,' 'tele-rehabilitation,' 'gait assessment.' To be included, articles had to be available in English; having data and measurements that suggest use or potential use of technique for in-home rehabilitation or physiotherapy. All design studies and all health condition and clinical populations were included. Reference lists from articles meeting the inclusion criteria were checked to ensure all relevant papers were included, and to search for additional studies using 'snowballing' method. Two reviewers used predefined inclusion criteria to select relevant published works and assess their quality using the GRADE - Grading of Recommendations Assessment, Development and Evaluation (www.gradeworkinggroup.org), and RE-AIM - Reach, Effectiveness, Adoption, Implementation and Maintenance (Glasgow, 2013). As the objective of the studies was not measuring the quality of the researches on the new treatment or therapy - for this PEDro scale (www.pedro.org.au) is commonly used - we decided to use a combination of GRADE and RE-AIM guidelines. NVivo10 software was used to manage the data. In our analysis, as trials and works on new technologies for in-home rehabilitation often at '*proof of concept state*' are included, the quality depend on other criteria than PEDro scale, as for example reliability of measurements, feasibility, long-term analysis of functionalities of developed technology, advantages comparing with other technologies, data on safety and adoption of technology. By using RE-AIM analysis of target population, effectiveness of the implemented technique, adoption by target population, staff, setting or institutions, implementation consistency, costs and adaptations made during delivery, maintenance of intervention effects in individuals and settings over time, can be carried out. Figure 2 presents a synthesis of the dimension and definitions of RE-AIM.

Decision on the quality of evidence was based on:

- Effectiveness;
- Potential harm;
- Diagnosis and prognosis potential of the implemented technique for in-home physiotherapy;
- Number of subjects included in the study and description of control condition;
- How clear was the description of the implemented system architecture and experimental protocol, reproducibility of measurements;
- Influence of confounding variables, risk of bias/study limitations;
- Consistency of results, precision of measurements and data reporting.

Figure 2. RE-AIM dimension and definitions
(Glasgow, 2013)

REACH

Participation rate among eligible;

Representativeness of settings participating individuals;

Representativeness of participants;

EFFICACY/EFFECTIVENESS

Effects on primary outcome of interest;

Impact on quality of life, negative outcomes;

ADOPTION

Participation rate among possible settings;

IMPLEMENTATION

Extent to which intervention was delivered as intended and adaptation made;

Time and costs of intervention;

than in hospital settings (ref);

MAINTENANCE

(Individual) Longer – term effects of intervention > 6 months;

(Individual) Impact of attrition on outcomes;

(Settings) Sustained delivery and modification of intervention.

For decision making on what physiotherapy intervention should be better in-home setting, a Boolean logic (strong evidence or no strong evidence) is more appropriate. Therefore, after multi-dimensional analysis with RE-AIM, the studies were grouped in fewer categories than with RE-AIM, using GRADE guidelines. In this evidence rating scale, the studies should be classified as:

- HLE (High Level of Evidence): further research is very unlikely to change the confidence in the estimate of accuracy of measurements;
- MLE (Moderate Level of Evidence): further research is likely to have an important impact on our confidence in the estimate of accuracy of measurement and may change the estimate;
- LLE (Low level of Evidence): further research is very likely to have an important impact on the confidence in the estimate of accuracy of measurement and is likely to change the estimate;
- VLE (Very Low Level of Evidence): any estimate of measurements is very uncertain.

Exclusion criteria for this work were: studies that did not go through a peer-review process for publication; studies published in conference and with a more complete version in a journal - the journal version was included and the conference version was discarded.

Main Evidence

In this chapter we present our results of what and when in-home physiotherapy based on RE-AIM and GRADE classification of 250 studies – pilot study/case report, randomized controlled trials, cohort/quasi-experimental studies related with in-home physiotherapy. Also, 26 review papers related with in-home rehabilitation or physiotherapy as well as 16 publications on future trials were analyzed for better understanding of the issue, controversies and research trend related with in-home physiotherapy. Systematic reviews and future trials were not included in GRADE and RE-AIM based analysis. In 165 studies, outcomes assessments were based on information and communication technologies – 72 for in-home exercises supervision and assessments, 25 for coordination of movement measurements, 39 for gait assessment and monitoring, 7 for balance assessments and monitoring, 6 for posture and muscle spasticity/rigidity evaluation, 16 for biofeedback (see list of definitions) based therapy.

Table 1 presents the frequency of the studies categorized as having high, moderate or low level of evidence on effectiveness of in-home exercises, where outcomes evaluation was made using scales.

Table 1. Visual representation of frequency of high, moderate or low level of evidence studies on effectiveness of in-home exercises where outcomes evaluation was made using scales.

		HLE				MLE				LLE		
			RE-AIM		RE-AIM		RE-AIM		RE-AIM			
		2013		2014		2013		2014		2013	2014	
		Number of Studies										Total
		17	17	8	8	23	23	16	16	8	8	80
Condition	Achilles Tendinopathy							1				1
	Ageing	3				5		2				11
	Alzheimer	1				2						3
	Ankylosis Spondylitis	1				1		1				3
	Cancer	1		1								2
	Cerebral Palsy					1						1
	Claudicants							1				1
	COPD					1						1
	Depression	2										2
	Hemofilia							1				1
	Hip Rehab			1		1						2
	Incontinence	2										2
	Ankle Sprain					1						1
	Knee Rehab	3		2		2		2				9
	Lower Limbs			1		1		1				3
	Multiple Sclerosis			2				3				5
	Neurogenic Claudication	1										1
	Neurological Physiotherapy					1						1
	Obesity					1		1				2
	Palliative Care			1								1
	Parkinson Disease					1						1
	Pelvic Girdle Pain	1										1
	Respiratory Rehab	1				1		1				2
	Stroke					2						2
	Temporomandibular Rehab							2				2
	Vascular Rehab	1				2						3

Most studies are related with measurements of in-home exercises effectiveness. Home-based training has shown to increase rehabilitation uptake, and to be safe and effective in improving short-term exercise capacity. Also, the long-term effect of in-home exercises on physical fitness and activity was studied in various clinical frameworks. Most are randomized and controlled studies and with exception of studies included in low level evidence category, they are compliant with RE-AIM criteria. One in 4 of these studies met the criteria for high level evidence and RE-AIM system. There is high level of evidence on effectiveness of tailored exercises for elderly population, for people with multiple sclerosis, Alzheimer disease, cancer, knee rehabilitation after knee arthroplasty (see Table 1).

Positive results were published on a program based on Lifestyle Functional Exercise (LiFE) to engage older people on physical exercising (Burton, Lewin, Clemson, & Boldy, 2013). By using exergame (see Sinclair, Hingston, & Masek, 2007), Nintendo Wii, video training (e.g. DVD video with comprehensive exercise, physiotherapist supervision via videoconferencing or tele-rehabilitation system), or wireless sensors (see Table 2 and Figure 3), the outcomes of in-home exercises were shown to be comparable to the standard in hospital or physiotherapy clinic rehabilitative approach.

This finding suggests that in-home physiotherapy for cardiac rehabilitation or management of functional decline in elderly people can be implemented effectively at home, mainly when co-administered with an integrated tele-rehabilitation service. In a recent study where 307 older adults were recruited from 83 towns, participants in DVD intervention condition demonstrated significant improvements in the Physical Performance Battery, lower extremity flexibility, and upper body strength (McAuley et al., 2013). Range of motion (ROM) for elbow and joint extension significantly increased at 1, 3, and 6 months, while for the wrists joint extension increased significantly at 1 months in comparison to baseline, with detailed one-to one instruction for home based functional training combined with botulin toxin type A injection in upper limb muscles, in a study with 190 post-stroke participants (Takekawa et al., 2013).

For better visualization of data, exergames based on Nintendo Wii, and Kinect technology are separately retrieved in Table 2 and Figure 4. High level of evidence exists on potential of mobile technologies for long term monitoring of Parkinson's disease motor symptom in-home setting (Mhatre et al., 2013; Tzallass et al., 2014). There are high and moderate level of evidence on effectiveness of wearable technologies (e.g. accelerometers, inertial measurement unit – IMU, force sensors) or contactless technologies (e.g. Kinect) for gait assessment and monitoring (see Figure 5). These low cost non-invasive or unobtrusive technologies might be used to deliver tailored in-home physiotherapy.

Table 2. Visual representation of frequency of the high, moderate or low level of evidence studies on effectiveness of in-home exercises where outcomes evaluation was made using various portable technologies.

		HLE				MLE				LLE		
			RE-AIM		RE-AIM		RE-AIM		RE-AIM			
		2013		2014		2013		2014		2013	2014	
		Number of Studies										Total
		2		6	6	12	12	10	10	1	7	38
Condition	Ageing			1	1			2	2			3
	Ankylosis spondilitis							1	1			1
	Braquial plexus injury							1	1			1
	Cancer					4	4					4
	Cardiac Rehab	2		3	3	1	1					6
	COPD					1	1	1	1			2
	Knee Rehab					1	1	1	1			2
	Metabolic Syndrom			1	1							1
	Parkinson's Disease			1	1	2	2	1	1			4
	Shoulder Rehab					1	1	1	1			2
	Transfemoral Amputation					1	1					1
	Vascular Rehab					1	1	2	2			3

Figure 3. Studies on physical exercises that can be performed in-home by using unobtrusive/contactless technologies

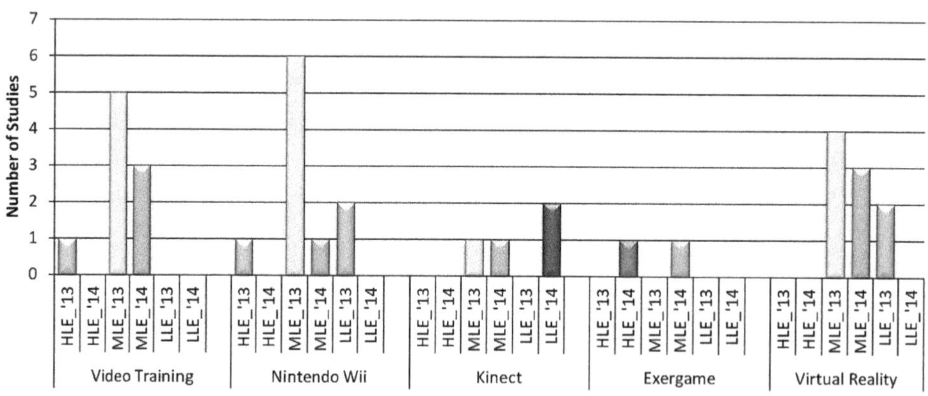

Figure 4. Studies on gait assessment using wearable technologies

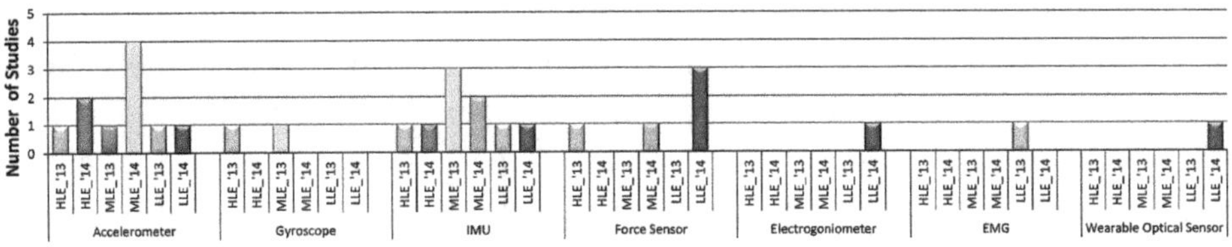

Figure 5. Studies on gait assessment using contactless technologies

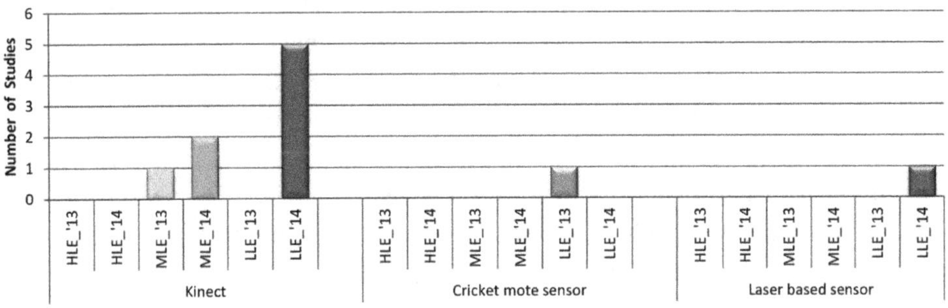

Small wearable or contactless technologies may greatly contribute for increase effectiveness of in-home physiotherapy both by accurate, real-time assessment and monitoring, as well as a tool for treatment. We include in the category of studies on biofeedback (Lee et al., 2013; Kent, Laird, & Haines, 2015) the development of new technologies for situation dependence cueing (auditory, vibratory or visual cueing) of gait, or freezing episode for Parkinson's disease episode (Zhao, Anhalt, Fietzek, & D'Angelo, 2013; Cinel, Poli, Citi, & Robertson, 2013; Rodger, Young, & Craig, 2014; Imbeault-Nepton & Otis, 2014; Cancela, Morano, Arredondo, & Bonato, 2014; Pepa, Ciabattoni, Verdini, Capecci, & Ceravolo, 2014).

These technologies might be applied in a variety of physiotherapy intervention plan (e.g. prevention of falls in elderly patient, training movements in people with cerebral palsy, Huntington diseases). Moreover, the potential of virtual reality (VR) technologies (see list of definitions) to assist and improve rehabilitation techniques and procedures was explored in various studies. VR has been used in several training exercises in-home setting, and has great potential to: incorporate the individual's visual, auditory, touch senses and proprioception for subject engagement; increased adherence to exercise; empowerment; and proactive participation of patients in rehabilitation.

Studies related with tremor evaluation, studies on development of technologies for coordination of movement assessment (e.g. tablet based software for evaluation of Parkinson' disease progression using alternate taping), studies having as main objective evaluation of limbs agility in various clinical context were included in the group of physiotherapy practice related with coordination of movement. New, interesting, techniques, mobile technologies based on accelerometer, inertial measurement unit (IMU), gyroscope, Wii Sports, Kinect are developed and tested for coordination of movement measurements. The majority of these studies are not compliant with RE-AIM (64%), testing being made only for short period of time (e.g. one session, or few days), in a small number of healthy subjects or patients.

By using ICT, physiotherapists can document the effects of interventions with valid outcome tools/instruments evaluation. However, in the implementation of ICT for tele-rehabilitation, it should be considered that patients with chronic diseases, and/or with disabilities might have greater than expected difficulties in using ICT often due to cognitive impairment or unfamiliarity with technology. Approaches described in the evaluated studies for dealing with such barriers (see Hoerbst & Ammenwerth, 2010; Kaye, Kokia, Shalev, Idar, & Chinitz, 2010; Irizarry, DeVito Dabbs, & Curran, 2015) include: suitable integration of solutions involving patient-caregiver dyads, integration of education to improve health and ICT literacy, better design of technology and careful attention to the safety of technology, adoption and maintenance (see table 3).

The evaluated studies suggest benefits of using ICT for various in-home physiotherapy interventions:

- Tailored program for experiential positions described in Patient Health Engagement Model (Graffigna & Barello, 2015) - blackout, arousal, adhesion and eudaimonic project - can be designed based on ICT, in order to induce a positive reaction in patients (Triberti & Riva, 2014a) and for cost-effective treatment;
- Context based practice and integration of physiotherapy intervention into real life of subject may be implemented;
- Physiotherapists and subjects can have greater choice over type, planning and progression of exercise activities;
- Shared decision making in care process;
- Subjects can receive personalized advices on home environment modification for safe and better quality of physiotherapy process;
- Family members or other caregivers might be involved directly or through positive technology as source of motivation, support and feedback in rehabilitation process.

Table 3. Visual representation of frequency of the high, moderate or low level of evidence studies on in-home physiotherapy interventions

		HL				ML				LL		
			RE-AIM		RE-AIM		RE-AIM		RE-AIM			
		2013		2014		2013		2014		2013	2014	
		Number of Studies										Total
Muscle		1	1			1	1			2	1	5
Spasticity/Rigidity	Scale	1								2		3
	Sensor					1					1	2
Posture						1		2			1	4
	Accelerometer							1				1
	IMU					1						1
	Kinect							1			1	2
Coordination		1	1	1	1	6	3	9	3	1	7	25
Balance						4	4	3	2	1	1	9
	Scale					1	1	1	1			2
	Nintendo Wii					3	3	1	1			3
	Kinect							1				1
	Virtual Reality									1		1
Biofeedback		1	1			6	4	6	6	1	2	16

FUTURE RESEARCH DIRECTIONS

Main issues that require future research are related with:

- Patient's experience in-home physiotherapy setting (see Triberti et al., 2014);
- Patient health and ICT literacy (see Irizarry et al., 2015);
- ICT literacy of health professionals (see Kaye et al., 2010);
- ICT usability (see Triberti & Riva, 2014b; Irizarry et al., 2015);
- Privacy and security of data (see Coulter & Magee, 2003) in implemented information system for in-home physiotherapy;
- Standards and technologies for integrated, interoperable information systems based on common specifications for technology and end to end services (see Hoerbst & Ammenwerth, 2010);
- Optimal model of physiotherapists endorsement.

Various trials were initiated and will bring within 3-4 years' new evidence for what and when in-home physiotherapy should be to meet personal and provider needs. The analysis of objectives and methodologies of these future trials may foster new research worldwide both for better integration of mobile health and tele-rehabilitation technologies in-home physiotherapy and advancement in physiotherapy practice.

- The potential *identification of functional decline of older adults* registered at the department of emergency for a minor health event, *through a telephone screening process* within four weeks after discharge are investigated (Grimner et al., 2013). This might contribute for early detection of health and medical risk, and identification of subjects for which preventive programs may be more effective.
- Effectiveness of *tailored home based exercise programs for fall prevention* in elderly population (Gschwind et al., 2013), dwelling older with cognitive impairments (Close et al., 2014) or older adults identified as having unsteadiness during turning (Giangregorio et al., 2014) are also ongoing.
- Efficacy and effectiveness of *therapies based on specification of patient participation in everyday activities,* such as therapeutic goal (Barzel et al., 2013), *Tai Chi based exercise program provided via tele-rehabilitation* (Tousignant et al., 2014), *or Nintento Wii Sports*™ (Adie et al., 2014) are studied in stroke patients.
- The potential of *ICT on behavioural physiotherapy* proposed by Broetz and Birbaumer (2013) for post stroke patients, in which goals, exercises and tasks - based on observation and analysis of daily activities - are setting and anticipated as a "self-control cue"- should be investigated.
- A study on the *engagement on physical exercise* of patients with multiple sclerosis and the feasibility of conducting a full scale clinical and cost-effectiveness trial of a home-based physiotherapist *supported by Wii intervention* ('Mii-vitaliSe') is ongoing (Thomas et al., 2014).
- The effectiveness of *robotic-assisted home therapy* compared with a home exercise program, on upper extremity motor recovery and health-related quality of life for stroke survivors in rural and underserved locations are investigated (Linder et al., 2013). In this trial are also explored whether initial degree of motor function of the upper limb may be a factor in predicting the extent to which patients with stroke may be responsive to home therapy approach.
- A randomized clinical trial evaluating the feasibility of *a home-based exercise program designed to increase physical activity (PA) and reduce the risk of cardiovascular disorders in subjects with human immunodeficiency virus (HIV)* was also initiated (Jaggers et al., 2013).

- *Internet-based multimodal program* - Move it to improve it (Mitii) comprising physical activity *for upper-limb and cognitive training* are evaluated in people with cerebral palsy (Boyd et al., 2013). In addition to better accessibility, the Mitii study aims to test the efficacy and cost-effectiveness of Mitii program for upper-limb function and motor planning, as well as to investigate neurovascular mechanisms related with upper limb motor function.
- A new program for *cardiac rehabilitation based on tele-guidance for improvement of self-management skills,* like self-efficacy and action planning for independent exercise and, consequently, for long-term engagement on physical fitness and physical activity, was designed and is evaluated (Kraal, Peek, van den Akker-Van Marle, & Kemps, 2013). This is in line with the new proposed model for better management of health care costs in which *quantified self* might be a tool for personalized health care and proactive participation of population in health decisions. In this context, *e-Patients* (see list of definitions) potential for improving quality of care is nowadays analyzed.
- An interesting new technology was described in an article published by Mortazavi et al. (2014) team in which *body-wearable sensors were used for exergame with near-realistic motions.* An enjoyable game is produced by technology that combines acquisition of data related with real world activities, realizes pattern recognition and uses algorithm for serious game. The designed classification algorithm in this work has precision of 77%, compared with 40% precision on current activity monitoring algorithms used for general daily living activities. It is not an optimal precision but it is an important direction of research that should be followed.
- An innovative, *computer-based gaming platform based on instrumentation with a motion-sense mouse which should transform broad range of common objects into therapeutic input devices* was designed and it is being evaluated (Srikesavan, Shay, Robinson, & Szturm, 2013). By using this technology, for control and play of any computer game, algorithm based on acquired movements that replicate common situation in everyday living, can be used. The system was designed for patients with rheumatoid arthritis, or osteoarthritis of the hand, for which training of graded finger mobility, strength, endurance or fine/gross dexterous functions may be realized using personalized objects. *This Internet of Things (IoT) based technology*(see Gubbi, Buyya, Marusic, & Palaniswami, 2013) is in line with trends on smart home technology (see representation from Figure 6, of the emergence, adoption, maturity, and impact on applications of specific technologies which is named *hype cycle,* for 2015). Connecting everyday existing objects and embedding intelligence in-home environment not only harvests information from the inhabitants and

Figure 6. Hype cycle for emerging technologies
(Gartner Inc., 2015)

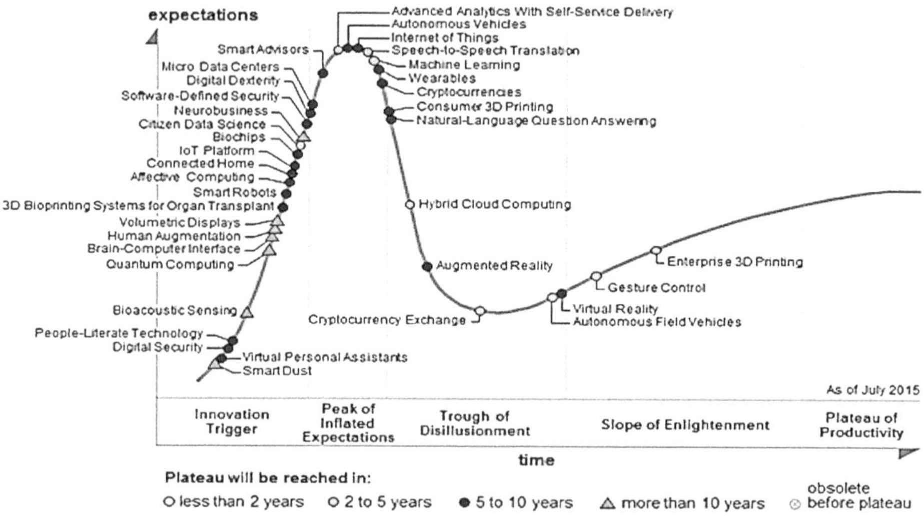

home environment, and allows augmented interaction with physical world, but also might provide a context awareness where the context is used to prevent information overload problem and to present *"the 'right' information, at the 'right' time, in the 'right' place, in the 'right' way to the 'right' person"* (Fischer, 2012).

Technology for in-home health care evolve towards continuous monitoring without any manual interventions, thus reducing provider patient interaction and cost while contributing to improvements in the quality of the data. For technology to disappear from the consciousness of the user (Gubbi et al., 2013) is required (1) a shared understanding of the situation of its users and their appliances, (2) software architectures and pervasive communication networks to process and convey the contextual information to where it is relevant, and (3) the analytics tools in the Internet of Things that aim for autonomous and smart behavior.

With move from www (static pages web) to web2 (social networking web) and to web3 (ubiquitous computing web) (Gubbi et al., 2013) health care services will need to adapt in order to create a new model of providing care. Real-time, face-to-face counseling with an expert health provider, and virtual meeting with support group might be provided in-home physiotherapy through ICT. For instance, *Doctor on Demand* lets people in U.S.A. to request a rapid video consultation with physician. Prescription can be sent electronically to the patient's nearest pharmacy. The cost for this video consultation can be as little as $40. *MDlive*, a competitor, in U.S.A., also offers quick video consultations, for $49. *Contact a Family* organization (www.cafamily.org.uk) has set up a virtual reality based on their own office where parents of disabled children meet, share information and provide support to each other.

IoT, context awareness, mobile technologies, e-Patients (Ferguson, 2007; Gee, Paterniti, Ward, & Soederberg, 2015; Bujnowska-Fedak & Kurpas, 2015), personal health records (PHRs) (Postolache, Girão, & Postolache, 2013), patient centered medical home (PCMH) (Stange et al., 2010) integrated in electronic health records (EHRs) (Williams & Samarth, 2011) will radically change home health care services, and until an optimal model will be found, cautions and in deep analysis of the advantages and drawbacks of various techniques is need.

It is desirable the development of cost-effective structural *solutions based on hierarchical and adaptive combination of low-cost, non-invasive and unobtrusive technologies capable of performing a wide array of multiple functions for training and care.* The basic idea is to design and develop a sort of 'fractal' and 'hierarchical' elements that can be easily put together to form higher level modules/components (module that build modules) for structural and functional sensing, and tailored rehabilitation. Several ongoing researches might contribute to this trend. The European project EASY-IMP has as main objective development of wearable meta-products for rehabilitation in which the functionalities will be configured by the end-users. This infrastructure will enable creation of new services for smartphone and for EASY users, and 'infinite applications in many target market'. In European research project CareStore an open and flexible infrastructure for facilitating seamless deployment and integration of assisted living devices and applications on heterogeneous platforms without requiring intervention from technical staff is in deployment (Wagner et al., 2013).

Promising, low cost, non-invasive, unobtrusive technologies are continuously presented and comprehensive researches on the effectiveness and large scale implementation of these technologies are required. Each year, many of innovative designs and technologies (e.g. many developed applications based on mobile applications for physiotherapy) with potential gains for health care disappear, as a consequences of low incentive for integration of new technologies, outdate risk-based regulatory framework, inefficient business model, and insufficient training of health professionals and general population for active search and integration of new technologies in daily life. Regulation and standardization of the new technologies for in-home health care is a slow process, and should be adapted to increase velocity of disruptive innovations in-home health care, in order to incorporate elements such as software reliance and cost-benefits analysis.

CONCLUSION

There is no lack of imagination for how to supply in-home physiotherapy and evidence exists on what and when physiotherapy intervention is more suited for better quality of service and cost-effectiveness of intervention. Small-scale efforts, pilot projects, and high level of evidence are increasing. There is a trend toward using feasible and acceptable in-home physiotherapy interventions combined with emerging ICT. Rigorous design of the in-home physiotherapy service incorporating ICT may lead to operational improvement and positive program outcome, augmented physiotherapists-patient relationships, autonomy and engagement of patients in regards to their healthcare. Also, this will provide environment for developing personalized, preventive, predictive and participatory physiotherapy, which will revolutionize healthcare management. ICT for in-home physiotherapy can contribute for integrated care programs (either vertically within healthcare system with continuing care, long-term care and self-management care or horizontal integration self-management care, nursing care, psychotherapy etc.). Training health care teams, informal caregivers and patients, to raise awareness and knowledge on information and communication technologies will greatly contribute for better in-home physiotherapy services and improve quality of life of patients receiving health care in-home setting. Researches should be made: for continuously description of what is known about the safety, feasibility and effectiveness of various in-home physiotherapy interventions; for dynamic adaptation of physiotherapy service in order to integrate multiple types of technologies for person-centered care in-home physiotherapy; and innovative financing mechanisms for in-home physiotherapy tools and services. Collaboration is needed (between public authorities, ICT providers, associations of physiotherapists and other health professionals, patient organizations, reimbursement scheme providers, insurer, medical devices and information technology regulatory organizations) for large-scale deployment of evidenced based in-home physiotherapy, and transferability of the results to other physiotherapy interventions.

REFERENCES

Adie, K., Schofield, C., Berrow, M., Wingham, J., Freeman, J., Humfryes, J., & Pritchard, C. (2014). Does the use of Nintendo Wii Sports improve arm function and is it acceptable to patients after stroke? Publication of the Protocol of the Trial of Wii in Stroke - TWIST. *International Journal of General Medicine*, *7*(1), 475–481. doi:10.2147/IJGM.S65379 PMID:25336985

Al-Jundi, W., Madbak, K., Beard, J. D., Nawaz, S., & Tew, G. A. (2013). Systematic review of home-based exercise programmes for individuals with intermittent claudication. *European Journal of Vascular and Endovascular Surgery*, *46*(6), 690–706. doi:10.1016/j.ejvs.2013.09.004 PMID:24076079

Alliance for Home Health Quality & Innovation. (2014). *The Future of Home Health Care Project*. Retrieved August, 2015, from http://www.ahhqi.org/images/pdf/future-whitepaper.pdf

Anderson, G., & Hussey, P. (2001). Comparing health system performance in OECD countries. *Health Affairs*, *20*(3), 219–232. doi:10.1377/hlthaff.20.3.219 PMID:11585171

Anderson, L., & Taylor, R. S. (2014). Cardiac rehabilitation for people with heart disease: An overview of Cohrane systematic reviews. *Cochrane Database of Systematic Reviews*, *12*, CD011273. PMID:25503364

Barello, S., & Graffigna, G. (2015). Patient engagement in healthcare: Pathways for effective medical decision-making. *Neuropsychological Trend*, *17*(17), 53–65. doi:10.7358/neur-2015-017-bare

Barzel, A., Ketels, G., Tetzlaff, B., Krüger, H., Haevernick, K., Daubmann, A., & Scherer, M. et al. (2013). Enhancing activities of daily living of chronic stroke patients in primary health care by modified constraint-induced movement therapy (HOMECIMT): Study protocol for a cluster randomized controlled trial. *Trials*, *14*, 334. PMID:24124993

Beratarrechea, A., Lee, A. G., Willner, J. M., Jahangir, E., Ciapponi, A., & Rubinstein, A. (2014). The impact of mobile health interventions on chronic disease outcomes in developing countries: A systematic review. *Telemedicine Journal and e-Health*, *20*(1), 75–82. doi:10.1089/tmj.2012.0328 PMID:24205809

Boyd, R. N., Mitchell, L. E., James, S. T., Ziviani, J., Sakzewski, L., Smith, A., & Scuffham, P. A. et al. (2013). Move it to improve it (Mitii): Study protocol of a randomised controlled trial of a novel web-based multimodal training program for children and adolescents with cerebral palsy. *BMJ Open*, *3*(4), 4. doi:10.1136/bmjopen-2013-002853 PMID:23578686

Broetz, D., & Birbaumer, N. (2013). Behavioral physiotherapy in post stroke rehabilitation. *NeuroRehabilitation*, *33*, 377–384. PMID:23949069

Bujnowska-Fedak, M. M., & Kurpas, D. (2015). The influence of online health information on the attitude and behavior of people Aged 50. *Advances in Experimental Medicine and Biology*, *861*, 1–17. doi:10.1007/5584_2015_130 PMID:26017724

Burton, E., Lewin, G., Clemson, L., & Boldy, D. (2013). Effectiveness of a lifestyle exercise program for older people receiving a restorative home care service: Pragmatic randomized controlled trial. *Clinical Interventions in Aging*, *8*, 1591–1601. doi:10.2147/CIA.S44614 PMID:24324331

Cancela, J., Moreno, E. M., Arredondo, M. T., & Bonato, P. (2014) Designing auditory cues for Parkinson's disease gait rehabilitation.*Proceedings IEEE Engineering in Medicine and Biology Society* (pp. 5852-5855).

Chan, Y., Wang, T., Chang, C., Chen, L., Chu, H., Lin, S., & Chang, S. (2015). Short-term effects of self-massage combined with home exercise on pain, daily activity, and autonomic function in patients with myofascial pain dysfunction syndrome. *Journal of Physical Therapy Science*, *27*(1), 217–221. doi:10.1589/jpts.27.217 PMID:25642077

Chien, C. L., Lee, C. M., Wu, Y. W., Chen, T. A., & Wu, Y. T. (2008). Home-based exercise increases capacity but not quality of life in people with chronic heart failure: A systematic review. *The Australian Journal of Physiotherapy*, *54*(2), 87–93. doi:10.1016/S0004-9514(08)70041-2 PMID:18491999

Cinel, C., Poli, R., Citi, L., & Robertson, D. (2013). An exploration of the effects of audio-visual entrainment on Parkinson's disease tremor.*Proceedings IEEE EMBS Conference on Neural Engineering* (pp. 1562-1565).

Close, J. C., Wesson, J., Sherrington, C., Hill, K. D., Kurrle, S., Lord, S. R., & Clemson, L. et al. (2014). Can a tailored exercise and home hazard reduction program reduce the rate of falls in community dwelling older people with cognitive impairment: Protocol paper for the i-FOCIS randomised controlled trial. *BMC Geriatrics*, *14*(89), 1–14. PMID:25128411

Coulter, A. (2005). What do patients and the public want from primary care? *BMJ (Clinical Research Ed.)*, *331*(7526), 1199–1201. doi:10.1136/bmj.331.7526.1199 PMID:16293845

Coulter, A., & Magee, H. (2003). *The European patient of the future*. McGraw Hill Education.

Coulter, C. L., Scarvell, J. M., Neeman, T. M., & Smith, P. N. (2013). Physiotherapist-directed rehabilitation exercises in the outpatient or home setting improve strength, gait speed and cadence after elective total hip replacement: A systematic review. *Journal of Physiotherapy*, *59*(4), 219–226. doi:10.1016/S1836-9553(13)70198-X PMID:24287215

Crocker, T., Young, J., Forster, A., Brown, L., Ozer, S., & Greenwood, D. C. (2013). The effect of physical rehabilitation on activities of daily living in older residents of long-term care facilities: Systematic review with meta-analysis. *Age and Ageing*, *42*(6), 682–688. doi:10.1093/ageing/aft133 PMID:24004604

Ferguson, T. (2007). *E-Patients: How they can help us heal healthcare.* Retrieved from http://e-patients.net/e-Patients_White_Paper.pdf

Fischer, G. (2012). Context-Aware Systems -The 'right' information, at the 'right' time, in the 'right' place, in the 'right' way, to the 'right' person. In G. Tortora, S. Levialdi, & M. Tucci (Eds.), *Proceedings of the Conference on Advanced Visual Interfaces (AVI 2012),*Capri, Italy (pp. 287-294). ACM.

Gartner Inc. (2015). *Gartner's 2015 hype cycle for emerging technologies identifies the computing innovations that organizations should monitor*. Retrieved from http://www.gartner.com/newsroom/id/3114217

Gee, P. M., Paterniti, D. A., Ward, D., & Soederberg Miller, L. M. (2015). e-Patients Perceptions of Using Personal Health Records for self-management Support of Chronic Illness. *Computers, Informatics, Nursing*, *33*(6), 229–237. doi:10.1097/CIN.0000000000000151 PMID:25899440

Giangregorio, L. M., Thabane, L., Adachi, J. D., Ashe, M. C., Bleakney, R. R., Braun, E. A., & Papaioannou, A. et al. (2014). Build better bones with exercise: Protocol for a feasibility study of a multicenter randomized controlled trial of 12 months of home exercise in women with a vertebral fracture. *Physical Therapy*, *94*(9), 1337–1352. doi:10.2522/ptj.20130625 PMID:24786946

Glasgow, R. E. (2013). *Reach, Effectiveness, Adoption, Implementation, and Maintenance (RE-AIM).* Retrieved from http://www.re-aim.hnfe.vt.edu/presentations/glasgow2013presentation.pdf

Grimmer, K., Luker, J., Beaton, K., Kumar, S., Crockett, A., & Price, K. (2013). Trialing individualized interventions to prevent functional decline in at-risk older adults (TRIIFL): Study protocol for a randomized controlled trial nested in a longitudinal observational study. *Trials*, *14*(1), 266. doi:10.1186/1745-6215-14-266 PMID:23962259

Gschwind, Y. J., Kressig, R. W., Lacroix, A., Muehlbauer, T., Pfenninger, B., & Granacher, U. (2013). A best practice fall prevention exercise program to improve balance, strength / power, and psychosocial health in older adults: Study protocol for a randomized controlled trial. *BMC Geriatrics*, *13*(1), 105. doi:10.1186/1471-2318-13-105 PMID:24106864

Gubbi, J., Buyya, R., Marusic, S., & Palaniswami, M. (2013). Internet of Things (IoT): A vision, architectural elements, and future directions. *Future Generation Computer Systems*, *29*(7), 1645–1660. doi:10.1016/j.future.2013.01.010

Gunn, H., Cattaneo, D., Finlayson, M., Freeman, J., & Sosnoff, J. J. (2014). Home or away? Choosing a setting for a falls-prevention program for people with multiple sclerosis. *International Journal of MS Care*, *16*(4), 186–191. doi:10.7224/1537-2073.2014-058 PMID:25694777

Hoerbst, A., & Ammenwerth, E. (2010). Electronic Health Records. A systematic review on quality requirements. *Methods of Information in Medicine*, *49*(4), 320–336. doi:10.3414/ME10-01-0038 PMID:20603687

Hood, L. E., & Galas, D. J. (2008). *P4 Medicine: personalized, predictive, preventive, participatory. A change of view that changes everything*. Washington: Computing Community Consortium. Retrieved from http://cra.org/ccc/wp-content/uploads/sites/2/2015/05/P4_Medicine.pdf

Imbeault-Nepton, I., & Otis, M. J. D. (2014). Synchronized walking cadence for TUG in perturbed environments: using Earcon or Tacton cues?*Proceedings of IEEE Internation Symposium on Haptic, Audio and Visual Environments and Games (HAVE)* (pp. 41-46). doi:10.1109/HAVE.2014.6954329

International Telecommunication Union. (2015). *The World Telecommunication/ICT Indicators Database*. Retrieved from http://www.itu.int/en/ITU-D/Statistics/Pages/stat/default.aspx

Irizarry, T., DeVito Dabbs, A., & Curran, C. R. (2015). Patient portals and patient engagement: A state of the science review. *Journal of Medical Internet Research*, *17*(6), e148. doi:10.2196/jmir.4255 PMID:26104044

Jaggers, J. R., Dudgeon, W., Blair, S. N., Sui, X., Burgess, S., Wilcox, S., & Hand, G. A. (2013). A home-based exercise intervention to increase physical activity among people living with HIV: Study design of a randomized clinical trial. *BMC Public Health*, *13*(1), 502. doi:10.1186/1471-2458-13-502 PMID:23706094

Jolly, K., Taylor, R., Lip, G. Y. H., Greenfield, S., Raftery, J., Mant, J., & Stevens, A. et al. (2007). The Birmingham Rehabilitation Uptake Maximisation Study (BRUM). Homebased compared with hospital-based cardiac rehabilitation in a multi-ethnic population: Cost-effectiveness and patient adherence. *Health Technology Assessment*, *11*(35), 1–118. doi:10.3310/hta11350 PMID:17767899

Jull, G., & Moore, A. (2013). Manual Therapy. *Manual Therapy*, *18*(6), 447–448. doi:10.1016/j.math.2013.09.006 PMID:24188381

Kaye, R., Kokia, E., Shalev, V., Idar, D., & Chinitz, D. (2010). Barriers and success factors in health information technology: A practitioner's perspective. *Journal of Management & Marketing in Healthcare*, *3*(2), 163–175. doi:10.1179/17533031 0X12736577732764

Kent, P., Laird, R., & Haines, T. (2015). The effect of changing movement and posture using motion-sensor biofeedback, versus guidelines-based care, on the clinical outcomes of people with sub-acute or chronic low back pain-a multicentre, cluster-randomised, placebo-controlled, pilot trial. *BMC Musculoskeletal Disorders*, *16*(1), 131. doi:10.1186/s12891-015-0591-5 PMID:26022102

Kraal, J. J., Peek, N., van den Akker-Van Marle, M. E., & Kemps, H. M. (2013). Effects and costs of home-based training with telemonitoring guidance in low to moderate risk patients entering cardiac rehabilitation: The FIT@Home study. *BMC Cardiovascular Disorders*, *13*(1), 82. doi:10.1186/1471-2261-13-82 PMID:24103384

Lee, H. N., Lee, S. Y., Lee, Y. S., Han, J. Y., Choo, M. S., & Lee, K. S. (2013). Pelvic floor muscle training using an extracorporeal biofeedback device for female stress urinary incontinence. *International Urogenicology Journal*, *24*(5), 831–838. doi:10.1007/s00192-012-1943-4 PMID:23052631

Linder, S. M., Rosenfeldt, A. B., Reiss, A., Buchanan, S., Sahu, K., Bay, C. R., & Alberts, J. L. et al. (2013). The home stroke rehabilitation and monitoring system trial: A randomized controlled trial. *International Journal of Stroke*, *8*(1), 46–53. doi:10.1111/j.1747-4949.2012.00971.x PMID:23280269

Lommi, M., Matarese, M., Alvaro, R., Piredda, M., & De Marinis, M. G. (2015). The experiences of self-care in community-dwelling older people: A meta-synthesis. *International Journal of Nursing Studies*, *52*(12), 1854–1867. doi:10.1016/j.ijnurstu.2015.06.012 PMID:26296653

McAuley, E., Wójcicki, T. R., Gothe, N. P., Mailey, E. L., Szabo, A. N., Fanning, J., & Mullen, S. P. et al. (2013). Effects of a DVD-delivered exercise intervention on physical function in older adults. *The Journals of Gerontology. Series A, Biological Sciences and Medical Sciences*, *68*(9), 1076–1082. doi:10.1093/gerona/glt014 PMID:23401566

Mehta, S. P., & Roy, J. S. (2011). Systematic revie of home physiotherapy after hip fracture surgery. *Journal of Rehabilitation Medicine*, *43*(6), 477–480. doi:10.2340/16501977-0808 PMID:21491074

Mhatre, P. V., Vilares, I., Stibb, S. M., Albert, M. V., Pickering, L., Marciniak, C. M., & Toledo, S. et al. (2013). Wii Fit balance board playing improves balance and gait in Parkinson disease. *PM & R*, *5*(9), 769–777. doi:10.1016/j.pmrj.2013.05.019 PMID:23770422

Mortazavi, B., Nyamathi, S., Lee, S. I., Wilkerson, T., Ghasemzadeh, H., & Sarrafzadeh, M. (2014). Near-realistic mobile exergames with wireless wearable sensors. *Biomedical and Health Informatics. IEEE Journal of*, *18*(2), 449–456.

Naylor, C., Parsonage, M., McDaid, D., Knap, M., Fossey, M., & Galea, A. (2012). *Long-term conditions and mental health. The cost of co-morbidities.* The Kings Fund Report. Retrieved from http://www.kingsfund.org.uk/sites/files/kf/field/field_publication_file/long-term-conditions-mental-health-cost-comorbidities-naylor-feb12.pdf

Nhavoto, J. A., & Gronlund, A. (2014). Mobile technologies and geographic information systems to improve health care systems: A literature review. *JMIR Mhealth and Uhealth*, *2*(2), e21. doi:10.2196/mhealth.3216 PMID:25099368

Novak, I. (2011). Effective home programme intervention for adults: A systematic review. *Clinical Rehabilitation*, *25*(12), 1066–1085. doi:10.1177/0269215511410727 PMID:21831927

Omran, A. R. (2005). First published 1971). The epidemiological transition: A theory of the epidemiology of population change. *The Milbank Quarterly*, *83*(4), 731–757. doi:10.1111/j.1468-0009.2005.00398.x PMID:16279965

Ontario, H. Q. (2013). In-home care for optimizing chronic disease management in the community: An evidence-based analysis. *Ontario Health Technology Assessment Series*, *13*(5), 1–65. PMID:24167539

Outpatient Service Trialists. (2004). Rehabilitation therapy services for stroke patients living at home: Systematic review of randomized trials. *Lancet*, *363*(9406), 352–356. doi:10.1016/S0140-6736(04)15434-2 PMID:15070563

Papalia, R., Vasta, S., Tecame, A., D'Adamio, S., Maffulli, N., & Denaro, V. (2013). Home-based vs supervised rehabilitation programs following knee surgery: A systematic review. *British Medical Bulletin*, *108*(1), 55–72. doi:10.1093/bmb/ldt014 PMID:23690452

Pepa, L., Ciabattoni, L., Verdini, F., Capecci, M., & Ceravolo, M. G. (2014). Smartphone based fuzzy logic freezing of gait detection in Parkinson's disease.*Proceeding IEEE/ASME Conference on Mechatronic and Embedded Systems and Applications (MESA)* (pp. 1-6).

Postolache, G., Girao, P. S., & Postolache, O. (2013). Requirements and barriers to pervasive health adoption. In S. C. Mukhopadhyay & O. A. Postolache (Eds.), *Pervasive and Mobile Sensing and Computing for Health Care. Technological and Social Issues* (pp. 315–352). Springer Verlag. doi:10.1007/978-3-642-32538-0_15

Rechel, B., Doyle, Y., Grundy, E., & McKee, M. (2009). *Policy brief. 10 Health system and policy analysis. How can health system respond to population ageing?* WHO Report. Retrieved from http://www.euro.who.int/__data/assets/pdf_file/0004/64966/E92560.pdf

Rodger, M. W., Young, W. R., & Craig, C. M. (2014). Synthesis of walking sounds for alleviating gait disturbances in Parkinson's. *IEEE Transactions on Neural Systems and Rehabilitation Engineering*, *22*(3), 543–548. doi:10.1109/TNSRE.2013.2285410 PMID:24235275

Siemonsma, P., Döpp, C., Alpay, L., Tak, E., van Meeteren, N., & Chorus, A. (2014). Determinants influencing the implementation of home-based stroke rehabilitation: A systematic review. *Disability and Rehabilitation*, *36*(24), 2019–2030. doi:10.3109/09638288.2014.885091 PMID:24520957

Sinclair, J., Hingston, P., & Masek, M. (2007). Considerations for the design of exergames.*Proceeding GRAPHITE'07 International Conference on Computer Graphics and Interactive Techniques in Australia and Southeast Asia* (pp. 289-295). doi:10.1145/1321261.1321313

Srikesavan, C. S., Shay, B., Robinson, D. B., & Szturm, T. (2013). Task-oriented training with computer gaming in people with rheumatoid arthritisor osteoarthritis of the hand: Study protocol of a randomized controlled pilot trial. *Trials*, *14*(1), 69. doi:10.1186/1745-6215-14-69 PMID:23497529

Stange, K. C., Nutting, P. A., Miller, W. L., Jaén, C. R., Crabtree, B. F., Flocke, S. A., & Gill, J. M. (2010). Defining and measuring the patient-centered medical home. *Journal of General Internal Medicine*, *25*(6), 601–612. doi:10.1007/s11606-010-1291-3 PMID:20467909

Takekawa, T., Abo, M., Ebihara, K., Taguchi, K., Sase, Y., & Kakuda, W. (2013). Long-term effects of injection of botulinum toxin type A combined with home-based functional training for post-stroke patients with spastic upper limb hemiparesis. *Acta Neurologica Belgica*, *113*(4), 469–475. doi:10.1007/s13760-013-0208-4 PMID:23716062

Thomas, M. J., Simpson, J., Riley, R., & Grant, E. (2010). The impact of home-based physiotherapy interventions on breathlessness during activities of daily living in severe COPD: A systematic review. *Physiotherapy*, *96*(2), 108–119. doi:10.1016/j.physio.2009.09.006 PMID:20420957

Thomas, S., Fazakarley, L., Thomas, P. W., Brenton, S., Collyer, S., Perring, S., & Hillier, C. et al. (2014). Testing the feasibility and acceptability of using the Nintendo Wii in the home to increase activity levels, vitality and well-being in people with multiple sclerosis (Mii-vitaliSe): Protocol for a pilot randomised controlled study. *BMJ Open*, *4*(5), e005172. doi:10.1136/bmjopen-2014-005172 PMID:24812193

Tousignant, M., Corriveau, H., Kairy, D., Berg, K., Dubois, M. F., Gosselin, S., & Danells, C. et al. (2014). Tai Chi-based exercise program provided via telerehabilitation compared to home visits in a post-stroke population who have returned home without intensive rehabilitation: Study protocol for a randomized, non-inferiority clinical trial. *Trials*, *15*(1), 42. doi:10.1186/1745-6215-15-42 PMID:24479760

Tractica. (2015). *Home health technologies, medical monitoring and management, remote consultations, eldercare, and health and wellness applications: Global market analysis and forecast*. Retrieved August, 2015, from https://www.tractica.com/research/home-health-technologies/

Triberti, S., Barello, S., Graffigna, G., Riva, G., Candelieri, A., & Archetti, F. (2014). Evaluating patient engagement and user experience of a positive technology intervention: the H-CIM case. In G. Graffigna, S. Barello, & S. Triberti (Eds.), *Patient Engagement. A consumer Centered Model to Innovate Healthcare* (pp. 66–77). De Gruyter Open.

Triberti, S., & Riva, G. (2014a). Positive technology for enhancing the patient engagement experiences. In G. Graffigna, S. Barello, & S. Triberti (Eds.), *Patient Engagement. A consumer Centered Model to Innovate Healthcare* (pp. 44–55). De Gruyter Open.

Triberti, S., & Riva, G. (2014b). Engaging users to design positive technologies for patient engagement: the perfect interaction model. In G. Graffigna, S. Barello, & S. Triberti (Eds.), *Patient Engagement. A consumer Centered Model to Innovate Healthcare* (pp. 56–65). De Gruyter Open.

Tzallas, A. T., Tsipouras, M. G., Rigas, G., Tsalikakis, D. G., Karvounis, E. C., Chondrogiorgi, M., & Fotiadis, D. I. et al. (2014). PERFORM: A system for monitoring, assessment and management of patients with Parkinson's disease. *Sensors (Basel)*, *14*(11), 21329–21357. doi:10.3390/s141121329 PMID:25393786

Valdes, K., Naughton, N., & Michlovitz, S. (2014). Therapist supervised clinic-based therapy versus instruction in a home program following distal radius fracture: A systematic review. *Journal of Hand Therapy*, *27*(3), 165–174. doi:10.1016/j.jht.2013.12.010 PMID:24508093

Wagner, S., Hansen, F. O., Pedersen, C. F., Memon, M., Aysha, F. H., Mathissen, M., & Wesby, O. L. et al. (2013). CareStore Platform for seamless deployment of ambient assited living applications and devices.*Proceedings of International Conference on Pervasive Computing Technologies for Healthcare and Workshops* (pp. 240-243).

Williams, T., & Samarth, A. (2011). *Electronic Health Records for Dummies*. Hobokem, NJ: Wiley Publishing, Inc.

Zhao, Y., Anhalt, F., Fietzek, U. M., & D'Angelo, L. T. (2013). Multi-cue unit: An independent device and actuator of a wearable system for gait-support in Parkinson patients.*Proceedings of IEEE International Conference on Microwaves, Communications, Antennas and Electronics Systems (COMCAS)* (pp. 1-5). doi:10.1109/COMCAS.2013.6685287

KEY TERMS AND DEFINITIONS

Biofeedback: Process that enables an individual to learn how to change body signals for the purposes of improving health and performance. It is necessary a precise measurement of body function and rapidly and accurately "feedback" information to the user. The presentation of this information supports desired function changes. Some recent examples of biofeedback use in physiotherapy are: extracorporeal biofeedback for female stress urinary incontinence, motion-sensor biofeedback in people with low back pain reduced pain and activity limitation.

E-Patients: Also known as Internet patient, is a health consumer who uses the Internet to gather information about a medical condition of particular interest to him, and who uses electronic communication tools (including Web 2.0 tools) in coping with medical conditions. The term encompasses both those who seek online guidance for their own ailments and the friends and family members (e-Caregivers) who go online on their behalf. Tom Ferguson have coined in 2007 E-Patients as individuals who are equipped, enabled, empowered and engaged in their health and health care decisions. E-Patients report two effects of their online health research – 'better health information and services, and different (but not always better) relationship with their doctors". PatientLikeMe, BrainTalk Communities, NeuroTalk are E-Patients social networks. The importance of E-Patients as consumer, curators and creators of information, are recently recognized and investigated. Understanding the frequency and characteristics of pronetariat (term coined by Joel de Rosnay, in 2005) in E-Patient group will be interesting.

Exergame: Term used for video games that are also a form of exercise. In context of health services, the term can be found also as Serious Game or Teragame – software or hardware based on interactive game, designed for the purpose of solving a problem, to train or educate users. Although serious games can be entertaining, their main purpose is more for training or education of the users. Serious game will sometimes deliberately sacrifice fun and entertainment in order to achieve a desired progress by the player. Exergames based on Nintendo Wii ™ technology were among the first games used on rehabilitation. Various games are now developed for Xbox Kinect technology, for smartphone (e.g. games apps from Google play and ITune store), or commercialized together with software for rehabilitation management (e.g. MIRARehab, BioGaming).

Information and Communication Technologies (ICT): Set of technologies that arise from information and advanced telecommunication and multi-media techniques which allow better communication means, information processing, storing, exchange and dissemination (adapted from OQLF/French wikipedia). ICT stresses the role of unified communications and the integration of telecommunications (telephone lines and wireless communication), Internet, multimedia, computers as well as necessary enterprise software, middleware, storage, and audio-visual systems, which enable users to access, store, transmit, and manipulate information through various means: text, video, audio, human-machine interface, etc.

Internet of Things (IoT): (Sometimes *Internet of Everything*). Was first coined by Kevin Ashton in 1999 in the context of supply chain management. However, in the past decade, the definition has been more inclusive covering wide range of applications like healthcare, utilities, transport, etc. Although the definition of 'Things' has changed as technology evolved, the main goal of making computer sense information without the aid of human intervention remains the same. It means a network of physical objects or "things" embedded with electronics, software, sensors and connectivity that enable it to achieve greater value and service by exchanging data with the manufacturer, operator and/or other connected devices based on the infrastructure of International Telecommunication Union's Global Standards Initiative. Each thing is uniquely identifiable through its embedded computing system, but is able to interoperate within the existing Internet infrastructure. Typically, IoT is expected to offer advanced connectivity of devices, systems, and services that goes beyond machine-to-machine communications (M2M) and covers a variety of protocols, domains, and applications. The interconnection of these embedded devices (including smart objects), is expected to usher in automation in nearly all fields, and expanding to the areas such as smart city.

PHRs: Health data and information related to the care of a patient is maintained by the patient. PHRs can be broadly described as a set of electronic tools that allow consumers to access, coordinate, and control appropriate parts of their health information. PHRs combine not only data, but knowledge and software tools, which motivate patients to become more involved in their healthcare. A PHR should typically present a comprehensive and precise review of the health and medical history of the individual patient through the collection of information from a variety of sources. PHRs, whether through patient portals, electronic downloads onto a personal USB drive, or through a company sponsored Web site (e.g. MyAlert, HealthKit iOS), allow patients timely access to their medical information. According HL7 standard PHRs shall: allow for historical clinical data and current state data management; assist the PHRs account holder to manage his or her compliance with medications and facilitate communication of his or her adherence to designed individuals; manage health education; support wellness, preventive medicine and self-care; support decision making; manage encounters with healthcare providers. Since it is retained, maintained and controlled by the consumer, the PHR positions the consumer at the core of the healthcare process, potentially fostering personal empowerment and facilitating self-management or quantified self, shared decision making and better clinical outcomes.

Virtual Reality (VT): Is computer based interactive, visual, and/or audio, and/or haptic (interaction involving touch), and/or immersive (providing information or stimulation for a number of senses, not only sight and sound, that deeply involve one's senses and may change mental state) simulation of real, imaginary or symbolic environment. The term virtual is used with meaning of digital, immaterial, 'quasi' real. There are many types of VR environments, from simple computer based games played on a computer, tablet, smartphone, TV screen with a mouse or other interface (e.g. MIRARehab, YouRehab, CoRehab, I Am a Dolphin apps developed by John Hopkins Hospital, PocketPhysio, Hand Rehab, Button Board apps for smartphone, Nintendo Wii, Xbox Kinect, PlayStation games, SecondLife) to life-like scenarios created in a large space in which the user sees the environment all around them (INJOY Quality Cooperation GmbH, Realyz-Mobilyz, CAVE, Icube, SASCube). By contrast, with virtual reality that replaces the real world with a simulated one in augmented reality, real, physical world can be seen directly or indirectly together with augmentation (computer-generation sensory input such as sound, video, graphics, GPS data). For instance, the developed software for Augmedix healthcare service, or Kinesio Capture apps for smartphone use augmented reality. Mixed Reality, a mix of the physical and virtual reality, refers to the merging of real and virtual worlds to produce new environments and visualizations where physical and digital objects co-exist and interact in real time. Windows Holographyc is a mixed reality computing platform developed by Microsoft. Various interfaces were developed for interaction with virtual reality – Leap Motion, Microsoft Kinect, Nimble from Intugine Technologies, Wii Remote, Wii Balance Board, iKids Interactive Zone, Gloveone, Fit Interactive's fitness system 3 Kick, Virtuix Omni, Oculos Rift, Samsung Gear VR, ZSpace, Google Cardboard, Epson Moverio BT-200, Microsoft Hololens).

Chapter 10
Healthy Avatars, Healthy People:
Care Engagement Through the Shared Experience of Virtual Worlds

Stefano Triberti
Catholic University of the Sacred Heart, Italy

Alice Chirico
Catholic University of the Sacred Heart, Italy

ABSTRACT

Recent literature shows that new technologies can be used to promote patient engagement. The present contribution focuses on Virtual Worlds (VWs), namely virtual environments that multiple users can experience together thanks to the use of avatars. Indeed, VWs offer interesting opportunities for patient engagement interventions on two levels. On the individual level, customized avatars are known to have relationships with users' inner experience and Self-conception, so that they may constitute a peculiar additional tool for psychological assessment. Moreover, they are able to promote healthy behaviors thanks to a strong vicarious reinforcement (Proteus effect). On the collective level, VWs constitute an ideal platform to support the emergence of collective flow states (Networked Flow) which are related to the patients' creative activity and well-being. The present contribution deepens these phenomena, presenting VWs as an innovative and interesting tool for the patient engagement interventions of the future.

DOI: 10.4018/978-1-5225-0663-8.ch010

INTRODUCTION

In this chapter we will discuss the role of new technologies for patient engagement, according to the model of patient engagement of Barello, Graffigna, Vegni and Bosio (2014), Graffigna and Barello (2015), Barello and Graffigna (2014). In details, we will focus on a specific virtual reality tool called Virtual Worlds (VWs), in order to show their implications for healthcare, from both an individual and a group perspective.

The model of patient engagement (PHE) (Graffina, Barello & Triberti, 2015) depicts a picture of the process in which a patient is involved during his/her everyday life experience of disease management. This process emerged as multi componential and dynamic because it regards the whole people's life, which is embraced in all its complexity.

In details, it is the conjunction of emotional (ability to cope with stress and negative emotions due to illness), cognitive (looking for adequate information regarding one's own illness and comprehending all its implications) and behavioral dimensions (adopting adaptive behaviors; adhering to treatment and medication) of people's lives that is responsible for their health engagement (Graffigna & Barello, 2015). The synergy among these dimensions influences patients' ability to adapt to the situation and to interpret personal disease as a normal experience of life which can be included in the broader perspective of existence.

Further, the model suggests that the above-mentioned process of patient engagement is composed of four phases whose synergy is necessary for a patient to benefit from all the resources provided by the healthcare system:

1. **Blackout:** It refers to the feeling of emotive, cognitive and behavioral blackout in which a patient is involved after the occurrence of a critical event, usually receiving the diagnosis.
2. **Arousal:** The name of this phase reflects its own main feature. Indeed, patients become more "activated", but as the terms "arousal" suggests, it is a general activation that does not lead to adopting adaptive coping strategies.
3. **Adhesion:** Even though the patients become more competent both regarding their health and the treatment rules they have to follow, they are still passive in complying with medical prescriptions because they don't understand deeply the meaning of the actions suggested by the medical professionals.
4. **Eudaimonic Project:** Patients are perfectly aware of their condition and accept it and all its implications. In other words, and in order to summarize this complex process, patient initially experience a state of complete disengagement,

then they move to a phase of activation (i.e., arousal), adhesion, in which they are still passive, to the building of their personal "eudaimonic project" in which the person is able to reframe disease into normal everyday life (Graffigna & Barello, 2015).

But, how can this model be so effective in healthcare contexts? Which is the added value that this model can provide?

First, the application of this model in health contexts allows facing the increased demand for health which concerns this period of time in which, thanks to the new discoveries and treatments in medicine, survival leading has been increased and there are more aged people than in the past (Graffigna, Barello, Wiederhold, Bosio, & Riva, 2013). This means that people are more likely to suffer for chronic diseases, a type of pathological situation which entails substantial costs for healthcare system.

According to this model, a chronic patient would become able to activate and maintain adaptive behaviors devoted to the management of the situation (behavioral component); to look for adequate information and cognitively structure both the management of the disease and the adherence to the therapy (cognitive component); to cope with the illness-related stress and negative emotions, and also to recover the ability to positively project his/her own life in the future (emotional component) (Barello et al., 2014; Graffigna, Barello, Libreri, & Bosio, 2014).

Moreover, engaging people in their healthcare helps them to co-build their own health together with healthcare professionals and to maintain social relationships and an active role inside their original community. In other words, people can become "advocates of good health" from a broader perspective.

Finally, one of the most relevant features of this model is its suitability to different types of chronic diseases, such as diabetes (Graffigna et al., 2014), cancer (Graffigna, Vegni, Barello, Olson, & Bosio, 2011), different types of addiction (Simpson, 2004) and chronic pain (Cracken, 2005).

Patients can be supported across all these phases in several ways. One of the most effective can be found in the use of new technologies to sustain patient's care experience (Graffigna & Barello, 2015; Graffigna, Barello, & Riva, 2013a, 2013b; Triberti & Riva, 2015a).

According to the positive technology paradigm (Botella et al., 2012; Riva, Baños, Botella, Wiederhold, & Gaggioli, 2012; Triberti & Riva, 2015a), new technologies can be used to structure, augment or even replace the features of an experience. Indeed, they are able to support the individuals in their daily routine and personal issues, contributing to a change in the perception of individuals' own life.

In details, new technologies can address this issue from three perspectives: Hedonic (using technologies to enhance or support the emerging of positive experiences); Eudaimonic (technologies are used as tools to sustain individuals' self-actualization); Social/interpersonal (technologies are used to promote connectedness among individuals) (Riva et al., 2012).

An interesting and still understudied example of the above-mentioned new technologies able to support the care experience and their level of engagement are Virtual Worlds.

NEW FRONTIERS FOR THE PROMOTION OF PATIENT ENGAGEMENT: THE NEW WORLD OF VIRTUAL WORLDS

As written above, new technologies constitute an interesting resource to foster and promote patient engagement. Indeed, recent literature shows how new technologies in general can be used in the context of interventions to this goal, for example, it is evidenced how a given technology can be used to promote the patient moving from a phase to another in the context of his/her own engagement development (Graffigna et al., 2013a, 2013b; Graffigna et al., 2014; Graffigna et al., 2013; Triberti & Riva, 2015a). However, studies focused on peculiar types of technological tools are still rare. In order to partially fill this gap, the present contribution focuses on Virtual Worlds (VWs), providing insights and examples of how they can be used in the context of patient engagement interventions.

Virtual Words are considered a sort of "successor" of Virtual Reality, in that they provide users with the possibility to share the experience of an interactive virtual environment through the creation, customization and use of avatars (Morie & Chance, 2011). In this sense, they combine the advantages of VR's three-dimensional immersive environments with the connectivity and peer support offered by social networks. On the other hand, VWs, compared to virtual reality, are characterized by persistence. In other words, these worlds do not stop existing and functioning after a participant has left. This property is specific to VWs and leads to new possibilities of interaction among users. Indeed, they allow shared activities among users through a synchronous communication modality (i.e., real time communication).

Famous examples of these peculiar media are *Second Life*, *Active Worlds* and *the Sims*.

VWs have been extensively used in the context of eLearning. According to the critical review by Loke (2015), VWs allow the users to learn knowledge and abilities at least in four ways. First, the users have the occasion to reflect on the events and the activities depicted in the virtual environment; second, they have the occasion to engage into verbal interactions with others, so they are able to share ideas and information; third, they are likely to perform cognitive processes (problem solving, decision making) if invited to resolve/cope with the virtually-simulated problems; fourth, they benefit of vicarious experiences and vicarious learning, in that they are able to see and imitate other people (or at least the digital representations of them) performing desirable actions and decisions.

In the context of learning studies, VWs showed to be more enjoyable, interesting and engaging than other tools and instruments (Pellas & Kazanidis, 2013; Tokel & İsler, 2013; Warburton, 2009).

Precisely, Pellas and Kazanidis (2013, 2014) analyzed the engagement promoted by VWs in users basing on a model entailing multiple factors, similar to the patient engagement which is of interest here. They noticed that the experience in VWs-for-learning features promising components such as the cognitive (self-regulation, investment in learning, learning goals…), the emotional (interest, identification, belonging, positive attitude…) and the behavioral ones (positive conduct, effort, participation…).

Basing on the first experiences as a resource for learning, VWs use made its way in the field of healthcare too. Precisely, both virtual reality and VWs have been used to train health professionals in their relational and communicational skills (Triberti & Liberati, 2014). For example, Sweigart and colleagues (Sweigart, Burden, Carlton, & Fillwalk, 2014) analyzed the effects of using a virtual clinic constructed inside *Second Life* to support nursing students' interviewing skills. The results showed the VW being a useful tool to recreate the setting for unfolding, multicultural, mu-tigenerational case studies. Similar conclusions are reported by other researchers (El Tantawi, Kashlan, & Saeed, 2013; Sweigart & Hodson-Carlton, 2013; Tiffany & Hoglund, 2014).

However, this intervention goal falls beyond the scope of the present chapter. Here, the focus will be on the possible uses of VWs as directed to patients, in particular in order to promote their engagement in the process of healthcare.

In the next sections, it will be showed how the experience of VWs may be of interest from two different (yet interdependent) viewpoints.

On the one hand, VWs allow the creation and customization of avatars, that are, digital representations of their users; on the individual level, this peculiar phenomenon presents interesting opportunities for healthcare projects.

On the other hand, VWs feature the possibility to build, maintain and transform relationship with others in the context of the virtual experience; rather than being "simply" a resource for social and relational benefits, this characteristic of VWs can be very interesting for patient engagement interventions in that it allows the promotion of shared experiences of knowledge and strategy/activity building.

The next two sections will deepen the above-mentioned aspects.

THE INDIVIDUAL LEVEL: AVATARS AND HEALTH

The word avatar comes from Sanskrit and originally referred to gods incarnating in humans. The word made its way through the field of New Media since the video game *Ultima Online – Quest of the Avatar* (Origin Systems, 1985), where it referred to a single fictional character. Later, this term was used to indicate any digital form or content that identifies the action and/or the communication by a human subject inside digital environments. In the context of video games and VWs, avatars are nearly always anthropomorphic figures.

While in video games it is possible to receive an avatar that is already designed by the game itself, in VWs avatars are often created and customized by the players.

Avatars are an interesting topic for cyber-psychology for at least two reasons.

First, they may have relationships with the identity and/or Self of their users; second, the research demonstrated that they are able to influence their users' behavior.

A debate exists about avatar constituting a more or less accurate representation of the users' Selves or not. According to the first theories (Gee, 2003; Kolko, 1998), when a VW (or video game) user create an avatar, he/she has to perform a "selection" among properties and features of his/her own Self representation, in order to "transfer" them in the avatar. The user can customize the appearance of the avatar resembling characteristics of his/her own appearance, and also artifacts and signs relating to interests, ideas, emotions and personality traits. In their customized features, user-created avatars showed to be sensitive also to age and gender (Martey et al., 2015; Villani, Gatti, Confalonieri, & Riva, 2012). According to these theories, avatars should be considered representations of identity.

Other researchers highlighted that not always users create avatars to represent themselves. One may create an avatar "just to try" to be a different person or even a different creature (Fox & Ahn, 2013); moreover, research showed that avatar creation may be sensitive to the context the avatar has to enter. For example (Vasalou & Joinson, 2009), users who expected to enter a dating-related VW created more attractive avatars.

Another field of research is the "avatar Self-discrepancy" one (Dunn & Guadagno, 2012; Jin, 2012), which sustains that users may create avatars to express *desired* renditions of the Selves. A perceived avatar-Self discrepancy has been associated with users' dissatisfaction with real life (Trepte & Reinecke, 2010) and users' intention to gain better mastery of the VW (Trepte, Reinecke, & Behr, 2009) .

Triberti and Argenton (2013) proposed an identity-construction model to show what identity and context materials are present for the user who want to create/customize an avatar, and what can guide his/her selection according to precise intentions.

The model crosses the theories of Social Identity (Tajfel & Turner, 2004) and Real/Ideal Self (Higgins, 1987). Figure 1 shows that the extremes of these theories are crossed to create four quarters.

The four quarters show possible avatars that can be created by a single user, depending on the virtual context and on his/her personal intentions.

Quarter 1 (Q1) and quarter 4 (Q4) show avatars created to resemble a personal idea of oneself, the first focusing on what the person thinks to be at the present moment, the second focusing on desired/prefigured renditions of the Self.

Quarter 2 (Q2) and quarter 3 (Q3) contains avatars that are created by a user who plan to enter a VW (or a multiplayer online game) where other people are present. These avatars may feature peculiar differences in order to be recognizable by others, or in order to communicate to them precise emotions, personality traits or ideas.

This model is useful to show how the creation of an avatar may be complex and related to one's own Self in many ways.

As said before, avatars not only have interesting relationship with Self and identity. They are also able to influence behavior.

Figure 1. Model for avatar identity construction
(adapted from Triberti & Argenton, 2013)

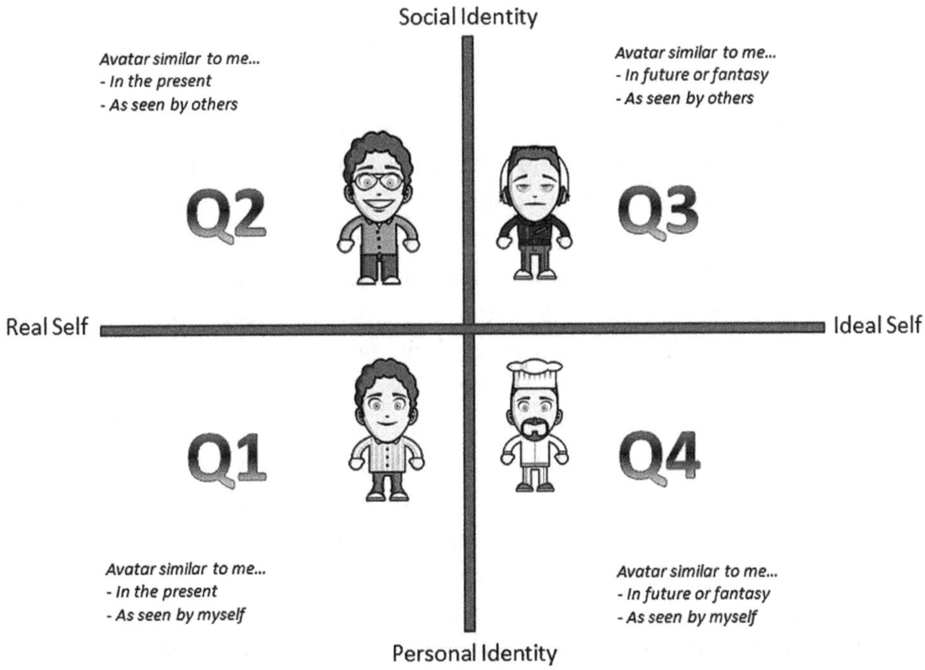

Basing on the mythological figure able to change his own form, researchers labeled *Proteus effect* (Fox, Bailenson, & Tricase, 2013; Yee, Bailenson, & Ducheneaut, 2009; Yee & Bailenson, 2007) the phenomenon of one's behavior modified by guiding a certain avatar. For example, guiding taller avatars moved users to behave more aggressively during virtual reality based negotiation games; using attractive avatars moved users to be more self-confident during virtual interactions.

In the next section, these phenomena will be deepened in the context of healthcare and patient engagement.

Avatars for Healthcare and Patient Engagement

After the brief introduction about avatars in the last paragraph, the present paragraph will deepen their utility as a resource for healthcare and for patient engagement interventions in particular.

As previously said, avatars maintain some kind of relationship with their users' Selves. Although this relation may be complex and influenced by different factors (e.g., avatars can be representation of the Self; just an identity experimentation; a desired rendition of the Self), it is clear that they can be considered as indicator of the inner experience of people.

Some studies already tested the possibility to use customized avatars as information about the users' characteristics, ranging from personality traits to stages of development (Fong & Mar, 2015; Villani et al., 2012). Other studies explored the virtual representation of life experiences through avatars customization and action inside VWs; for example, Lomanowska and Guitton (2014) analyzed the virtual re-enactment of pregnancy, birth and maternity inside *Second Life*.

Patient engagement, or more precisely, the phase of care engagement a given patient is in, is known to have peculiar influences on his/her own conception of the Self (Barello & Graffigna, 2014). For example, a chronic patient in the blackout phase is living the experience of the establishing of a diagnosis, which means he/she is struggling with the emotional shock deriving from realizing he/she is now a person with a disease: for this reason, the patient perceives him/herself as a "ill body", and is completely absorbed in the illness experience. Differently, the last stages of the patient engagement process allow one to recover his/her own life project despite the presence of the disease and the need to daily adhere to treatment and comply with caregivers and health professionals advices. Again according to Barello and Graffigna (2014), the patient now understands that the "patient self" is only one of the possible Selves, so that he/she is able to recognize his/her internal resources as useful to project satisfactory life trajectories for the future (Barello et al., 2015).

On this basis, if used in conjunction with other assessment tools, the avatar can be considered as a resource to analyze a patient's inner experience, in terms of what he/she thinks to be, or what he/she desires to become/achieve in the future. For example, it is possible to assume that patients in early stages of the engagement process may be driven to represent themselves with a limited number of features, or they may represent themselves highlighting visual features related to the disease or to the emotionally-difficult situation they are living. Differently, patients who start recovering positive conceptions of the Selves projected in the future may customize avatars with a higher number of features identifying passions and interests. In this sense, when imagining a patient engagement intervention which makes use of VWs for patients, the customization of avatars may be a supplemental tool for psychological analysis and assessment, and also a tool to guide patients' interviews deepening their evolving Self-conception.

With regard to the second interesting aspect of avatar, namely their ability in modifying behavior, it has been already used in the context of healthcare interventions.

For example, Murray and colleagues (Murray, Hardy, Spruijt-Metz, Hekler, & Raij, 2013) proposed a classification of avatars' features (physical, behavioral and environmental, that is modification of the environment where the avatar resides) to provide feedback to patients about their progress in disease treatment; for instance, avatar's strength in lifting objects may be an indication of the user's empowered ability due to rehabilitation exercises.

According to Kim and Sundar (2012), participants who created their avatars resembling ideal Selves then obtained positive outcomes (in terms of promotion and prevention-focused Self-regulatory strategies) for health management.

Another experiment (Fox & Bailenson, 2009) showed that participants who saw a digital representation of themselves doing physical exercise then performed more physical exercise comparing with participants who saw a digital representation of another person, due to a stronger effect of vicarious reinforcement. Surveys showed that the effect resisted in a follow-up.

In this sense, both the characteristics and the behavior of an avatar emerged as having an effect on the behaviour of their users. The Proteus effect (Yee & Bailenson, 2007) already demonstrated to be useful in the context of healthcare, so it is possible to prefigure the use of avatars also in order to influence patients in their journey, across the process of activation/engagement in their own care. For example, watching one's own avatar participating in VW-based simulation of medical consultation and gaining positive outcomes from it may positively influence the patient's motivation to recover the consultation also in daily life.

The Social Level: Relationships in Virtual Worlds and Networked Flow

In order to support a patient during all the engagement process, important aspects are personal relationships with care providers, family and also people who are suffering from the same disease.

As above-mentioned, VWs are a powerful tool to support patient engagement also at the level of social relationships.

For example, they are useful tools to share information and experiences regarding healthcare with others. Moreover, they can be used also to gain social support, to find clear guidelines to follow with regard to a specific disease and much more (Suomi, Mäntymäki, & Söderlund, 2014). In other words, they are able to connect people in a new way.

Indeed, considering patients with difficulty in walking or simply in moving, it would be very expensive and almost impossible to help them to keep constantly in contact with other people. On the other hand, the experience of being a part of a group is crucial in order to share emotions, thoughts, coping strategies, receive social support which can have positive health effects (Berkman & Syme, 1979; Bandura, 2001; Buunk, Gibbons, & Buunk, 1997/2013; Cantisano, Rimé, & Muñoz-Sastre, 2013; Cohen & Wills, 1985; Cohen & Syme, 1985). Indeed, first, social support can be both emotional (e.g., emotions sharing) and cognitive (e.g., simple information sharing) (Richmond, Ross, & Egeland, 2007; Buunk et al., 1997/2013; Lin, Dean, & Ensel, 2013) and generally, being part of a group has a great impact on our Self (Suls & Wheeler, 2000).

Therefore, even though the link between the experience in VWs and the real life need to be further analyzed (Beard, Wilson, Morra, & Keelan, 2009), VWs are undoubtedly able (Cohen & Syme, 1985) to create a bridge between these patients and the world outside the hospital, and to give rise to the feeling of being part of a group. VWs allow patients to reframe their Selves as persons and not only as patients.

Therefore the added value provided by VWs is that they allow people with different kinds of disabilities and from a great distance, to become again owners of their lives, moving from a patient-condition to a person-condition (Graffigna & Barello, 2015). This is crucial to engage patients towards their healthcare because it helps them to become active co-builders of their own health, assuming responsibility for it.

In the next paragraph, we will show that being a part of a group can lead not only to all the above mentioned benefits, but also to the emerging of a positive optimal group experience of engagement.

Indeed, recently, according to the model of Networked Flow (Gaggioli, Riva, Milani, & Mazzoni, 2013), it has been found that when a group is entirely focused on a specific activity, it is possible that a positive optimal group experience of engagement emerges, both in a real and in a virtual setting. Sawyer (2003) was the first who investigate this phenomenon which was labeled "group flow". Each time group members are involved in a specific task, it is possible that this experience occurs and it is responsible for optimal group performances and a maximum level of engagement among members.

The potentialities of this optimal group experience to promote patients' active participation towards their healthcare will be discussed in the next paragraph.

A New Way to Engage Patients: From Group Flow to Networked Flow Experience

As said in the previous paragraph, engaging patients in their own healthcare is necessary to help them adapt to the situation and to interpret personal disease as a normal experience of life which can be included in the broader perspective of existence.

However, not all the patients can be easily engaged. Take chronic patients, in particular those who suffer from physical disease (e.g., patients who can't walk). The healthcare system can difficulty bear the costs necessary to engage them.

Therefore, we suggest a new way of supporting patient engagement which can be affordable, amusing and available for all the patients. VWs are the key to address this issue. With this regard, they provide benefits both at an individual level and at a group level. While the first (i.e., individual level) was addressed in the previous paragraphs, the second level will be detailed and discussed in the following.

As we mentioned before, taking part in a group is a fertile field to engage patients in their own care management, showing a double advantage for each member:

1. These group experiences provide social support and sharing of coping strategies, and can support both individual and group well-being through the promotion of connectedness (Ryff & Singer, 2000; Buunk et al., 1997/2013; Cantisano et al., 2013; Cohen & Wills, 1985; Cohen & Syme, 1985).
2. These group experiences can lead people to experience a sense of total absorption in the task so that they feel fully engaged in what they are doing (Gaggioli et al., 2013; Riva et al., 2012; Riva, Milani, & Gaggioli, 2010). Moreover, working together on the same task, patients can be motivated to produce new resources (artifacts, practices, strategies) useful to manage together their own common experience of disease and illness.

While the first aspect has been discussed in the last section of the previous paragraph, the second one deserves to be further explained.

Recently, a new model on group creativity has been developed by Gaggioli and colleagues (Gaggioli et al., 2013), namely, the Networked Flow model. According to this frame, when a group is entirely focused on a specific activity, it is possible that a positive optimal group experience of engagement emerges, both in a real and in a virtual setting.

With the term "optimal group experience", we refer to the phenomenon of *group flow* which was first investigated by Sawyer (2003).

He highlighted that each time group members are involved in a specific task, it is possible that this experience occurs and it is responsible for optimal group performances and a maximum level of engagement among members.

In order to clarify the implications of living this optimal group experience for patient engagement, it is necessary to better introduce this phenomenon, its history and its peculiarities.

First, the domain in which group flow has been first investigated is creativity. In details, the existence of group flow was discovered several years before the development of the Networked Flow model that can be considered as a more general frame in which group flow is included.

As we explained previously, Sawyer (2003, 2006, 2008) was the first to introduce the concept of "group flow" and to investigate it deeply.

Starting from the analysis of improvisational groups engaged in public performances (jazz bands and theaters), he noticed the emergence of a peculiar group optimal experience, closely related to high performances, and highest level of group engagement, which he labeled "group flow". Group flow, far from being the sum of individual optimal experiences of each member (Csikszentmihalyi, 1975; Csikszentmihalyi, 2000), can be considered as an emergent property of group itself, as a sort of "collective state of mind" (p. 43). People feel as a part of a unique body, moving in unison and sharing the same intentions. This phenomenon emerges from the interactions occurring within a group and is able to positively influence overall performance.

He found also several group features able to support the emerging of this experience:

1. The presence of *shared objectives.*
2. The ability to *listen carefully to each other.*
3. *Deep concentration* on the task.
4. *Perception of control* on individual actions, autonomy and personal competence.
5. *Blending egos* so that members feel as if they were a unique body.
6. *Equal participation* among members.
7. **Familiarity:** Members should know the performance of colleagues.

8. *Clear and free communication* among group members.
9. The ability to *build on other's ideas.*
10. *Possibility of failure* must be clear in members' mind.

Other researches confirmed the relevance of these dimensions to trigger group flow experience (Hart & Di Blasi, 2013; Sawyer, 2008), even though this phenomenon should be explored more deeply in order to discover all its potentialities.

An important integration of this initial perspective towards group engagement is provided by the Networked Flow model which considers group creative collaboration, not only in dynamic terms, but also in structural terms. Therefore, also group structure and artifacts produced need to be considered as a part of the same "creative network".

In other words, the change of perspective occurs from "creative groups" to "creative networks" (Gaggioli et al., 2013) where not only people but also the environment in which creative process takes place and the artifacts produced deserve to be considered.

To better clarify this issue and the implications for patient engagement, the Networked Flow model will be discussed in details.

First, the name of this model itself reminds its main features which are:

1. The presence of *an optimal group experience among members* (i.e., group flow) closely related to the most creative group performances
2. The importance of *group structure and social pre-existing environment.*

According to this model, group flow is more than a simple sum of individual interactions (Sawyer, 2003, 2006, 2008), and it can be reached only after the achievement of a "collaborative zone of proximal development" (Gaggioli, Mazzoni, Milani, & Riva, 2015). This condition is characterized by the reach of a balance between individual and group actions which allows the emerging of a sense of Social Presence (i.e., the sensation that we are together in the same place with other Selves in a real or virtual environment) (Biocca & Harms, 2003; Harms & Biocca, 2004; Riva, 2008; Riva et al., 2010).

Simply, when group members feel closely connected to each other and fully absorbed by the group task, even though they are not in the same place, a fertile collaboration field is established and groups are able to achieve their best performance and to create products with a great potential impact on the wider society.

Therefore, this model highlights that this maximum level of group engagement can be reached also in a virtual environment.

The second pilaster of this model refers to the importance that is attributed to group structure, considering also artifacts which emerge from group performance. This feature is due to the "stigmergic" nature of group collaborative processes, namely, each mark left by a member is a trigger for the performance of a next action by the same or by another individual (Elliot, 2006; Grassé, 1959).

Therefore, creativity itself is distributed in the minds, interactions and artifacts of a group. Creativity is not only a matter of people but also concerns artifacts produced by individuals which contribute to create a network, namely a creative network (Gaggioli et al., 2013).

Therefore, in order to engage patients at a group level also artifacts are essential, as it will be detailed.

According to the Networked Flow model, this optimal experience (i.e., networked flow) emerges as a complex phenomenon in which not only the dimension of process but also the structural one is considered. This experience arises concurrently with a process of group creativity which emerges in six stages:

1. **Meeting and Persistence:** From an initial cultural and socio-economical frame, some individuals recognize reciprocal intentions directed towards the present, and something similar to a group begins to emerge.
2. **Reducing the Distance:** People, who recognize to have similar intentions, reduce distance and start to interact more frequently. They start to act as a minority with regard to the original frame.
3. **The Liminality-Parallel Action:** The boundaries of the new subgroup become clearer and definite; therefore the group acts to differentiate itself from the pre-existing frame.
4. **Networked Flow:** This phase is characterized by the emerging of the optimal group experience of Networked Flow in which mainly, individuals' intentions are blended together into group' ones and the new frame becomes explicit.
5. **Creation of the Artifact:** This is the phase in which group's intentions are embedded in one or more artifacts which are, however, used and considered relevant only by the group itself and not by the whole frame. It emerges clearly now the "distributed" nature of optimal creative group process which is not only dependent on individuals but also on artifacts made. Definitely, it is possible to say that group intentions are embedded in the group artifact.
6. **Application of the Artifact:** At this phase, artifacts meet the pre-existing framework. Therefore, "optimal creative group process" does not finish with the creation of the artifact, but with its introduction in the whole pre-existing network.

These phases underline the distributed nature of group creativity which is not only in the mind of group members but also in the produced artifacts (Inghilleri, Riva, & Riva, 2014).

The role of artifacts can now be more clarified.

Indeed, according to the Networked Flow model, during group flow, people are extremely engaged and concentrated on group task which has the delicate function of creating an artifact in which all group's intentions are incorporated. Therefore, also the artifact is part of group collaboration process and represents group identity.

It is now clear how these experiences can affect patients' attitude towards their healthcare by promoting their engagement through group creative tasks: being a part of a group who is involved in the creation of an artifact relevant for all the group members, can lead to a maximum level of group engagement, namely, group flow.

Because this experience (i.e., group flow) can occur both in natural and in virtual environments (Gaggioli et al., 2013; Riva et al., 2012; Riva et al., 2010; Sawyer, 2003, 2006, 2007, 2008), VWs are particularly suitable to promote these experience.

At this point, also the link between the process of patients' engagement, new technologies (in this case VWs) and group flow, emerges clearly.

Given that VWs are democratic tools able to extend the possibility of social interaction also to patients who, differently, could not have been connected with other people; and, according to the frame of Networked Flow, group collaboration can lead to the emergence of a group optimal experience also in mediated environments, and patients can be effectively engaged also through VWs. Indeed, they can be involved in group creative activities and can be motivated to produce new resources (artifacts, practices, strategies) useful to manage together their own common experience of disease. Social interactions through VWs can be another way to gain social support. Moreover, the experience of being able to create useful artifacts is closely related also to people's self-efficacy and self-esteem, which are key components of well-being (Bandura, 1982, 2001; Brown, Hoye, & Nicholson, 2012; Kernis, 2013; Thoits, 2013; Wu et al., 2012). Indeed, our efficacy beliefs are linked to our sense of engagement regarding a task, both at an individual and at a group level (Simbula, Guglielmi, & Schaufeli, 2011; Vera, Le Blanc, Taris, & Salanova, 2014).

Both group flow and Networked Flow are extremely engaging experiences, in which each member of a group is fully concentrated and absorbed by the group task. But, which kind of task can be effective for the emerging of group flow and networked flow? In other words, which task can better sustain patients' engagement with regard to their healthcare? If we analyze the literature regarding VWs and patients' engagement, one of the most used VW platforms is *Second Life* (Beard et al., 2009; Suomi et al., 2014). *Second Life* is an online VW in which it is possible to interact with other people by means of avatars. Despite the high number of health-related interventions on Second Life (informative, supportive, training, or recruiting for researches), Suomi et al. (2014) evidenced that little social interactions occur in this environment. Even though users have many opportunities of interacting with each other also through non verbal communication cues, it seemed that no intervention was really able to support this social interaction feature. For this reason we suggest group creative activities in which users (i.e., patients) can build together one or more artifacts that have an impact also on the real world. Indeed, the high sense of presence and social presence that users can experience during the execution of tasks, even in a VW, are able to support their engagement and sense of self-efficacy. In other words, thanks to the features of Second Life platform, patients can feel as if others were actually present with them in that environment. Patients can actually work in group creating something meaningful for them and also for the entire society. Doing so, in this mediated environment, patients would be able to enter a state of flow which could enable them to feel more engaged in their own care management giving them the opportunity of feeling again owners and active co-builder of their own lives (Csikszentmihalyi, 1997; Riva, Castelnuovo, & Mantovani, 2006).

Consider the example of a chronic patient who is never going to be able to walk, or who can only moves fingers on a keyboard. This person may feel not competent to do something useful for his own condition, experiencing his own dependency by caregivers and care providers every day. A patient engagement plan may be particularly difficult when directed to patients who, due to a peculiar pathological condition, are actually impaired in basic functions. VWs such as Second Life offer the possibility of overcoming these hindrances and make also people who suffer from severe chronic disease able to become again owner of their healthcare and of some aspects of their everyday life. Imagine that chronic patients unable to move, except of their fingers and heads, are asked to think and realize a project for other people who are experiencing their same conditions. They are invited to share their personal backgrounds in order to make something useful and meaningful for other real people, and also for themselves. Therefore, they can participate and contribute to the design of new projects of healthcare. Finally, also a completely different task as managing a virtual place (say: a facility in which new patients' avatars may be welcomed when entering the VW) can foster the emerging of a group flow experience. Creativity is the first step requested to healthcare professionals, but it is not the only one. Care providers have to be sensitive towards the intrinsic patient's needs, giving voice to them in an innovative way, until patients will be able to do it by their own. The combination between patients' actual needs and patients' expectations towards the future will be the bases of the fascinating architecture of patient engagement in VWs. With this regard, VWs can actually become worlds in which everything is possible and with an impact on the real life too (Beard et al., 2009).

An example in this direction can be found in the system of online support groups (Shopler & Galinsky 2014). Patients suffering from cancer benefited of online support groups, reducing symptomatology, distress and promoting wellbeing. The dimension of sharing provided by this typology of intervention is easily reproducible trough VWs, which could also put distant patients in contact and could offer the possibility for a complete anonymity too. Finally, we suggest that some kinds of disease force patient to social isolation (e.g., immunodeficiency), so VWs could help to overcome this hindrance.

A final example in this direction is the research protocol proposed by Gaggioli et al. (2014), who evidenced the possible positive implications of group reminiscence therapy for institutionalized elderly adults in terms of increased self-esteem, life satisfaction, quality of life and decreased depressive symptoms. Among the different possible reminiscence modalities (Haber, 2006) we suggest here the one based on "life review" that seems the most suitable approach to promote the reach of an Eudaimonic project, according to the model of patient engagement. Indeed, this approach allows patient to concentrate on both positive and negative life time memories, in order to help patient to achieve ego integrity again. This could be a powerful tool to reframe disease in to normal everydaylife. Further, the positive implications of reminiscence interventions could be enriched by the social dimension of sharing provided by VWs also for those patients unable to move.

CAVEATS

Despite the relevant and extraordinary possibilities provided by new technologies in healthcare, there is also a "dark side" regarding the use of these tools for patient engagement. In this contribution we have focused on the positive outcomes that could be originated by the use of VWs only. Nevertheless, there are also some negative aspects which should be considered regarding the use of new technologies. Indeed, some possible negative outcomes are related to the patient engagement phase the patient is involved in. For example, according to the PHE model, at the beginning (blackout phase) patients are not prepared to effectively face the disease, and they are not aware of the situation. Therefore, it could be really difficult to use technologies such as VWs in this phase. In this context, the main challenges are (i) to make patients aware of the fact that they are not alone while facing their own illness; (ii) to make them aware of the most important information they should know concerning their illness. Therefore, it could be difficult to persuade them of the add value of new technologies regarding the two above-mentioned aspects. Instead, some patients may prefer traditional procedures, such as talking with their own doctor or directly with their own family.

For what regards the following phases, it is important to guarantee that patients are not considering VWs as a video game or "just fun". Otherwise, it should be made clear that they are using a healthcare tool. Moreover, both medical professionals and patients could not feel enough competent regarding the use of VWs which would be perceived as hindrances instead of facilitators, able to help patients to adequately face their own disease and its implications. Finally, patients suffering from cognitive deficits should be accompanied in the exploration of WVs by medical assistants, since the use of some virtual reality-based technology requires attention and cognitive abilities.

FUTURE RESEARCH DIRECTIONS

In light of the above-mentioned literature and observations made before, a possible future challenge for researchers in this field could be investigating the long-term effects of avatars for users. For example, can avatars be able to (i) change over time offering useful feedback to patients about their own body changes and (ii) to help them better understand their own health situation (for example, aging avatars, or avatars visibly recovering from disease symptoms)? To this purpose, a possible way could be to adopt longitudinal perspective of analysis. Further, almost all features of WVs can be manipulated. Therefore, this aspect opens the possibility of building infinite types of VWs, so that customization emerges as the main feature of these environments. Moreover, it is possible to modify a pre-existing environment provided, for example, by the *Second Life* platform, in order to reach a specific therapeutic goal. On the other hand, this potentiality deserves to be further investigated with regard to the implications of manipulating some features with respect to others. To address this issue, it could be very useful to adopt a multidisciplinary approach towards VWs design, in order to improve all their potentialities and understanding the implications due to some choices regarding designs with respect to others. For example, User-Centered Design, as a design based on a prior research/analysis of users' needs and intentions, has been already associated to the use of new technologies for patient engagement and patient centered medicine (Triberti & Liberati, 2014; Triberti & Riva, 2015b).

Other possible future research directions relate to the current development of virtual reality technologies, which may be adapted to Virtual Worlds too in the future. Total immersion inside computer-generates experiences is today more and more reachable. For example, research on the so-called body-swapping illusion (Petkova & Ehrsson, 2008; Riva, in press; Serino et al., 2015) suggest that it is possible to induce the sensation to own a virtual body, even different from the real one. The relevance of this technology is evident in the field of diseases characterized by alteration of bodily self-consciousness, which can be manipulated according to patient's needs. These new scenarios expand the potentialities of virtual reality-based tools of generating meaningful experiences for their users.

Finally, virtual reality is moving to mobile devices and it is becoming more affordable. New head-mounted displays are available on the market, such as Google Cardboard, able to adapt mobile phones for the fruition of virtual reality-based contents. Therefore, everyone can experience an immersive VR environment with a low economic investment. Since these VR devices are intuitive and easy to use, they constitute a concrete opportunity to expand actual possibilities in the healthcare field.

CONCLUSION

To conclude, the model of patient engagement offers a picture of the process patients go through during their everyday life experience of disease management. The final expected outcome is the reaching of a complete awareness towards their own disease with the assumption of an active role in managing their healthcare.

New technologies are one of the best ways to support patients across all the phases of this complex process. They can be used to structure, augment or even replace the features of an experience. Indeed, they are able to support the individuals in their daily routine and personal issues, contributing to a change in the perception of individuals' own life.

An example of new technologies which emerges as effective tools for patient engagement are Virtual Words.

Their impact can be seen both at an individual level, relating to the utilization of an avatar, and at a group level. Indeed, avatars can be used as an assessment tool in that they have relationships with the users' inner experience and Self-conception. Moreover, the opportunities provided by VWs are mainly two: (i) the democratic nature of this tool which can be used also by people unable to move and living from a great distance; (ii) the economic benefits due to the fact that the majority of VWs platforms are free.

Moreover, at a group level, VWs can be used to foster optimal group experiences responsible for high levels of engagement and group performance. This experience emerges when all group members are involved in a specific task relevant for each of them. There are many examples of task that groups of patients can do in a virtual world. Therefore, all patients can feel engaged towards their healthcare using VWs.

We suggest deepening the analysis of the opportunities for patient engagement provided by these kinds of digital environments, so that the people suffering from different diseases could benefit from their use regarding their own healthcare.

VWs can be actually considered "unexplored worlds" for what regards their social dimension; therefore, we hope that future researchers and web developers would be interested in deepening VWs tools as a resource to promote patient engagement and well-being.

REFERENCES

Bandura, A. (1982). Self-efficacy mechanism in human agency. *The American Psychologist*, *37*(2), 122–147. doi:10.1037/0003-066X.37.2.122

Bandura, A. (2001). Social cognitive theory: An agentic perspective. *Annual Review of Psychology*, *52*(1), 1–26. doi:10.1146/annurev.psych.52.1.1 PMID:11148297

Barello, S., & Graffigna, G. (2014). Engaging patients to recover life projectuality: An Italian cross-disease framework. *Quality of Life Research: An International Journal of Quality of Life Aspects of Treatment, Care and Rehabilitation*, *24*(5), 1087–1096. doi:10.1007/s11136-014-0846-x PMID:25373927

Barello, S., Graffigna, G., Vegni, E., & Bosio, A. (2014). The challenges of conceptualizing patient engagement in healthcare: A lexicographic literature review. *Journal of Participatory Medicine*, *6*, e9.

Barello, S., Graffigna, G., Vegni, E., Savarese, M., Lombardi, F., & Bosio, A. C. (2015). 'Engage me in taking care of my heart': A grounded theory study on patient–cardiologist relationship in the hospital management of heart failure. *BMJ Open*, *5*(3), e005582. doi:10.1136/bmjopen-2014-005582 PMID:25776041

Beard, L., Wilson, K., Morra, D., & Keelan, J. (2009). A survey of health-related activities on second life. *Journal of Medical Internet Research*, *11*(2), e17. doi:10.2196/jmir.1192 PMID:19632971

Berkman, L. F., & Syme, S. L. (1979). Social networks, host resistance, and mortality: A nine-year follow-up study of Alameda County residents. *American Journal of Epidemiology*, *109*(2), 186–204. doi:10.4236/health.2012.49087 PMID:425958

Biocca, F., & Harms, C. (2003). *Guide to the Networked Minds Social Presence Inventory v. 1.2: Measures of co-presence, social presence, subjective symmetry, and intersubjective symmetry*. Michigan State University. Retrieved from http://cogprints.org/6743/

Botella, C., Riva, G., Gaggioli, A., Wiederhold, B. K., Alcaniz, M., & Banos, R. M. (2012). The present and future of positive technologies. *Cyberpsychology, Behavior, and Social Networking*, *15*(2), 78–84. doi:10.1089/cyber.2011.0140 PMID:22149078

Brown, K. M., Hoye, R., & Nicholson, M. (2012). Self-esteem, self-efficacy, and social connectedness as mediators of the relationship between volunteering and well-being. *Journal of Social Service Research*, *38*(4), 468–483. doi:10.1080/01488376.2012.687706

Buunk, B. P., Gibbons, F. X., & Buunk, A. (1997/2013). *Health, coping, and well-being: Perspectives from social comparison theory*. Mahwah, NJ: Erlbaum.

Cantisano, N., Rimé, B., & Muñoz-Sastre, M. T. (2013). The social sharing of emotions in HIV/AIDS: A comparative study of HIV/AIDS, diabetic and cancer patients. *Journal of Health Psychology*, *18*(10), 1255–1267. doi:10.1177/1359105312462436 PMID:23129833

Cohen, S., & Wills, T. A. (1985). Stress, social support, and the buffering hypothesis. *Psychological Bulletin*, *98*(2), 310–357. doi:10.1037/0033-2909.98.2.310 PMID:3901065

Cohen, S. E., & Syme, S. (1985). *Social support and health*. New York: Academic Press.

Csikszentmihalyi, M. (1975). *Beyond boredom and anxiety*. San Francisco, CA: Jossey-Bass.

Csikszentmihalyi, M. (1997). *Finding flow: The psychology of engagement with everyday life*. New York: Basic Books.

Csikszentmihalyi, M. (2000). *Beyond boredom and anxiety*. San Francisco: Jossey-Bass.

Dunn, R. A., & Guadagno, R. E. (2012). My avatar and me–Gender and personality predictors of avatar-self discrepancy. *Computers in Human Behavior*, *28*(1), 97–106. doi:10.1016/j.chb.2011.08.015

El Tantawi, M. M., El Kashlan, M. K., & Saeed, Y. M. (2013). Assessment of the Efficacy of Second Life, a Virtual Learning Environment, in Dental Education. *Journal of Dental Education*, *77*(12), 1639–1652. PMID:24319136

Elliot, M. (2006). Stigmergic collaboration: The evolution of group work. *journal of media and culture*, *9*(2).

Fong, K., & Mar, R. A. (2015). What Does My Avatar Say About Me? Inferring Personality From Avatars. *Personality and Social Psychology Bulletin*, *41*(2), 237–249. doi:10.1177/0146167214562761 PMID:25576173

Fox, J., & Ahn, S. J. (2013). Avatars: Portraying, Exploring, and Changing Online and Offline Identities. In R. Luppicini (Ed.), *Handbook of Research on Technoself: Identity in a Technological Society* (Vol. 1, pp. 255–271). Hershey: IGI Global. doi:10.4018/978-1-4666-2211-1.ch014

Fox, J., & Bailenson, J. N. (2009). Virtual self-modeling: The effects of vicarious reinforcement and identification on exercise behaviors. *Media Psychology*, *12*(1), 1–25. doi:10.1080/15213260802669474

Fox, J., Bailenson, J. N., & Tricase, L. (2013). The embodiment of sexualized virtual selves: The Proteus effect and experiences of self-objectification via avatars. *Computers in Human Behavior*, *29*(3), 930–938. doi:10.1016/j.chb.2012.12.027

Gaggioli, A., Mazzoni, E., Milani, L., & Riva, G. (2015). The creative link: Investigating the relationship between social network indices, creative performance and flow in blended teams. *Computers in Human Behavior*, *42*, 157–166. doi:10.1016/j.chb.2013.12.003

Gaggioli, A., Riva, G., Milani, L., & Mazzoni, E. (2013). *Networked Flow: Towards an Understanding of Creative Networks*. Heidelberg: Springer. doi:10.1007/978-94-007-5552-9

Gaggioli, A., Scaratti, C., Morganti, L., Stramba-Badiale, M., Agostoni, M., Spatola, C. A., & Riva, G. et al. (2014). Effectiveness of group reminiscence for improving wellbeing of institutionalized elderly adults: Study protocol for a randomized controlled trial. *Trials*, *15*(1), 408. doi:10.1186/1745-6215-15-408 PMID:25344703

Gee, J. P. (2003). *What videogames have to teach us about learning and literacy* (2nd ed.). New York: Palgrave Macmillan.

Graffigna, G., & Barello, S. (2015). Modelling Patient Engagement in Healthcare: Insight for Research and Practice. In G. Graffigna, S. Barello, & S. Triberti (Eds.), *Patient Engagement: A consumer-centered model to innovate healthcare*. Berlin: DeGruyter Open. doi:10.1515/9783110452440-004

Graffigna, G., Barello, S., Libreri, C., & Bosio, C. A. (2014). How to engage type-2 diabetic patients in their own health management: Implications for clinical practice. *BMC Public Health*, *14*(1), 648. doi:10.1186/1471-2458-14-648 PMID:24966036

Graffigna, G., Barello, S., & Riva, G. (2013a). How to make health information technology effective: The challenge of patient engagement. *Archives of Physical Medicine and Rehabilitation*, *94*(10), 2034–2035. doi:10.1016/j.apmr.2013.04.024 PMID:24075414

Graffigna, G., Barello, S., & Riva, G. (2013b). Technologies for patient engagement. *Health Affairs (Project Hope)*, *32*(6), 1172. doi:10.1377/hlthaff.2013.0279 PMID:23733998

Graffigna, G., Barello, S., & Triberti, S. (2015). *Patient Engagement: A consumer-centered model to innovate healthcare*. Berlin: DeGruyter Open. doi:10.1515/9783110452440

Graffigna, G., Barello, S., Triberti, S., Wiederhold, B. K., Bosio, A. C., & Riva, G. (2014). Enabling eHealth as a pathway for patient engagement: A toolkit for medical practice. *Studies in Health Technology and Informatics*, *199*, 13–21. PMID:24875682

Graffigna, G., Barello, S., Wiederhold, B. K., Bosio, A. C., & Riva, G. (2013). Positive technology as a driver for health engagement. *Studies in Health Technology and Informatics*, *191*, 9–17. PMID:23792833

Graffigna, G., Vegni, E., Barello, S., Olson, K., & Bosio, C. A. (2011). Studying the social construction of cancer-related fatigue experience: The heuristic value of Ethnoscience. *Patient Education and Counseling*, *82*(3), 402–409. doi:10.1016/j.pec.2010.12.017 PMID:21292426

Grassé, P. P. (1959). La reconstruction du nid et les coordinations interindividuelles chezBellicositermes natalensis et Cubitermes sp. la théorie de la stigmergie: Essai d'interprétation du comportement des termites constructeurs. *Insectes Sociaux*, *6*(1), 41–80. doi:10.1007/BF02223791

Haber, D. (2006). Life review: Implementation, theory, research, and therapy. *International Journal of Aging & Human Development*, *63*(2), 153–171. doi:10.2190/DA9G-RHK5-N9JP-T6CC PMID:17137032

Harms, C., & Biocca, F. (2004). Internal Consistency and Reliability of the Networked Minds - Measure of Social Presence.*Proceedings of the Seventh Annual International Workshop: Presence*. Valencia, CA: Universidad Politecnica de Valencia press.

Hart, E., & Di Blasi, Z. (2015). Combined flow in musical jam sessions: A pilot qualitative study. *Psychology of Music, 43*(2), 275-290. doi:0305735613502374.

Higgins, E. T. (1987). Self-discrepancy: A theory relating self and affect. *Psychological Review*, *94*(3), 319–340. doi:10.1037/0033-295X.94.3.319 PMID:3615707

Inghilleri, P., Riva, G., & Riva, E. (2014). *Enabling Positive Change: Flow and Complexity in Daily Experience*. Berlin: De Gruyter Open.

Jin, S. A. A. (2012). The virtual malleable self and the virtual identity discrepancy model: Investigative frameworks for virtual possible selves and others in avatar-based identity construction and social interaction. *Computers in Human Behavior*, *28*(6), 2160–2168. doi:10.1016/j.chb.2012.06.022

Kernis, M. H. (2013). *Self-esteem issues and answers: A sourcebook of current perspectives*. New York: Psychology Press.

Kim, Y., & Sundar, S. S. (2012). Visualizing ideal self vs. actual self through avatars: Impact on preventive health outcomes. *Computers in Human Behavior*, *28*(4), 1356–1364. doi:10.1016/j.chb.2012.02.021

Kolko, B. E. (1998). Representing bodies in virtual space: The rhetoric of avatar design. *The Information Society*, *15*(3), 177–186. doi:10.1080/019722499128484

Lin, N., Dean, A., & Ensel, W. M. (2013). *Social support, life events, and depression*. New York: Academic Press.

Loke, S.-K. (2015). How do virtual world experiences bring about learning? A critical review of theories. *Australasian Journal of Educational Technology*, *31*(1), 112–122.

Lomanowska, A. M., & Guitton, M. J. (2014). My avatar is pregnant! Representation of pregnancy, birth, and maternity in a virtual world. *Computers in Human Behavior*, *31*, 322–331. doi:10.1016/j.chb.2013.10.058

Martey, R. M., Stromer-Galley, J., Consalvo, M., Wu, J., Banks, J., & Strzalkowski, T. (2015). Communicating age in Second Life: The contributions of textual and visual factors. *New Media & Society*, *17*(1), 41–61. doi:10.1177/1461444813504270

Morie, J. F., & Chance, E. (2011). Extending the reach of health care for obesity and diabetes using virtual worlds. *Journal of Diabetes Science and Technology*, *5*(2), 272–276. doi:10.1177/193229681100500211 PMID:21527093

Murray, T., Hardy, D., Spruijt-Metz, D., Hekler, E., & Raij, A. (2013). Avatar interfaces for biobehavioral feedback. In A. Marcus (Ed.), *Design, User Experience, and Usability. Health, Learning, Playing, Cultural, and Cross-Cultural User Experience* (pp. 424–434). Heidelberg: Springer. doi:10.1007/978-3-642-39241-2_47

Pellas, N., & Kazanidis, I. (2013). On the value of Second Life for students' engagement in blended and online courses: A comparative study from the Higher Education in Greece. *Education and Information Technologies*.

Pellas, N., & Kazanidis, I. (2014). Engaging students in blended and online collaborative courses at university level through Second Life: Comparative perspectives and instructional affordances. *New Review of Hypermedia and Multimedia, 20*(2), 123–144. doi:10.1080/13614568.2013.856958

Petkova, V. I., & Ehrsson, H. H. (2008). If I were you: Perceptual illusion of body swapping. *PLoS ONE, 3*(12), e3832. PMID:19050755

Richmond, C. A., Ross, N. A., & Egeland, G. M. (2007). Social support and thriving health: A new approach to understanding the health of indigenous Canadians. *American Journal of Public Health, 97*(10), 1827–1833. doi:10.2105/AJPH.2006.096917 PMID:17761564

Riva, G. (2008). *Psicologia dei nuovi media*. Bologna: Il Mulino.

Riva, G. (in press) Embodied Medicine: What Human-Computer Confluence Can Offer to Health Care. In A. Gaggioli, A. Ferscha, G. Riva, S. Dunne, and I. Viaud-Delmon (Eds.), Human Computer Confluence: Transforming Human Experience Through Symbiotic Technologies, Berlin: De Gruyter Open

Riva, G., Banos, R. M., Botella, C., Wiederhold, B. K., & Gaggioli, A. (2012). Positive technology: Using interactive technologies to promote positive functioning. *Cyberpsychology, Behavior, and Social Networking, 15*(2), 69–77. doi:10.1089/cyber.2011.0139 PMID:22149077

Riva, G., Castelnuovo, G., & Mantovani, F. (2006). Transformation of flow in rehabilitation: The role of advanced communication technologies. *Behavior Research Methods, 38*(2), 237–244. doi:10.3758/BF03192775 PMID:16956100

Riva, G., Milani, L., & Gaggioli, A. (Eds.). (2010). Networked Flow: comprendere e sviluppare la creatività di rete. Milano, IT: LED.

Ryff, C. D., & Singer, B. (2000). Interpersonal flourishing: A positive health agenda for the new millennium. *Personality and Social Psychology Review, 4*(1), 30–44. doi:10.1207/S15327957PSPR0401_4

Sawyer, R. K. (2003). *Group creativity: Music, theater, collaboration*. Mahwah, NJ: LEA.

Sawyer, R. K. (2006). Group creativity: Musical performance and collaboration. *Psychology of Music, 34*(2), 148–165. doi:10.1177/0305735606061850

Sawyer, R. K. (2007). *Group genius: The creative power of collaboration*. New York: Basic Books.

Sawyer, R. K. (2008). *Group genius: The creative power of collaboration* (2nd ed.). New York: Basic Books.

Schopler, J., & Galinsky, M. (2014). Expanding our view of support groups as open systems. In M. Galinsky & J. Schopler (Eds.), *Support groups: Current perspectives on theory and practice* (pp. 3–10). New York: The Haworth Press, Inc.

Serino, S., Pedroli, E., Keizer, A., Triberti, S., Dakanalis, A., Pallavicini, F., & Riva, G. et al. (2015). Virtual Reality Body Swapping: A Tool for Modifying the Allocentric Memory of the Body. *Cyberpsychology, Behavior, and Social Networking*. doi:10.1089/cyber.2015.0229 PMID:26506136

Simbula, S., Guglielmi, D., & Schaufeli, W. B. (2011). A three-wave study of job resources, self-efficacy, and work engagement among Italian schoolteachers. *European Journal of Work and Organizational Psychology*, *20*(3), 285–304. doi:10.1080/13594320903513916

Simpson, D. D. (2004). A conceptual framework for drug treatment process and outcomes. *Journal of Substance Abuse Treatment*, *27*(2), 99–121. doi:10.1016/j.jsat.2004.06.001 PMID:15450644

Suls, J., & Wheeler, L. (Eds.). (2000). *Handbook of social comparison*. New York: Kluwer Academic/Plenum. doi:10.1007/978-1-4615-4237-7

Suomi, R., Mäntymäki, M., & Söderlund, S. (2014). Promoting Health in Virtual Worlds: Lessons From Second Life. *Journal of Medical Internet Research*, *16*(10), e229. doi:10.2196/jmir.3177 PMID:25313009

Sweigart, L., Burden, M., Carlton, K. H., & Fillwalk, J. (2014). Virtual simulations across curriculum prepare nursing students for patient interviews. *Clinical Simulation in Nursing*, *10*(3), e139–e145. doi:10.1016/j.ecns.2013.10.003

Sweigart, L., & Hodson-Carlton, K. (2013). Improving student interview skills: The virtual avatar as client. *Nurse Educator*, *38*(1), 11–15. doi:10.1097/NNE.0b013e318276df2d PMID:23222623

Tajfel, H., & Turner, J. C. (2004). The Social Identity Theory of Intergroup Behavior. In J. T. Jost, & J. Sidanius (Eds.), Political Psychology: Key Readings (pp. 276–293). New York: Psychology Press.

Thoits, P. A. (2013). Self, identity, stress, and mental health. In C. S. Aneshensel, J. C. Phelan, & A. Bierman (Eds.), *Handbook of the sociology of mental health*. New York: Springer. doi:10.1007/978-94-007-4276-5_18

Tiffany, J. M., & Hoglund, B. A. (2014). Facilitating Learning Through Virtual Reality Simulation: Welcome to Nightingale Isle. In Virtual, Augmented Reality and Serious Games for Healthcare 1 (pp. 159-174). Springer Berlin Heidelberg.

Tokel, S. T., & İsler, V. (2013). Acceptance of virtual worlds as learning space. *Innovations in Education and Teaching International.*

Trepte, S., & Reinecke, L. (2010). Avatar creation and video game enjoyment: Effects of life-satisfaction, game competitiveness, and identification with the avatar. *Journal of Media Psychology: Theories, Methods, and Applications*, *22*(4), 171–184. doi:10.1027/1864-1105/a000022

Trepte, S., Reinecke, L., & Behr, K.-M. (2009). Creating virtual alter egos or superheroines? Gamers' strategies of avatar creation in terms of gender and sex. *International Journal of Gaming and Computer-Mediated Simulations*, *1*(2), 52–76. doi:10.4018/jgcms.2009040104

Triberti, S., & Argenton, L. (2013). *Psicologia dei videogiochi.* Milano: Apogeo.

Triberti, S., & Liberati, E. G. (2014). Patient centered virtual reality: an opportunity to improve the quality of patient's experience. In P. Cipresso & S. Serino (Eds.), *Virtual Reality Technologies, Medical Applications and Challenges* (pp. 1–30). New York: Nova Science.

Triberti, S., & Riva, G. (2015a). Positive Technology for Enhancing the Patient Engagement Experiences. In S. Barello, G. Graffigna, & S. Triberti (Eds.), *Patient Engagement: a comsumer- centered model to innovate healthcare*. Berlin: De Gruyter Open. doi:10.1515/9783110452440-005

Triberti, S., & Riva, G. (2015b). Engaging Users to Design Positive Technologies for Patient Engagement: the Perfect Interaction Model. In S. Barello, G. Graffigna, & S. Triberti (Eds.), *Patient Engagement: a comsumer- centered model to innovate healthcare*. Berlin: De Gruyter Open. doi:10.1515/9783110452440-006

Vasalou, A., & Joinson, A. N. (2009). Me, myself and I: The role of interactional context on self-presentation through avatars. *Computers in Human Behavior*, *25*(2), 510–520. doi:10.1016/j.chb.2008.11.007

Vera, M., Le Blanc, P. M., Taris, T. W., & Salanova, M. (2014). Patterns of engagement: The relationship between efficacy beliefs and task engagement at the individual versus collective level. *Journal of Applied Social Psychology*, *44*(2), 133–144. doi:10.1111/jasp.12219

Villani, D., Gatti, E., Confalonieri, E., & Riva, G. (2012). Am I my avatar? A tool to investigate virtual body image representation in adolescence. *Cyberpsychology, Behavior, and Social Networking*, *15*(8), 435–440. doi:10.1089/cyber.2012.0057 PMID:22823468

Warburton, S. (2009). Second Life in higher education: Assessing the potential for and the barriers to deploying virtual worlds in learning and teaching. *British Journal of Educational Technology*, *40*(3), 414–426. doi:10.1111/j.1467-8535.2009.00952.x

Wu, L. M., Austin, J., Hamilton, J. G., Valdimarsdottir, H., Isola, L., Rowley, S., & Rini, C. et al. (2012). Self-efficacy beliefs mediate the relationship between subjective cognitive functioning and physical and mental well-being after hematopoietic stem cell transplant. *Psycho-Oncology*, *21*(11), 1175–1184. doi:10.1002/pon.2012 PMID:21739524

Yee, N., & Bailenson, J. (2007). The Proteus effect: The effect of transformed self-representation on behavior. *Human Communication Research*, *33*(3), 271–290. doi:10.1111/j.1468-2958.2007.00299.x

Yee, N., Bailenson, J., & Ducheneaut, N. (2009). The proteus effect: Implications of transformed digital self-sepresentation on online and offline behavior. *Communication Research*, *36*(2), 285–312. doi:10.1177/0093650208330254

KEY TERMS AND DEFINITIONS

Avatar: Any representation of a human user's action and/or communication inside a digital environment. In VWs and video games, these are typically 3d graphical representations.

Group Flow: An optimal group experience of fully engagement often described as sense of "*collective mind*" by people who experienced it.

Networked Flow model: An innovative framework to understand networks creativity which is seen as a process culminating in the generation and sharing of an artifact.

Patient Engagement: A process of disease/illness management which culminates in patients' experience of feeling responsible for their own healthcare and able to manage it adequately. At the highest level, patients recover a positive life project despite the presence of a chronic disease.

PHE Model: A theoretical model explaining the evolutionary phases of the patient engagement process.

Positive Technology: A theoretical, research and design paradigm that consider new technologies a resource to improve the quality of people's personal experience by structuring, augmenting or even replacing its features.

Proteus Effect: The phenomenon of avatars modifying the behavior of their own users.

Virtual Words: Internet-based virtual environments where people can interact by means of their avatars.

Chapter 11
Waiting for Health Care Services

Stefan Janzek-Hawlat
Vienna University of Technology, Austria

Hilda Tellioğlu
Vienna University of Technology, Austria

ABSTRACT

Waiting for health care services have impact on people from several perspectives. First of all, seen from patients' point of view, due to psychologically and physically burden short waiting times are an indication of quality. Second, seen from health care systems' point of view, short waiting times can be a competitive advantage for health care providers. Finally, short-waiting times can contribute to a more effective system applied in health care. In this chapter, the impact of waiting times of patients are analyzed on all three levels based on quantitative and qualitative study carried out by the authors as well as on the foregoing literature review. The situation of patients and their requirements are shown, strategies to reduce waiting times are presented by also considering the role of information and communication technologies, and several relevant questions raised are answered.

INTRODUCTION

A new kind of patient has entered the healthcare sector (Carpman, Grant, & Simmons, 1986; Marberry, 2006; Marsh, 1993), an active one who wants to participate directly in healthcare decisions and is therefore increasingly responsible for his or her own health (Wallner, 2013). At the same time, this new patient demands service

DOI: 10.4018/978-1-5225-0663-8.ch011

quality and person-centred care that causes a paradigm shift in the understanding of healthcare and in the definition and perception of services provided for it. One of the impacts is to move the focus of healthcare in many western societies from a paternalistic approach to a shared decision making process, in which the needs of the patient are central (Emanuel & Emanuel, 1992; Gillon, 1994). In such a setting patient-participation and informed consent are fundamental rights (Kizer, 2001). Another impact is creating a more patient-friendly environment in hospitals and at resident physicians (Mangold, Peintinger, & Kopetzki, 2010).

Increasing requirements to service quality and focusing on person-centred services have also impact on the healthcare sector as any other business sector. In healthcare patients – in this context they are the consumers – demand the right to safety, to information, to choose among alternatives, and the right to be heard (Kennedy, 1962). However, healthcare is different than the other business areas; it is a highly complex field. It is not always easy for consumers to contract or consent, sometimes because of their current health condition (e.g., in case of mentally ill patients or patients in a coma), sometimes because of the complexity of the medical situation and related diagnosis or treatment procedures.

Nevertheless, patients' autonomy has become more important in the last few decades. The US-Institute of Medicine, for example, states patient-centeredness as one of the six aims for increasing general healthcare quality provided (Adams, Greiner, & Corrigan, 2004). The World Health Organization World Alliance for Patient Safety (2005) highlights the determinant of including patients and their family into the healthcare decisions (Pittet, Allegranzi, Storr, & Donaldson, 2005). Increasing patient participation in processes and health-related decision-making as well as the changing role of patients to consumers can improve the quality of care and through this the healthcare system in general (Longtin et al., 2010; Lancet, 2005). In the "Vienna Recommendations on Health Promoting Hospitals" from 1997, the WHO, sub-organisations, and their member states announced official documents that confirmed the same statement and furthermore claimed that it would also improve the efficiency of healthcare systems (World Health Organization [WHO], 1997; Committee on Patient Safety and Quality Improvement, 2005; General Medical Council [GMC], 2013; Nursing & Midwifery Council [NMC], 2015; Brink-Muinen et al., 2006). About 15 years after "Vienna Recommendations", the Austrian government has included "patient empowerment" in the on-going healthcare reform (Grazie & Wimmer-Puchinger, 2014). One of its ten targets is to increase health literacy by improving the involvement of the citizens in their own health issues.

Due to the demographic changes in Europe, the frequency of the use of healthcare services increases (Statistik Austria, 2015a, 2015b). Putting the needs of patients in the centre, Austria shows good numbers in the quality and quantity of healthcare services provided. On the one hand, 7.7 hospital beds and 4.75 doctors per 1,000 inhabitants as well as a life expectancy of 80 years paint a favourable picture of a high quality healthcare system in Austria[1] (Mundi Index, 2012). Looking at the number of healthy life years (60 years)[2] and the health expenditure of 10.8% of the GDP (Gross Domestic Product)[3], the Austrian healthcare system is in the midfield of the European Union (WHO, 2015). But, there is further place for improvement. Several surveys show the most potential for improvement lies in the waiting times in hospitals and at resident doctors: The main problem is still the waiting for meeting a physician and a "two-tier healthcare system"[4]. The question is how to reduce the waiting times, how to focus on health instead of illness, and how to strengthen the patient-centred approach (Deloitte, 2011).

So far, waiting for healthcare services have got only little public attention in Austria. There is almost no data available. A questionnaire published in 2009 showed that the average waiting time at general practitioners (GP) is 34 minutes and at specialists 28 minutes (Fischer, 2009). The question whether electronic appointment systems lower waiting times of patients was not studied. This chapter aims to evaluate and analyse waiting process and waiting environment on an organisational and structural level, and tries to find solutions to decrease waiting times as they have negative impact on citizens (Bailey, 1952), support infections (Eck, DeBaun, & Pugliese, 2001), and are a financial burden for patients, clinics, and the Austrian healthcare and economy system in general (Fleischer, 2011).

In this chapter, findings of a study done at the Vienna University of Technology are presented (Janzek-Hawlat, 2015). Besides showing the reasons and the duration of waiting times, the main part focuses on the study of ICT based tools, which are able to reduce waiting times by increasing patient engagement and participation. This paper aims to answer the following research questions:

- What are the reasons for waiting in outpatient clinics and at hospitals?
- How long is the average waiting time for patients at general practitioners and at hospital ambulances?
- How are waiting times perceived by patients?
- Are there any convincible improvements to decrease the burden of waiting and make waiting more comfortable for patients?
- Are there differences in waiting times at healthcare institutions with and without electronic appointment systems?
- How can ICT based solutions help decrease waiting times by increasing patient participation?

Waiting for healthcare services has effects on different levels. First of all, from the patients' point of view (Bailey, 1952; Eck et al., 2001), short waiting times are an indication of quality and are able to reduce the psychologically and physically burden which likely occur due long waiting times (Arneill & Devlin, 2002). Second, seen from a healthcare system's point of view, short waiting times can be a competitive advantage for healthcare providers. Finally, short-waiting times can contribute to a more effective and efficient system applied in healthcare (Fleisher, 2013). To sum up, in this chapter the impact of waiting for healthcare services is analysed on all these three levels based on our quantitative and qualitative study and the literature review. The situation of the patients and their requirements are shown, strategies to reduce waiting times are presented, and the questions listed above are answered and discussed.

The next section summarises the relevant state of the art literature related to waiting for healthcare services. After introducing the methodology applied for this research work, results are presented, structured in four areas: the origin of waiting, waiting times per se, perception of waiting, solutions for reducing waiting times. The chapter is finalised with a conclusion including future work.

WAITING IN HEALTH CARE

In the healthcare sector, there are in general two kinds of waiting. First, patients wait in waiting rooms of doctors' offices or hospital ambulances to meet the physician. Second, there is waiting for appointments, diagnostic procedures like MRT, surgeries, or transplantation of organs. Both issues are important and currently important topics of public discussions (Laschet, 2014; Staeck, 2014; Lammers, 2014), but only the first will be the subject of interest in this chapter.

Long waiting and queues in healthcare services are associated with several negative impacts. First, waiting is usually associated with being non-productive. Second, due to the unpredictability of waiting times, waiting often delays one's follow-up activities, which might be business or spare-time related. Third, waiting cause stress, frustration, and anger to the people waiting (Wijayasinghe, 2013). Furthermore, while waiting in waiting rooms of healthcare facilities patients might be infected by others also waiting in the same area (Eck et al., 2001). This leads to the paradox situation that long waiting can decrease the patients' health condition.

When patients wait for healthcare services they decrease the idle time of physicians. Professionals' time has been found 37.5 times more valuable than patients' time (Bailey, 1952). A peculiarity of waiting for healthcare is that the patient can change the service provider only under considerable expense. The patient has in general no access to information about waiting times in other healthcare providing institutions. Especially in hospitals and clinics, it can be psychologically difficult to change the physician, once a patient is already in treatment. Even the change of a family doctor is associated with effort because, for instance, the new GP might not have access to necessary previous healthcare data.

There are several studies on waiting for healthcare services. Norman and Bailey took a closer look on waiting times and appointment systems at outpatient clinics based on data from the Nuffield Provincial Hospital (Bailey, 1952). Due to the use of mathematical models, they examined a series of 50 hypothetical clinics, each with 25 patients. They found out that the best appointment interval is between 5 and 5.5 minutes as the average waiting time and the consultant's time wasted is about 7 to 8 minutes. However, they also showed that the increase of patient's waiting time clearly decreases the consultant's average wasted time. For instance, when patients wait about 17 minutes, the consultant's wasted idle time is reduced between 1 to 2 minutes. Furthermore, they showed that the waiting times of patients have a positive skew. Within the mentioned study 30% of the patients were waiting up to 5 minutes, 25% between 5 and 10 minutes, 15% between 10 and 15 minutes, 12% had no waiting times, and the rest more than 15 minutes. They concluded that a suitable appointment system decreases waiting times without increasing the idle time of physicians. The best situation is when appointments at regular intervals are equal to the average consultation time, and the arrival of the physician is at the same time as the second patient. Miceli and Wolosin (2004) found out that longer waiting times correlate negatively with satisfaction with healthcare services. But they also showed that good communication and a strong relationship between the healthcare provider and the patient is able to reduce those negative effects. So, transparency and being aware of waiting times including their origin are important for patients' satisfaction. Becker and Douglass categorise the waiting process in an ambulatory waiting room into three steps (Becker & Douglass, 2008): 1) time for pre-process which is the arrival time of the patient till the patient is taken into the exam room; 2) time for in-process that is the time between entering and leaving the exam room; and 3) time for post-process that is the remaining time from leaving the exam room till exiting the building. In this chapter slightly different categories are used: 1) waiting for the administrative work at the administrative desk; 2) waiting in waiting area; and 3) time for in-process.

There has only been little research about the correlation of real waiting times, perceived waiting times, and attractiveness of the waiting area. De Man et al. (2005) showed that the perceived waiting time correlates with the perception of the quality of service in nuclear medicine. The perceived waiting time was higher than the actual waiting time. The time inside the exam room was found too short. If patients are given information about the reasons for their waiting the difference between perceived and actual waiting time decreases. Arneill and Devlin (2002) confirmed de Man's results and they detected a relationship between the quality of care, perceived waiting times, anxiety, staff-patient interaction, and attractiveness of the physical setting for patients in an out-patient facility. Based on a study in emergency care departments (Becker & Douglass, 2008) patients tend to overestimate shorter waiting times and underestimate longer waiting times. 23% of the patients thought that they waited 0-5 minutes. In fact, only 15% of them waited 0-5 minutes. 11% of the patients thought they waited over 30 minutes. Actually, 25% of them waited over 30 minutes. Furthermore, they found out that in more attractive environments patients experienced a larger difference between actual and perceived times.

Taylor states two kinds of psychological and physiological responses to waiting can be observed: 1) uncertainty including annoyance, irritability, stress; and 2) anger (Taylor, 1994). Entertainment programs such as providing TV or magazines, outdoor views, refreshments as well as giving patients a choice what they can do while waiting could dramatically reduce those negative implications (Haggard & Hosking, 2003).

Becker and Douglass (2008) found a strong significant correlation between the level of anxiety and the attractiveness of a clinic. A well-designed environment is able to reduce stress and psychological harm of waiting patients. Arneill and Devlin (2002) emphasised how the design of outpatient waiting rooms influences the perception of the quality of healthcare services. More comfortable designed waiting areas are associated with greater perception of provided healthcare (Devlin, 2008; Marberry, 2006). Furthermore, healthcare staff can also perform better after small design changes of their work environment (Becker & Poe, 1980). So, there is a relation between the design of the environment, performance and attitude of healthcare staff, and patients' satisfaction with the healthcare services. This paper takes up this issue and asks the patients how the environment could be changed to make the waiting more comfortable. However, this question includes only comparable small changes like a water dispenser or more magazines. It does not include general redesigns of buildings, as this would often be impossible.

The result of more than 7,000 questionnaires filled in by German physicians to study the adherence to schedules of patients (Hartmannbund, 2014) was that in 1 in 10 appointments at GPs and in 1 in 7 appointments at specialist patients did not show up at all.

This chapter takes up those points within a questionnaire by asking the waiting patients how the waiting process in a certain institution is perceived (possible answers are "long", "ok", and "short"), and how one feels while waiting (possible answers are "comfortable", "neutral", and "uncomfortable"). This distinction enables to search for a correlation between those two factors. We study waiting times of an emergency hospital ambulance for follow-up examination and treatment. The focus lies on the waiting inside the waiting room and the administrative desk. We chose a hospital for our study because hospitals are places where the healthcare chain can be followed. It is the "the chain of operations that need to be performed to produce a particular health service" (Vissers & Beech, 2005). Defining such an effective healthcare chain enables the creation of strategic management tools to allocate resources to increase operational effectiveness and linking organisational objectives with operational processes to increase patients' satisfaction (Armistead, 1999).

METHODOLOGY

There are two research traditions, which differ in regard to the approach, data, aim, and usage (Erzberger, 1998). The objective tradition (1) on the one hand aims to verify correlations. Following a positivistic, quantitative, and rational approach, it tries to check hypothesis for explorative empirical science. The subjective tradition (2) on the other hand aims to find new correlations. It follows an interpretative and qualitative approach using qualitative data to generate hypothesis. Both research traditions have their place in the scientific community and also in the research presented in this chapter.

Figure 1 points out that we used mixed method research approach in our study. On the one hand, each step depends on one or more previous steps (Przyborski & Wohlrab-Sahr, 2010; Gläser & Laudel, 2009; Mayring, 2002; Girtler, 2001). On the other, we combined quantitative data with qualitative to first setup the quantita-

Figure 1. Mixed method research approach shows the process flow with activities and results of our methodology

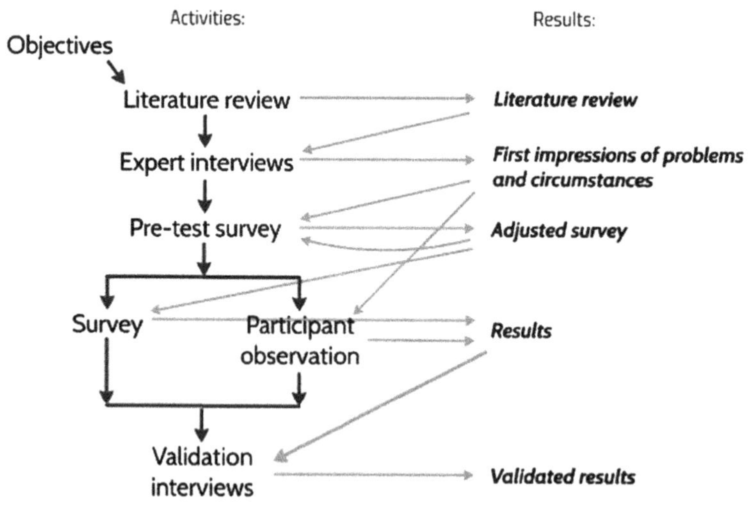

tive data inquiry parameters and then to explain the quantitative data gathered by putting it into context.

Within the first step of our methodology, the objectives were defined. Then the literature was used firstly to get an insight into the study area and secondly to define a proper methodology. Based on the results from the literature review, semi-structured, guideline-based, problem-centred expert interviews (Strauss, 1998) were conducted to get detailed insight and knowledge concerning the topic of waiting at the chosen physicians and the hospital ambulances. Based on the expert interviews, the questionnaire for the patients was designed. Before handing out, it was pre-tested several times till the questions were comprehensible and understandable. After the pre-tests, the questionnaire was handed out to the patients at the waiting rooms of a hospital ambulance and several GP offices. Parallel to and shortly after the survey phase, participant observation took place to examine the processes, which lead to waiting times, the environment of the waiting areas, and how the patients acted during the waiting time. Finally, the results were discussed with and validated through a subset of the resident physicians included in the study. The data was presented and physicians were given the opportunity to comment and reflect. The method was again a semi-structured, guideline-based, problem-centred expert interview.

We captured the quantitative data at two different kinds of environments (Janzek-Hawlat, 2015): at 4 GPs offices and at a hospital ambulance. In a first expert interview with the GPs the study was introduced and explained, the procedure was clarified, and the questions were asked. The semi-structured open interview was recorded, a participant observation was scheduled and questionnaires at the GP's waiting room were set up. In total there were 63 questionnaires filled in at GPs' offices. The head of the occupational medicine at the hospital was the expert interviewed. We spent a whole day for observation at the hospital's ambulance for follow-up care. This particular ambulance was chosen because the patients were normally not severely injured, had usually time and the ability to fill out the questionnaire that was given. In sum, there were 60 questionnaires filled in at the hospital.

In the following section, we present our empirical material and our findings. First, we show some relevant quantitative data. Second, we put the empirical data into context by using the evidence from the qualitative inquiry and discussing it. We derive results and discussion points based on our study.

SOME FIGURES FROM OUR STUDY

Our study showed that the majority of the patients at the hospital ambulance had an appointment between 9 a.m. and 9:29 a.m. *Figure 2* shows the distribution of ap-

Figure 2. Distribution of the appointments at the hospital ambulance within our study

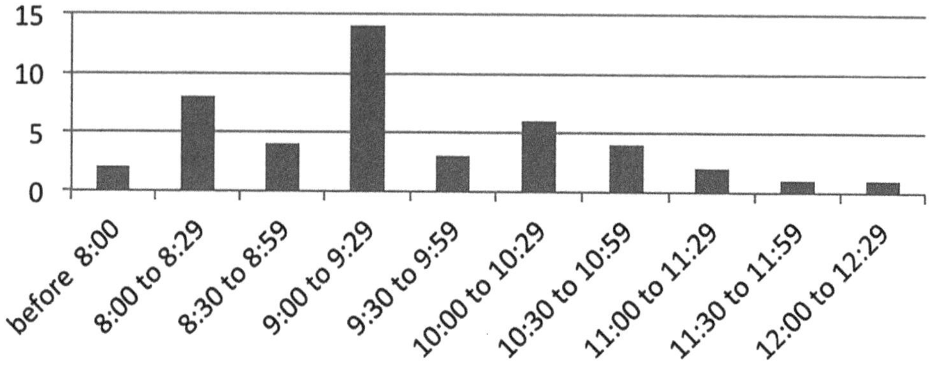

pointments made in our study. This example also shows that the scheduling process (with or without an appointment system) must be truly integrated in the workflow of a healthcare provider. Otherwise it causes additional waiting time for its patients.

There is no significant difference between waiting times at the administrative desk at the hospital ambulance and at resident physicians. While the majority of the patients were waiting less than six minutes in all these environments, some patients wait more than 11 minutes. In all the observed offices there was only one person working at the administrative desk. Questions like extension of long-term medications or the writing of sick notes might increase the waiting time at administrative desks. Some patients suggested providing an additional desk for administrative services. On the other hand, physicians in our study said that they couldn't afford to employ additional administrative persons. They calculate these additional costs in terms of patients: "Another employee is not affordable. One hour *(of an administration staff)* costs around 10-20 patients. Hiring another employee would make it necessary to have more patients, what decreases the time I have for each patient."

Patients at the hospital ambulance for follow-up care normally get an appointment calculated by the computer. The computer system is supposed to assign an appointment every 15 minutes. This allocation is not displayed in the system. Patients' appointments were at 8:00 (5 times out of 47 surveys), 9:00 (12 times out of 47 surveys) or 10:00 (6 times out of 47 surveys). Some patients even got an appointment at 9:20, which would be impossible according to the computer system. So either the right appointment time does not reach the patient due to false communication or the system is flawed. 60% of patients at the hospital ambulance for follow-up care waited between 60 and 120 minutes (see *Figure 3*). 8% were waiting less than 30 minutes, 20% waited more than 120 minutes. The median was 90 minutes.

Figure 3. Distribution of the waiting times at the hospital ambulance studied

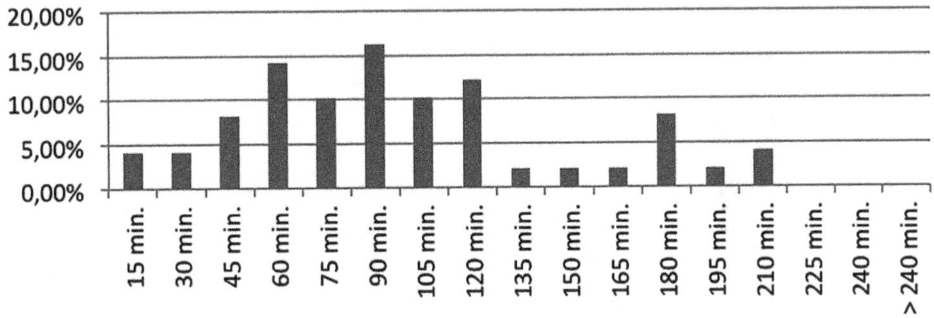

The median waiting time at resident physicians with an electronic appointment system was 17 minutes, at physicians without any electronic appointment system 64 minutes. Waiting times at physicians using appointment systems are clearly lower than at physicians not using one. However, both numbers are clearly lower than waiting times at the hospital. *Figure 4* shows the distribution of waiting times for hospital ambulance patients and patients at resident physicians studied.

Within the study the question asked to the patients was: "How do you perceive the waiting time?" The results show a clear tendency (see *Figure 5*). The shorter the waiting time, the more comfortable the patients feel, which is obvious. While 66.7% of the patients at the physicians using an electronic appointment system (EAS) feel comfortable, only 25% of the patients at physicians without an EAS and 10.2% of the patients at the hospital feel comfortable in their waiting environment.

Figure 4. Distribution of waiting times for hospital ambulance patients and patients at resident physicians studied

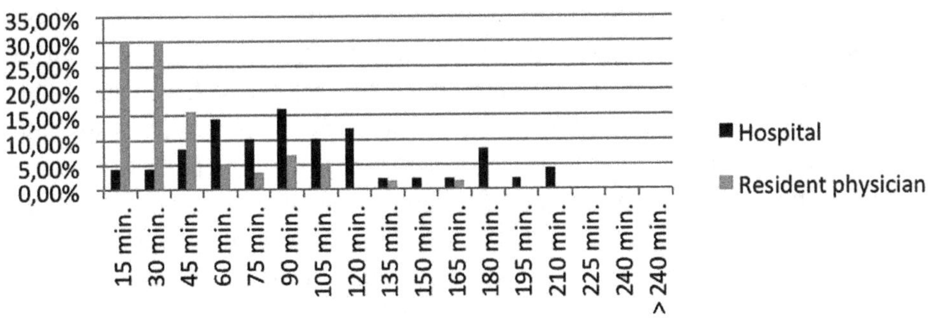

Figure 5. Perception of the waiting time by patients in the study (EAS=Electronic Appointment System)

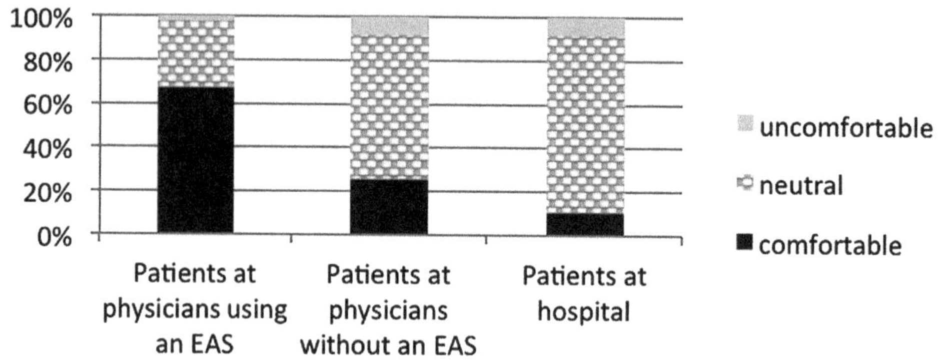

DISCUSSION

This section contains results and findings from the analysis of the collected qualitative and quantitative data supplemented by key results from the related work. Before presenting patient participation tools which target the reduction of waiting times, the issue of waiting will be described and discussed from different point of views including the reasons for waiting times and their average length. The section is structured by the questions asked in the introduction of the chapter.

The Origin for Waiting in Health Care

One approach to detect the causes of waiting in healthcare is process-oriented modelling of the healthcare flows. Modelling the physician-patient-interaction as well as the business processes of the doctor's office and the hospital ambulance makes possible to identify waiting situations. In this research the processes are not modelled because of the complexity of generalising for different healthcare providers: Some physicians claim that "there is no medical process" and that it is "difficult to standardise a medical process". The process starting from the first contact with the patients and ending with their diagnoses and treatment are found very inhomogeneous especially if the office organisation of a GP or specialist is considered. A process from one medical institution cannot be compared to the process of another one. Designing such a process would lead to an either very complex or inaccurate outcome. Also the research literature confirms that a standardisation of medical processes is hard to achieve. A study concludes that the incalculable medical everyday life, e.g., that a call from another institution concerning a patient during the office hours can lead to longer waiting times (Wijayasinghe, 2013), or an emergency patient arrives and the whole waiting list must be rearranged (Chan, 2013).

Patients normally call before visiting the physicians' office. During these calls patients are asked to state the medical issues, so a certain suitable time slot can be reserved for them. That is not always doable with all patients. Some patients might be able to express themselves others might not. This kind of problems is related to health literacy. Health literacy is a function of the interaction between individuals in health context, which they are opposed to. This applies to the patient, physician but also to the administrative personnel such as the receptionists or nurses. A lack of health literacy concerns especially the lower social classes (Nielsen-Bohlman, Panzer, & Kindig, 2004). However, the improvement of scheduling systems is one of the main claims of the patients studied.

One cannot imagine running a healthcare institution without using an electronic appointment system. However, there are some shortcomings in the application of such systems: If a system is not flexible enough to vary the duration of the time slot reserved for a patient later on and this patient does not appear at the right time, gaps in the schedule occur. If the next patient is not available, the time until s/he arrives is wasted time. A survey from the Hartmannbund (2014) in Germany states that one in seven patients misses an appointment at resident specialist and one in ten patients misses an appointment at GPs. The problem becomes bigger if a patient comes later than the appointment. This causes even longer waiting times (Hartmannbund, 2014). At the hospital of this study, the majority of patients (45 out of 60) had an appointment and 24.4% of them came late (11 out of 45). These numbers show that coming late to an appointment is quite often the case. For that reason and to prevent idle time, physicians overbook their appointment schedule as they expect – based on their own experiences – a certain amount of patients to come late or not to show up. So, they might reserve shorter time slots for the patients, so that the gap is not that big or that the next patient is already waiting and can be treated first, if another patient comes late. Norman and Bailey showed that long waiting times decrease the consultants' average time wasted (Bailey, 1952). Such systems fail when more patients come on schedule than estimated. This could then lead to the situation that the schedule falls apart and patients have to wait although having an appointment. Consequently, patients feel that appointments are not working well and start disregarding them.

Waiting Time Per Se

Waiting times captured in this study are comparable to the results from other studies (Dansky & Miles, 1997; Becker & Douglass, 2008). Within their survey in an emergency care department, Dansky and Miles (1997) found out that patients waited on average 55 minutes in the waiting area before entering the exam room. Becker and Douglass (2008) included different kinds of waiting times into their study such as total time in clinic, time spent with doctor, and time spent in the examination room. The average total time in the clinic was 63 minutes, the total waiting time was 48 minutes, and the time spent with a physician was 13 minutes.

Only one third of the participants of our survey perceived the waiting time at the hospital ambulance as "long". Almost two thirds thought the waiting time was "ok". This perception of waiting times is similar to the perception of waiting times at the GPs without an electronic appointment system. However, the waiting at the hospital triggered most often "neutral" (more than 80%) sensations. This indicates that people are used to long waiting times at hospitals and that is why they are neutral to their occurrence.

To overcome the physical and psychological burden of waiting (Taylor, 1994), hospitals often offer some kind of entertainment program such as TV or magazines in the waiting area. However, two fundamental issues are not provided to the patient: First, information about the waiting time or their position in the waiting line. Second, giving people the opportunity to leave the waiting room for some time, as they have to wait in front of the exam rooms so they do not miss their call (Haggard & Hosking, 2003). More than 60% of the patients of the hospital (37 out of 60) would have liked to know how much longer they had to wait. Forwarding this information to the patients would boost the perceived involvement of the patient into the administrative processes. It would not only enable a better understanding for long waiting times, but also dissolve the stress and tension of patients, as they are not able to estimate the time till they can see a doctor.

To increase the attractiveness and consequently decrease the anxiety of patients (Becker & Douglass, 2008) the following improvements were suggested by the patients: They would like to have more magazines and medical journals to read and to have more space in the waiting area. But the most important thing for them was to know how long they have to wait. To comply with this request, it would be necessary to show the waiting queue on the available screens in the waiting area. Then patients would know the approximate waiting time. This would reduce stress and tenseness of patients drastically as they could, e.g., go to the restrooms without having the feeling that they might miss their call.

It is interesting to see that physicians without electronic appointment systems (EAS) estimate the time that patients wait for them quite well, while physicians with an EAS overestimate this time. 50% of the patients of physicians without an EAS state that the duration of the waiting was "ok", but 41.7% considered they were waiting too "long". In contrast, 51.4% of the patients of physicians with an EAS regarded the time they waited for the physician as "ok" and 48.6% said that they waited a "short" time. The majority of patients at physicians without an EAS felt "neutral" concerning waiting. This result is similar to the hospital results, where most of the patients had also a "neutral" feeling towards waiting. Again, the results differ from the results of physicians with an EAS. There, two thirds of the patients considered waiting as "comfortable".

Improvements required by patients for waiting areas at the resident physicians are similar to the improvements required in the hospital setting. Here patients would like to have more magazines and more medical journals as well. They also would like to have a drink dispenser. It is interesting to see that some patients request more space than others. The need to know how much longer they have to wait is not as high as in the hospital, but was addressed by some patients explicitly. Due to a smaller and more individual system at the resident physicians compared to the hospital, it is not easy to display and explain the queue mechanisms. However, small improvements like a drink dispenser or magazines are acceptable for the resident physicians. The validation interviews showed that physicians are under certain conditions willing to apply the suggested improvements, e.g., provide water or more magazines. On the contrary, costly improvements such as drink dispenser or displaying waiting times are not accepted due to financial reasons.

Perception of Waiting

The impact of waiting on patients and physicians is completely different. Patients are affected directly as they lose the waiting time immediately. Physicians are affected in a different way. First of all, they feel the pressure of patients waiting and therefore they may reduce the treatment time per single patient. Furthermore, they face the anger and impatience once the long waiting patient is treated (Becker & Douglass, 2008). Second, the longer the waiting queue, the larger the waiting room has to be. Third, the probably biggest effect for physicians is that they have a bad reputation on online platforms about rating physicians and their services.

Our study showed that the median waiting time at resident physicians using an EAS has been lower than any other. Patients at physicians with an EAS perceive waiting times as shorter and more pleasant. Long waiting times in combination with an EAS increase patients' dissatisfaction drastically. Patients at the hospital ambulance in this study had to wait much longer and felt much less comfortable in the provided waiting environment.

Solutions for Reducing Waiting Times

The question regarding Electronic Appointment Systems (EASs) was to find out whether they have positive or negative impact on waiting times. Resident physicians have two ways of organising their office: to use an EAS, reserve time slots, and process patients within the reserved time; or to call one patient after the other and give them as much time as they need. The results of our study show that waiting times are lower at physicians with an EAS. The average waiting time is between 10 and 20 minutes at physicians with an EAS and 23.5 and 77.5 minutes at physicians without an EAS.

Our findings show that there are some problems for administrative staff if a physician introduces an EAS to the office. This occurs because the work type and workload of administrative staff changes through the EAS. A lot of administrative work is shifted from the physician to the administrative personnel when using an EAS.

The survey included several questions concerning the general acceptance of the tools suggested in the literature. Besides the implementation of ICT based tools, the possibility of changes within the intra-institutional processes, which are developed in cooperation with physicians and administrative personnel, are evaluated.

A topic, which has been of much debate lately in literature but also in the public, is the emergence of online doctors. Within such a setting, a patient sits at home in front of the computer connected to the doctor via camera and microphone. On the one hand, this tool enables the patient to wait at home in a familiar surrounding which makes the waiting time much more comfortable. On the other hand, it gives the physicians independence from space. Online medical consulting provides patients the possibility to choose time and place of the consultation. Patients are able to communicate with their physicians from home or from another convenient place. This topic has been of much debate in the literature lately because there have already been several providers, which offer online consultations.

The acceptance of online doctors within our study is miscellaneous. About two thirds of the waiting patients participating in the survey at one resident physician's office can imagine visiting their doctor online. The majority of the patients at the other resident physician's office cannot imagine visiting their doctor online. To find out the reasons for this, further studies are necessary. Patients at the hospital, who had to wait much longer than patients at resident physicians, were torn. 47.4% can imagine visiting their doctor online, 52.6% cannot. Those results correspond to the results from a study in Germany, where up to 44% of patients can imagine visiting a doctor online (Techniker Krankenkasse [TK], 2014). It is interesting to see that the higher the education level of patients, the more they are willing to see their physician online.

Remarkably, the question of visiting an online doctor is not related to waiting. People who are waiting longer do not tend to visit doctors online. It is rather depending on the way the physician works and maybe also depending on demographic factors like age or being a digital native or not. The results clearly show the importance of the Internet in the healthcare sector and correspond with the results from a study by Google (2012), which says that the Internet (meaning mainly the hospitals' websites) is the most frequented resource prior to a healthcare consumption. The fact that more than 60% of the patients visit two or more hospital websites before visiting a healthcare institution shows how important the online presence of healthcare institutions is.

Another idea for reducing waiting time by using ICT solutions is publishing waiting times online to enable patients to choose either when to visit a certain healthcare facility or to choose one out of several reachable healthcare facilities (Chan, 2013). There have been several attempts to publish waiting times online in different countries. Several hospital departments use the platform *twitter* and other social media platforms to publish waiting times. *Figure 6* shows on the left side an example of the Progress West Hospital in St. Louis Missouri (USA), which tweets the waiting times of the emergency department. Public hospitals in Vancouver (Canada) chose another way. They founded a platform where the waiting times from all emergency departments are published centrally, shown on the right side of *Figure 6*. Based on this information, patients have the possibility to choose where to go. It is then their choice.

Publishing waiting times online has two positive effects (Dansky & Miles, 1997; Miceli & Wolosin, 2004; De Man et al., 2005): First, by giving patient information about internal processes and the reasons how long they will wait, which increases acceptance of waiting times. Second, publishing waiting times online has the power to equalise the distribution of patients and healthcare facilities over time and place. The willingness of the patients to look at published waiting times has also

Figure 6. Online published waiting times of the Progress West Emergency Department in Missouri, USA [accessed 10.11.2014] (left); Canadian online platform showing waiting times online [accessed 06.07.2015 17:32] (right).

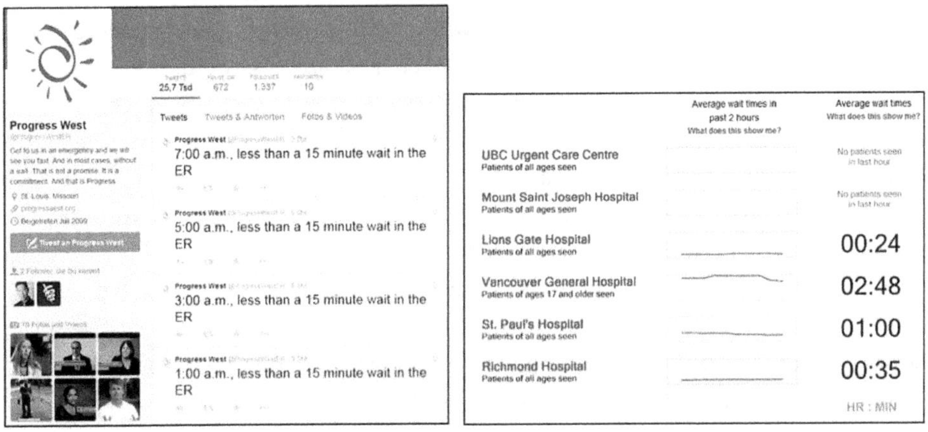

been one of the subjects of the questionnaire in our study. The majority of the patients (79,3% of the patients at the hospital, 58,7% of the patients at resident physicians) who took part in the study are in favour of seeing waiting times online. Furthermore, 83% of the patients at hospitals and 73,8% of the patients at resident physicians, who would like to see waiting times online, would also plan their visit according to this information.

CONCLUSION

The question of whether patients want to participate in healthcare processes at all is an ambiguous one. Several studies have been done on this question and the results are diverse (Guadagnoli & Ward, 1998; Levinson, Kao, Kuby, & Thisted, 2005; Strull, Lo, & Charles, 1984; Little et al., 2001; Say, Murtagh, & Thomson, 2006; Mandell, Poses, Kazis, & Duefield, 2000). Naturally the willingness for participation is highly dependent on the subject (Longtin et al., 2010). Decisions, which are less or not dependent on medical knowledge or expertise, should involve patients more than issues which are highly complex, especially in medical terms (Little et al., 2001). Waiting is a good example. Patients could be included in dealing with the problems of waiting for healthcare and finding out ways to overcome these problems. No special medical knowledge is necessary to be involved in this challenge and it has in fact impact to everyone.

In this chapter after studying waiting times for patients and physicians at hospitals and outpatient clinics the impact of waiting is analysed on three levels based on our quantitative and qualitative study and literature review: from patients' point of view, from healthcare providers' point of view, and from the healthcare system's point of view. The situation of the patients and their requirements are shown, strategies to reduce times, especially for waiting for the administrative work at the administrative desk, for waiting in waiting area and for waiting for in-process, are presented, and the questions listed in the introduction of the chapter are answered.

One of the main results is that waiting times depend very much on the fact whether the doctor has an electronic appointment system (EAS) or not. The study shows that waiting times can be decreased substantially by using an EAS. While patients visiting doctors not using an EAS had to wait 64 minutes in median, the median was only 17 minutes at doctors with an EAS. However, there is of course room for improvement concerning the allocation of the time slots for each patient at an EAS. Some patients find it very hard to describe what kind of medical condition they want to discuss with the doctor on the telephone while making the appointment. One of the reasons for that is the lack of health literacy.

Another finding is that the majority of patients are willing to use ICT based tools, which are supposed to decrease waiting times. Patients are willing to visit their doctor online or plan the hospital or doctors' visit according to published waiting times of certain healthcare institutions. The implementation of such tools would not only decrease waiting times, they would also increase patient empowerment and the involvement in healthcare service consumption, which again could increase health literacy. Better health literacy would then lead to a better communication between healthcare providers and consumers. Appointments could then be planned easier or more efficiently, which would in then increase the patients' flow.

The question on what kind of patients is more likely to use ICT tools, for instance, for reducing waiting times still remains. Factors such as age or socioeconomic levels obviously influence patients' participation remarkably and should therefore be considered in future work to identify technological or organisational ways to reduce waiting for patients in healthcare sector (Levinson et al., 2005; Say et al., 2006; Gaston & Mitchell, 2005; McKinstry, 2000; Rosen, Anell, & Hjortsberg, 2001; Cassileth, Zupkis, Sutton-Smith, & March, 1980; Rothenbacher, Lutz, & Porzsolt, 1997).

The most obvious reason for waiting for healthcare services is that there are too many patients and too few doctors or hospitals (Blake, 2006). Hiring more physicians at a hospital by increasing the quantity of the healthcare provided, shifting work from physicians to other healthcare staff, or distributing patients better over existing healthcare providers might help solving this problem. These issues have a political, financial, and economic dimension that cannot be dealt with in this chapter. As a next step the EASs and other (online) information systems need to be designed and adapted that help provide patients the above-mentioned functionality like showing the reasons for waiting or how much time left to meet the doctor or get the treatment. These need to be evaluated again "in the wild" to improve the circumstances that cause waiting times and so to reduce waiting for patients.

REFERENCES

Adams, K., Greiner, A. C., & Corrigan, J. M. (2004). *1st Annual Crossing the Quality Chasm Summit: A Focus on Communities*. Washington, DC: National Academies Press.

Armistead, C. (1999). Knowledge management and process performance. *Journal of Knowledge Management*, *3*(2), 143–157. doi:10.1108/13673279910275602

Arneill, A. B., & Devlin, A. S. (2002). Perceived Quality of Care: The Influence of the Waiting Room Environment. *Journal of Environmental Psychology*, *22*(4), 345–360. doi:10.1006/jevp.2002.0274

Bailey, N. T. (1952). A Study of Queues and Appointment Systems in Hospital Out-Patient Departments, with Special Reference to Waiting-Times. *Journal of the Royal Statistical Society. Series B. Methodological, 14*(2), 185–199.

Becker, F., & Douglass, S. (2008). The ecology of the patient visit: Physical attractiveness, waiting times, and perceived quality of care. *The Journal of Ambulatory Care Management, 31*(2), 128–141. doi:10.1097/01.JAC.0000314703.34795.44 PMID:18360174

Becker, F., & Poe, D. B. Jr. (1980). The effects of user-generated design modifications in a general hospital. *Journal of Nonverbal Behavior, 4*(4), 195–218. doi:10.1007/BF00986197

Blake, H. (2006). *Waiting Line Models,* Retrieved from http://www.csus.edu/indiv/b/blakeh/mgmt/documents/OPM101SupplC.pdf

Brink-Muinen, V. D., Van Dulmen, S. M., De Haes, H. C., Visser, A. P., Schellevis, F. G., & Bensing, J. M. (2006). Has patients' involvement in the decision-making process changed over time? *Health Expectations, 9*(4), 333–342. doi:10.1111/j.1369-7625.2006.00413.x PMID:17083560

Carpman, J. R., Grant, M. A., & Simmons, D. A. (1986). *Design that cares: planning health facilities for patients and visitors*. Chicago: American Hospital Pub.

Cassileth, B. R., Zupkis, R. V., Sutton-Smith, K., & March, V. (1980). Information and participation preferences among cancer patients. *Annals of Internal Medicine, 92*(6), 832–836. doi:10.7326/0003-4819-92-6-832 PMID:7387025

Chan, K. (2013). *Going to the ER? Real-time hospital emergency wait times now online*. Retrieved from http://www.vancitybuzz.com/2013/04/hospital-emergency-room-wait-times-online/

Committee on Patient Safety and Quality Improvement. (2005). ACOG Committee Opinion No. 320: Partnering with patients to improve safety. *Obstetrics and Gynecology, 106*(5), 1123–1128. doi:10.1097/00006250-200511000-00057 PMID:16260544

Dansky, K. H., & Miles, J. (1997). Patient satisfaction with ambulatory healthcare services: Waiting time and filling time. *Hospital & Health Services Administration, 42*(2), 165–177. PMID:10167452

De Man, S., Vlerick, P., Gemmel, P., De Bondt, P., Matthys, D., & Dierckx, R. (2005). Impact of waiting on the perception of service quality in nuclear medicine. *Nuclear Medicine Communications, 26*(6), 541–547. doi:10.1097/00006231-200506000-00010 PMID:15891598

Deloitte. (2011). *Umfrage 2011 zum Gesundheitswesen in der Schweiz. Wichtigste Ergebnisse, strategische Auswirkungen.*

Devlin, A. S. (2008). Judging a Book by Its Cover: Medical Building Facades and Judgments of Care. *Environment and Behavior*, *40*(3), 307–329. doi:10.1177/0013916507302242

Eck, E. K., DeBaun, B., & Pugliese, G. (2001). *The Contagious Patient: Identifying, Containing, and Treating Appropriately.* Retrieved http://www.infectioncontroltoday.com/articles/2001/12/the-contagious-patient.aspx

Emanuel, E. J., & Emanuel, L. L. (1992). Four models of the physician-patient relationship. *Journal of the American Medical Association*, *267*(16), 2221–2227. doi:10.1001/jama.1992.03480160079038 PMID:1556799

Erzberger, C. (1998). *Zahlen und Wörter: Die Verbindung quantitativer und qualitativer Daten und Methoden im Forschungsprozeß*. Dt. Studien-Verlag.

Fischer, T. (2009). *Die ärztliche Versorgung im niedergelassenen Bereich aus dem Blickwinkel der Patienten: Schlaglichter auf ein vernachlässigtes Gebiet der Gesundheitspolitik.*

Fleisher, J. (2013). Hospitals Duel Over Wait Times. *The Wall Street Journal.*

Gaston, C. M., & Mitchell, G. (2005). Information giving and decision-making in patients with advanced cancer: A systematic review. *Social Science & Medicine*, *61*(10), 2252–2264. doi:10.1016/j.socscimed.2005.04.015 PMID:15922501

General Medical Council. (2013). *Good Medical Practice.* Retrieved from http://www.gmc-uk.org/guidance/news_consultation/20477.asp

Gillon, R. (1994). Medical ethics: Four principles plus attention to scope. *BMJ (Clinical Research Ed.)*, *309*(6948), 184–188. doi:10.1136/bmj.309.6948.184 PMID:8044100

Girtler, R. (2001). *Methoden der Feldforschung*. Stuttgart: UTB GmbH.(in German)

Gläser, J., & Laudel, G. (2009). *Experteninterviews und qualitative Inhaltsanalyse: als Instrumente rekonstruierender Untersuchungen.* Wiesbaden: VS Verlag für Sozialwissenschaften.

Google (2012). *The Digital Journey to Wellness: Hospital Selection Infographic.*

Grazie, D., & Wimmer-Puchinger, B. (2014). Rahmen-Gesundheitsziel 3 - Gesundheitskompetenz der Bevölkerung stärken, Bericht der Arbeitsgruppe. Bundesministerium für Gesundheit, Editor (in German).

Guadagnoli, E., & Ward, P. (1998). Patient participation in decision-making. *Social Science & Medicine*, *47*(3), 329–339. doi:10.1016/S0277-9536(98)00059-8 PMID:9681902

Haggard, L., & Hosking, S. (2003). *Healing the Hospital Environment: Design, Management and Maintenance of Healthcare Premises*. London: Taylor & Francis.

Hartmannbund. (2014). *Umfrage „Termintreue" – Datenbasis*. Retrieved from http://www.hartmannbund.de/uploads/Landesverb%C3%A4nde/Niedersachsen/2014-07-09_Handout-Presse.PDF (in German).

Janzek-Hawlat, S. (2015). *Impact of waiting times in health care* [Master Thesis]. Faculty of Informatics, Vienna University of Technology.

Kennedy, J. F. (1962). *Special message to Congress on protecting consumer interest*. Presidential Papers. President's Office Files.

Kizer, K. W. (2001). Establishing healthcare performance standards in an era of consumerism. *The New England Journal of Medicine*, *286*(10), 1213–1217. PMID:11559267

Lammers, W. M. (2014). *So lässt sich die Wartezeit in der Praxis reduzieren*. ÄrzteZeitung. (in German)

Lancet, T.The Lancet. (2005). Will consumerism lead to better health? *Lancet*, *366*(9483), 343. doi:10.1016/S0140-6736(05)66999-1 PMID:16060053

Laschet, H. (2014). *Kommentar zur Wartezeit-Umfrage: Säumige Patienten?* ÄrzteZeitung. (in German)

Levinson, W., Kao, A., Kuby, A., & Thisted, R. A. (2005). Not all patients want to participate in decision making. A national study of public preferences. *Journal of General Internal Medicine*, *20*(6), 531–535. doi:10.1111/j.1525-1497.2005.04101.x PMID:15987329

Little, P., Everitt, H., Williamson, I., Warner, G., Moore, M., Gould, C., & Payne, S. et al. (2001). Preferences of patients for patient centred approach to consultation in primary care: Observational study. *BMJ (Clinical Research Ed.)*, *322*(7284), 468–540. doi:10.1136/bmj.322.7284.468 PMID:11222423

Longtin, Y., Sax, H., Leape, L. L., Sheridan, S. E., Donaldson, L., & Pittet, D. (2010). Patient Participation: Current Knowledge and Applicability to Patient Safety. *Mayo Clinic Proceedings*, *85*(1), 53–62. doi:10.4065/mcp.2009.0248 PMID:20042562

Mangold, M., Peintinger, M, & Kopetzki, C. (2010). Behandlungsablehnung trotz vitaler Indikation. RdM - Recht der Medizin 2010/4. (in German)

Mansell, D., Poses, R. M., Kazis, L., & Duefield, C. A. (2000). Clinical factors that influence patients' desire for participation in decisions about illness. *Archives of Internal Medicine*, *160*(19), 2991–2996. doi:10.1001/archinte.160.19.2991 PMID:11041908

Marberry, S. O. (2006). *Improving Healthcare with Better Building Design*. Chicago, IL: Health Administration Press.

Marsh, G. E. Jr. (1993). Hospital Interior Architecture: Creating Healing Environments for Special Patient Populations. *The New England Journal of Medicine*, *328*(12), 894–895. doi:10.1056/NEJM199303253281224

Mayring, P. (2002). *Einführung in die qualitative Sozialforschung*. Weinheim: Beltz. (in German)

McKinstry, B. (2000). Do patients wish to be involved in decision making in the consultation? A cross sectional survey with video vignettes. *BMJ (Clinical Research Ed.)*, *321*(7265), 867–871. doi:10.1136/bmj.321.7265.867 PMID:11021866

Miceli, J., & Wolosin, R. J. (2004). *You're running late - now what? Patient satisfaction, wait time and physician behavior.* Orlando, Florida: World organization of national colleges, academies and academic associations of General Practitioners/ Family Physicians.

Mundi Index. (2012). *Land Vergleich > Krankenhausbetten pro Einwohner*. Retrieved from http://www.indexmundi.com/g/r.aspx?v=2227&l=de

Nielsen-Bohlman, L., Panzer, A. M., & Kindig, D. A. (2004). *Health literacy: A prescription to end confusion*. Washington, D.C.: National Academies Press.

Nursing & Midwifery Council. (2015). *The code - Professional standards of practice and behaviour for nurses and midwives*. Retrieved from http://www.nmc.org.uk/standards/code/

Pittet, D., Allegranzi, B., Storr, J., & Donaldson, L. (2005). 'Clean Care is Safer Care': The Global Patient Safety Challenge 2005–2006. *International Journal of Infectious Diseases*, *10*(6), 419–424. doi:10.1016/j.ijid.2006.06.001 PMID:16914344

Przyborski, A., & Wohlrab-Sahr, M. (2010). *Qualitative Sozialforschung: Ein Arbeitsbuch*. München: Oldenbourg Wissenschaftsverlag. (in German)

Rosen, P., Anell, A., & Hjortsberg, C. (2001). Patient views on choice and participation in primary health care. *Health Policy (Amsterdam)*, *55*(2), 121–128. doi:10.1016/S0168-8510(00)00122-6 PMID:11163651

Rothenbacher, D., Lutz, M. P., & Porzsolt, F. (1997). Treatment decisions in palliative cancer care: Patients' preferences for involvement and doctors' knowledge about it. *European Journal of Cancer*, *33*(8), 1184–1189. doi:10.1016/S0959-8049(97)00034-8 PMID:9301440

Say, R., Murtagh, M., & Thomson, R. (2006). Patients' preference for involvement in medical decision making: A narrative review. *Patient Education and Counseling*, *60*(2), 102–114. doi:10.1016/j.pec.2005.02.003 PMID:16442453

Staeck, F. (2014). *Wartezeiten-Debatte: Regierung gegen Vergleich von PKV mit GKV*. ÄrzteZeitung. (in German)

Statistik Austria. (2015a). *Demographie*. Retrieved from http://www.statistik.at/web_de/statistiken/soziales/gender-statistik/demographie/

Statistik Austria. (2015b). *Stationäre Aufenthalte*. Retrieved from http://www.statistik.at/web_de/statistiken/gesundheit/stationaere_aufenthalte/index.html

Strauss, A. L. (1998). *Grundlagen qualitativer Sozialforschung: Datenanalyse und Theoriebildung in der empirischen soziologischen Forschung*. Fink. (in German)

Strull, W. M., Lo, B., & Charles, G. (1984). Do patients want to participate in medical decision making? *Journal of the American Medical Association*, *252*(21), 2990–2994. doi:10.1001/jama.1984.03350210038026 PMID:6502860

Taylor, S. J. (1994). Waiting for Service: The Relationship between Delays and Evaluations of Service. *Journal of Marketing*, *58*(2), 56–69. doi:10.2307/1252269

Techniker Krankenkasse. (2014). *TK-Meinungspuls Gesundheit 2014*. Retrieved from http://www.tk.de/tk/themen/meinungspuls-gesundheit-oktober-2014/meinungspuls-gesundheit-oktober-2014-studienband/660168

Vissers, J., & Beech, R. (2005). *Health operations management: Patient flow logistics in health care. Routledge health management series*. London, NY: Routledge.

Wallner, J. (2013). Rechtsethischer Anspruch und faktische Grenzen von Patienteaufklärung und Informed Consent.[in German]. *Zeitschrift für Gesundheitspolitik*, *2013*(4).

Wijayasinghe, D. S. (2013). *I arrive on time but end up waiting to see my doctor. Why?* The Globe and Mail.

World Health Organization. (1997). The Vienna Recommendations on Health Promoting Hospitals.

World Health Organization. (2015). *Health expenditure, total (% of GDP)*. Retrieved from http://www.who.int/gho/health_financing/total_expenditure/en/

KEY TERMS AND DEFINITIONS

Electronic Appointment System: A piece of software to book appointments online, here for healthcare institutions.

Health Literacy: Ability to read, understand, describe and use healthcare information that is needed for health decisions or treatment.

Mixed Method Research Approach: Research approach applying mixed (qualitative and quantitative) methods in which each step depends on one or more previous steps.

Outpatient Clinics: A clinic, department or ward of a hospital that provides diagnosis and care for patients not staying overnight.

Qualitative Research: Exploratory research for understanding reasons of phenomena inquired quantitatively.

Waiting Time: The time patients have to wait for a physician or for appointments, diagnostic procedures in hospitals or at resident doctors.

ENDNOTES

1. http://www.indexmundi.com/g/r.aspx?v=2227&l=de
2. http://epp.eurostat.ec.europa.eu/statistics_explained/index.php/Healthy_life_years_statistics/de
3. http://www.statistik.at/web_de/presse/073804
4. https://www.gesundheit.gv.at/Portal.Node/ghp/public/content/gesundheitsbarometer.html

APPENDIX

Interview Guideline at the Resident Physician and Hospital

Part A

A1: What are the main patient processes?
A2: What are the reasons for waiting times?
- **A2.1:** Are there inner organisational reasons?
- **A2.2:** Are there external reasons?

A3: How long is the average waiting time?
A4: Are there any possibilities to decrease waiting times?
- **A4.1:** Are there inner organisational possibilities to decrease waiting times?
- **A4.2:** Are there possibilities outside the organisation to decrease waiting times?
- **A4.3:** Are there IT-based solutions, which could decrease waiting times?

A5: Are you using an appointment system?
- **A5.1:** What is the percentage of your patients using your appointment system?
- **A5.2:** What is the percentage of your patients who could use your appointment system?
- **A5.3:** Are appointment systems in general decreasing waiting times?

Part B

B1: How is the office/hospital equipped?
- **B1.1:** At the reception
- **B1.2:** In the waiting area

B2: Are there any entertainment facilities within the waiting area?

Questionnaire for Patients Waiting in the Hospital Waiting Area or Resident Physician

Part A: "Waiting"

A1: At what time did you arrive in the waiting area?
A2: How long was the waiting time at the administrative desk?
A3: Do you have an appointment?
- Yes | no
- **A3.1:** If yes, at what time?

A4: How do you sense the length of the waiting time here normally?
- Long | ok | short

A5: How do you sense the waiting in the waiting area?

Pleasant | neutral | unpleasant

A6: What would it need to make the waiting time more pleasant (multiple answers)?

Books and magazines | more media entertainment | more space | increase cleanness | new design of the waiting area | water dispenser | more informative literature | I would like to know how much longer I have to wait | others…

A7: Are you coming alone or in company?

Partner | friend | child/children | other … | I'm here alone

A7.1: If you are coming in company, what would this person do if he or she wouldn't be here?

Working | free time | homework | others…

A7.2: If you are coming with a child, is there enough entertainment provided for the child?

Yes | no

A8: What would you do if you wouldn't be here?

Working | free time | homework | cure at home | other…

Part B: Decrease Waiting Time

B1: Could you imagine visiting your doctor online?

Yes | no

B2: Would you like to see waiting times online?

Yes | no

B2.1: Would you plan your visit according to the online waiting times?

Yes | no

B3: Do you prefer a strict appointment system?

Yes | no

B4: Do you have other suggestions to decrease the waiting time?

Part C: Demographics

C1: Please state your age

C2: What is your sex?

Compilation of References

Aakhus, E., Granlund, I., Oxman, A., & Flottorp, S. (2015). Tailoring interventions to implement recommendations for the treatment of elderly patients with depression: a qualitative study. *International journal of mental health systems, 9*(1), 1-24.

Abdoolatiff, S., & Narod, F. B. (2009). Investigating the effectiveness of computer simulations in the teaching of "atomic structure and bonding". In *Chemistry Education in the ICT Age* (pp. 85-100).

Adams, K., Greiner, A. C., & Corrigan, J. M. (2004). *1st Annual Crossing the Quality Chasm Summit: A Focus on Communities*. Washington, DC: National Academies Press.

Adeseun, G. A., Bonney, C. C., & Rosas, S. E. (2012). Health literacy associated with blood pressure but not other cardiovascular disease risk factors among dialysis patients. *American Journal of Hypertension, 25*(3), 348–353. doi:10.1038/ajh.2011.252 PMID:22237154

Adibi, S. (2015). Introduction. In S. Adibi (Ed.), *mHealth Multidisciplinary Verticals* (pp. 1–10). London: CRC Press, Taylor & Francis Group.

Adie, K., Schofield, C., Berrow, M., Wingham, J., Freeman, J., Humfryes, J., & Pritchard, C. (2014). Does the use of Nintendo Wii Sports improve arm function and is it acceptable to patients after stroke? Publication of the Protocol of the Trial of Wii in Stroke - TWIST. *International Journal of General Medicine, 7*(1), 475–481. doi:10.2147/IJGM.S65379 PMID:25336985

Agree Collaboration. (2001). Appraisal of guidelines for research & evaluation (AGREE) instrument.

Ahern, D., Phalen, J. M., & Eaton, C. B. (2008). The role of eHealth in patient engagement and quality improvement. In M. C. Gibbons (Ed.), *eHealth solutions for healthcare disparities* (pp. 75–92). New York: Springer. doi:10.1007/978-0-387-72815-5_9

Ahleit, B. D. (1995). Interventions for clients with lower respiratory problems. In D. D. Ignatavicius, M. L. Workman, & M. A. Mishler (Eds.), *Medical surgical nursing: a nursing process approach* (2nd ed., pp. 673–728). Philadelphia: Saunders WB.

Ahmad, F. S., Metlay, J. P., Barg, F. K., Henderson, R. R., & Werner, R. M. (2013). Identifying hospital organizational strategies to reduce readmissions. *American Journal of Medical Quality*, *28*(4), 278–285. doi:10.1177/1062860612464999 PMID:23118202

Ajzen, I. (1971). Attitudinal vs. normative messages: An investigation of the differential effects of persuasive communications on behavior. *Sociometry*, *34*(2), 263–280. doi:10.2307/2786416

Ajzen, I. (1988). *Attitudes, personality, and behavior*. Chicago, IL: Dorsey.

Ajzen, I. (1991, December). (199I). The theory of planned behavior. *Organizational Behavior and Human Decision Processes*, *50*(2), 179–211. doi:10.1016/0749-5978(91)90020-T

Ajzen, I. (2002). Perceived Behavioral Control, Self-Efficacy, Locus of Control, and the Theory of Planned Behavior. *Journal of Applied Social Psychology*, *32*(4), 665–683. doi:10.1111/j.1559-1816.2002.tb00236.x

Ajzen, I., & Albarracen, D. (2007). *Predicting and changing behavior: A reasoned action approach*. Mahwah, NJ: Lawrence Erlbaum Associates Publishers.

Ajzen, I., Czasch, C., & Flood, M. G. (2009). From Intentions to Behavior: Implementation Intention, Commitment, and Conscientiousness1. *Journal of Applied Social Psychology*, *39*(6), 1356–1372. doi:10.1111/j.1559-1816.2009.00485.x

Aldred, H., Gott, M., & Gariballa, S. (2005). Advanced heart failure: Impact on older patients and informal carers. *Journal of Advanced Nursing*, *49*(2), 116–124. doi:10.1111/j.1365-2648.2004.03271.x PMID:15641944

Al-Jundi, W., Madbak, K., Beard, J. D., Nawaz, S., & Tew, G. A. (2013). Systematic review of home-based exercise programmes for individuals with intermittent claudication. *European Journal of Vascular and Endovascular Surgery*, *46*(6), 690–706. doi:10.1016/j.ejvs.2013.09.004 PMID:24076079

Alliance for Home Health Quality & Innovation. (2014). *The Future of Home Health Care Project*. Retrieved August, 2015, from http://www.ahhqi.org/images/pdf/future-whitepaper.pdf

Alwan, A., MacLean, D. R., Riley, L. M., d'Espaignet, E. T., Mathers, C. D., Stevens, G. A., & Bettcher, D. (2010). Monitoring and surveillance of chronic noncommunicable diseases: Progress and capacity in high-burden countries. *Lancet*, *376*(9755), 1861–1868. doi:10.1016/S0140-6736(10)61853-3 PMID:21074258

American Diabetes Association. (2013). American Diabetes Association releases new research estimating annual cost of diabetes at $ 245 billion. Retrieved from http://www.diabetes.org/for-media/2013/annual-costs-of-diabetes-2013.html?loc=cost-of-diabetes

Amrhein, P. C., Miller, W. R., Yahne, C. E., Palmer, M., & Fulcher, L. (2003). Client Commitment Language During Motivational Interviewing Predicts Drug Use Outcomes. *Journal of Consulting and Clinical Psychology*, *71*(5), 862–878. doi:10.1037/0022-006X.71.5.862 PMID:14516235

Anderson, G., & Hussey, P. (2001). Comparing health system performance in OECD countries. *Health Affairs*, *20*(3), 219–232. doi:10.1377/hlthaff.20.3.219 PMID:11585171

Anderson, L., & Taylor, R. S. (2014). Cardiac rehabilitation for people with heart disease: An overview of Cohrane systematic reviews. *Cochrane Database of Systematic Reviews*, *12*, CD011273. PMID:25503364

Anderson, W. G., Kools, S., & Lyndon, A. (2013). Dancing Around Death Hospitalist–Patient Communication About Serious Illness. *Qualitative Health Research*, *23*(1), 3–13. doi:10.1177/1049732312461728 PMID:23034778

Armistead, C. (1999). Knowledge management and process performance. *Journal of Knowledge Management*, *3*(2), 143–157. doi:10.1108/13673279910275602

Arneill, A. B., & Devlin, A. S. (2002). Perceived Quality of Care: The Influence of the Waiting Room Environment. *Journal of Environmental Psychology*, *22*(4), 345–360. doi:10.1006/jevp.2002.0274

Assal, J. P. (1999). Revisiting the approach to treatment of long-term illness: From the acute to the chronic state. A need for educational and managerial skills for long-term follow-up. *Patient Education and Counseling*, *37*(2), 99–111. doi:10.1016/S0738-3991(98)00109-8 PMID:14528538

Atkin, C. (1994). Designing persuasive health messages. *Effective dissemination of clinical health information*, 95-0015.

Azoulay, E., Chevret, S., Leleu, G., Pochard, F., Barboteu, M., Adrie, C., & Schlemmer, B. et al. (2000). Half the families of intensive care unit patients experience inadequate communication with physicians. *Critical Care Medicine*, *28*(8), 3044–3049. doi:10.1097/00003246-200008000-00061 PMID:10966293

Baca-Motes, K., Brown, A., Gneezy, A., Keenan, E. A., & Nelson, L. D. (2013). Commitment and Behavior Change: Evidence from the Field. *The Journal of Consumer Research*, *39*(5), 1070–1084. doi:10.1086/667226

Bacigalupo, R., Cudd, P., Littlewood, C., Bissell, P., Hawley, M. S., & Buckley Woods, H. (2013). Interventions employing mobile technology for overweight and obesity: An early systematic review of randomized controlled trials. *Obesity Reviews*, *14*(4), 279–291. doi:10.1111/obr.12006 PMID:23167478

Badcott, D. (2005). The expert patient: Valid recognition or false hope? *Medicine, Health Care, and Philosophy*, *8*(2), 173–178. doi:10.1007/s11019-005-2275-7 PMID:16215797

Bailey, N. T. (1952). A Study of Queues and Appointment Systems in Hospital Out-Patient Departments, with Special Reference to Waiting-Times. *Journal of the Royal Statistical Society. Series B. Methodological*, *14*(2), 185–199.

Bain, L. L., Wilson, T., & Chaikind, E. (1989). Participant perceptions of exercise programs for overweight women. *Research Quarterly for Exercise and Sport*, *60*(2), 134–143. doi:10.1080/02701367.1989.10607428 PMID:2489834

Bandura, A. (1982). Self-efficacy mechanism in human agency. *The American Psychologist, 37*(2), 122–147. doi:10.1037/0003-066X.37.2.122

Bandura, A. (2001). Social cognitive theory: An agentic perspective. *Annual Review of Psychology, 52*(1), 1–26. doi:10.1146/annurev.psych.52.1.1 PMID:11148297

Bao, H., Wang, J., Zhou, D., Han, Z., Zhang, Y., Su, L., & Li, Q. et al. (2015). Community Physician-Guided Long-Term Domiciliary Oxygen Therapy Combined with Conventional Therapy in Stage IV COPD Patients. *Rehabilitation Nursing*, (Sep): 10. PMID:26354385

Barello, S., & Graffigna, G. (2014). Engaging patients to recover life projectuality: an Italian cross-disease framework. *Quality of Life Research,* 24(5), 1087-1096. doi:10.1007/s11136-014-0846-x

Barello, S., & Graffigna, G. (2014). Engaging patients to recover life projectuality: An Italian cross-disease framework. [Epubaheadofprint]. *Quality of Life Research: An International Journal of Quality of Life Aspects of Treatment, Care and Rehabilitation.* doi:10.1007/s11136-014- 0846-x PMID:25373927

Barello, S., & Graffigna, G. (2015). Engagement-sensitive decision making: training doctors to sustain patient engagement in medical consultations. In G. Graffigna, S. Barello, & S. Triberti (Eds.), *Patient Engagement: A Consumer-Centered Model to Innovate Healthcare* (pp. 78–93). Berlin: De Gruyter Open. doi:10.1515/9783110452440-008

Barello, S., & Graffigna, G. (2015). Patient engagement in healthcare: Pathways for effective medical decision-making. *Neuropsychological Trend, 17*(17), 53–65. doi:10.7358/neur-2015-017-bare

Barello, S., Graffigna, G., Savarese, M., & Bosio, A. C. (2014a). Engaging patients in health management: Towards a preliminary theoretical conceptualization. *Psicologia Della Salute, 3*(3), 11–33. doi:10.3280/PDS2014-003002

Barello, S., Graffigna, G., & Vegni, E. (2012). Patient engagement as an emerging challenge for healthcare services: Mapping the literature. *Nursing Research and Practice, 2012*, 905934. doi:10.1155/2012/905934 PMID:23213497

Barello, S., Graffigna, G., Vegni, E., & Bosio, A. C. (2014). The challenges of conceptualizing patient engagement in healthcare: A lexicographic literature review. *Journal of Participatory Medicine, 6*, e9.

Barello, S., Graffigna, G., Vegni, E., & Bosio, A. C. (2014b). The challenges of conceptualizing patient engagement in health care: A lexicographic literature review. *Journal of Participatory Medicine, 6*, e9.

Barello, S., Graffigna, G., Vegni, E., Savarese, M., Lombardi, F., & Bosio, A. C. (2015). 'Engage me in taking care of my heart': A grounded theory study on patient–cardiologist relationship in the hospital management of heart failure. *BMJ Open, 5*(3), e005582. doi:10.1136/bmjopen-2014-005582 PMID:25776041

Barnes, S., Gardiner, C., Gott, M., Payne, S., Chady, B., Small, N., & Halpin, D. et al. (2012). Enhancing patient-professional communication about end-of-life issues in life-limiting conditions: A critical review of the literature. *Journal of Pain and Symptom Management*, *44*(6), 866–879. doi:10.1016/j.jpainsymman.2011.11.009 PMID:22819438

Barzel, A., Ketels, G., Tetzlaff, B., Krüger, H., Haevernick, K., Daubmann, A., & Scherer, M. et al. (2013). Enhancing activities of daily living of chronic stroke patients in primary health care by modified constraint-induced movement therapy (HOMECIMT): Study protocol for a cluster randomized controlled trial. *Trials*, *14*, 334. PMID:24124993

Bear, D. M., & Jain, Y. (2011). *U.S. Patent No. 8060249*. Washington, DC: U.S. Patent and Trademark Office.

Beard, L., Wilson, K., Morra, D., & Keelan, J. (2009). A survey of health-related activities on second life. *Journal of Medical Internet Research*, *11*(2), e17. doi:10.2196/jmir.1192 PMID:19632971

Bear, R. A., & Stockie, S. (2014). Patient engagement and patient-centred care in the management of advanced chronic kidney disease and chronic kidney failure. *Canadian Journal of Kidney Health and Disease*, *1*(1), 24. Published online21October2014. doi:10.1186/s40697-014-0024-7 PMID:25780613

Beatty, A. L., Fukuoka, Y., & Whooley, M. A. (2013). Using mobile technology for cardiac rehabilitation: A review and framework for development and evaluation. *Journal of the American Heart Association*, *2*(6), e000568. doi:10.1161/JAHA.113.000568 PMID:24185949

Becker, F., & Douglass, S. (2008). The ecology of the patient visit: Physical attractiveness, waiting times, and perceived quality of care. *The Journal of Ambulatory Care Management*, *31*(2), 128–141. doi:10.1097/01.JAC.0000314703.34795.44 PMID:18360174

Becker, F., & Poe, D. B. Jr. (1980). The effects of user-generated design modifications in a general hospital. *Journal of Nonverbal Behavior*, *4*(4), 195–218. doi:10.1007/BF00986197

Becker, H. S. (1960). Notes on the Concept of Commitment. *American Journal of Sociology*, *66*(1), 32–40. doi:10.1086/222820

Bélanger, E., Rodríguez, C., Groleau, D., Légaré, F., Macdonald, M. E., & Marchand, R. (2014). Initiating decision-making conversations in palliative care: An ethnographic discourse analysis. *BMC Palliative Care*, *13*(1), 63. doi:10.1186/1472-684X-13-63 PMID:25859161

Bellardita, L., Graffigna, G., Donegani, S., Villani, D., Villa, S., Tresoldi, V., & Valdagni, R. (2012). Patient's choice of observational strategy for early-stage prostate cancer. *Neuropsychological Trends*, *12*, 107–116. doi:10.7358/neur-2012-012-bell

Bender, J., Yue, R., To, M., Deacken, L., & Jadad, A. (2013). A lot of action, but not in the right direction: Systematic review and content analysis of smartphone applications for the prevention, detection, and management of cancer. *Journal of Medical Internet Research*, *15*(12), e287. doi:10.2196/jmir.2661 PMID:24366061

Bennett, H. D., Coleman, E. A., Parry, C., Bodenheimer, T., & Chen, E. H. (2010). Health coaching for patients. *Family Practice Management, 17*(5), 24–29. PMID:21121566

Beratarrechea, A., Lee, A. G., Willner, J. M., Jahangir, E., Ciapponi, A., & Rubinstein, A. (2014). The impact of mobile health interventions on chronic disease outcomes in developing countries: A systematic review. *Telemedicine Journal and e-Health, 20*(1), 75–82. doi:10.1089/tmj.2012.0328 PMID:24205809

Bergs, D. (2002). "The hidden client"- women caring for husbands with COPD: Their experience of quality of life. *Journal of Clinical Nursing, 11*(5), 613–621. doi:10.1046/j.1365-2702.2002.00651.x PMID:12201888

Berkman, L. F., & Syme, S. L. (1979). Social networks, host resistance, and mortality: A nine-year follow-up study of Alameda County residents. *American Journal of Epidemiology, 109*(2), 186–204. doi:10.4236/health.2012.49087 PMID:425958

Berkman, N. D., Davis, T. C., & McCormack, L. (2010). Health literacy: What is it? *Journal of Health Communication, 15*(sup2Suppl. 2), 9–19. doi:10.1080/10810730.2010.499985 PMID:20845189

Berkman, N. D., DeWalt, D. A., Pignone, M. P., Sheridan, S. L., Lohr, K. N., Lux, L., & Bonito, A. J. et al. (2004). *Literacy and health outcomes (AHRQ Publication No. 04-E007-2)*. Rockville, MD: Agency for Healthcare Research and Quality.

Berkman, N. D., Sheridan, S. L., Donahue, K. E., Halpern, D. J., & Crotty, K. (2011). Low health literacy and health outcomes: An updated systematic review. *Annals of Internal Medicine, 155*(2), 97–107. doi:10.7326/0003-4819-155-2-201107190-00005 PMID:21768583

Berkowitz, L., & Cottingham, D. R. (1960). The interest value and relevance of fear arousing communications. *Journal of Abnormal and Social Psychology, 60*(1), 37–43. doi:10.1037/h0045247 PMID:13799520

Bero, L. A., Grilli, R., Grimshaw, J. M., Harvey, E., Oxman, A. D., & Thomson, M. A. (1998). Closing the gap between research and practice: An overview of systematic reviews of interventions to promote the implementation of research findings. *BMJ (Clinical Research Ed.), 317*(7156), 465–468. doi:10.1136/bmj.317.7156.465 PMID:9703533

Berwick, D. M. (2010). *What patient-centered care should mean*. Retrieved from http://patientprivacyrights.org/wp-content/uploads/2010/02/What-Patient-Centered-Should-Mean.pdf

Berwick, D. M., Nolan, T. W., & Whittington, J. (2008). The triple aim: Care, health, and cost. *Health Affairs, 27*(3), 759–769. doi:10.1377/hlthaff.27.3.759 PMID:18474969

Bettoncelli, G., Blasi, F., Brusasco, V., Centanni, S., Corrado, A., De Benedetto, F., & Sanguinetti, C. M. et al. (2014). The clinical and integrated management of COPD. *Sarcoidosis, Vasculitis, and Diffuse Lung Diseases, 31*, 3–21. PMID:24820963

Bickmore, T. W., & Paasche-Orlow, M. K. (2012). The role of information technology in health literacy research. *Journal of Health Communication, 17*(3), 23–29. doi:10.1080/10810730.2012.712626 PMID:23030559

Bickmore, T., Pfeifer, L., Byron, D., Forsythe, S., Henault, L., Jack, B., & Paasche-Orlow, M. et al. (2010). Usability of conversational agents by patients with inadequate health literacy: Evidence from two clinical trials. *Journal of Health Communication, 15*(2), 197–210. doi:10.1080/10810730.2010.499991 PMID:20845204

Bigi, S., & Rossi, M. G. (2015). Comunicare (nel)la cronicità [Communicating (within) chronic care]. *MeDIA. Aggiornamento e Formazione in Diabetologia e Malattie Metaboliche, 15*(3).

Bigi, S., Rossi, M. G., Barello, S., Graffigna, G., Mulas, M. F., & Musacchio, N. (2015). *Speaking wisely: pratiche dialogiche appropriate in diabetologia* [Speaking wisely: appropriate dialogical practices in diabetes care]. Paper presented at XX Congresso Nazionale AMD, L'Evoluzione della Diabetologia alla luce del Piano Nazionale Diabete, Genova, Italy.

Bigi, S. (2014). Key components of effective collaborative goal setting in the chronic care encounter. *Communication & Medicine, 11*(2), 103–115. doi:10.1558/cam.v11i2.21600 PMID:26596119

Bigi, S., & Macagno, F. (Manuscript submitted for publication). From types of dialogue to dialogue moves - The case of doctor-patient interaction as a communicative practice. *Discourse Processes.*

Bigi, S., Macagno, F., & Mayweg-Paus, L. (Manuscript submitted for publication). Medical consultation as a type of dialogical practice. *Patient Education and Counseling.*

Biocca, F., & Harms, C. (2003). *Guide to the Networked Minds Social Presence Inventory v. 1.2: Measures of co-presence, social presence, subjective symmetry, and intersubjective symmetry.* Michigan State University. Retrieved from http://cogprints.org/6743/

Black, P., & Penson, D. (2006). Prostate cancer on the Internet-information or misinformation? *The Journal of Urology, 175*(5), 1836–1842. doi:10.1016/S0022-5347(05)00996-1 PMID:16600774

Blake, H. (2006). *Waiting Line Models,* Retrieved from http://www.csus.edu/indiv/b/blakeh/mgmt/documents/OPM101SupplC.pdf

Blue, L., Lang, E., McMurray, J. J., Davie, A. P., McDonagh, T. A., Murdoch, D. R., & Morrison, C. E. et al. (2001). Randomised controlled trial of specialist nurse intervention in heart failure. *BMJ (Clinical Research Ed.), 323*(7315), 715–718. doi:10.1136/bmj.323.7315.715 PMID:11576977

Bodenmann, G. (2005). Dyadic coping and its significance for marital functioning. In T. A. Revenson, K. Kayser, & G. Bodenmann (Eds.), *Couples coping with stress: Emerging perspectives on dyadic coping* (pp. 35–50). Washington, DC: American Psychological Association. doi:10.1037/11031-002

Boren, S. A. (2009). A review of health literacy and diabetes: Opportunities for technology. *Journal of Diabetes Science and Technology, 3*(1), 202–209. doi:10.1177/193229680900300124 PMID:20046666

Borgmann, H., Wölm, J., Vallo, S., Mager, R., Huber, J., Breyer, J., & Tsaur, I. et al. (2015). Prostate Cancer on the Web-Expedient Tool for Patients' Decision-Making? *Journal of Cancer Education*. PMID:26234650

Botella, C., Riva, G., Gaggioli, A., Wiederhold, B. K., Alcaniz, M., & Banos, R. M. (2012). The present and future of positive technologies. *Cyberpsychology, Behavior, and Social Networking*, *15*(2), 78–84. doi:10.1089/cyber.2011.0140 PMID:22149078

Boulware, L. E., Carson, K. A., Troll, M. U., Powe, N. R., & Cooper, L. A. (2009). Perceived susceptibility to chronic kidney disease among high-risk patients seen in primary care practices. *Journal of General Internal Medicine*, *24*(10), 1123–1129. doi:10.1007/s11606-009-1086-6 PMID:19711135

Boulware, L. E., Hill-Briggs, F., Kraus, E. S., Melancon, J. K., Falcone, B., Ephraim, P. L., & Powe, N. R. et al. (2013). Effectiveness of educational and social worker interventions to activate patients' discussion and pursuit of preemptive living donor kidney transplantation: A randomized controlled trial. *American Journal of Kidney Diseases*, *61*(3), 476–486. doi:10.1053/j.ajkd.2012.08.039 PMID:23089512

Bourbeau, J. (2004). Self-management interventions to improve outcomes in patients suffering from COPD. *Expert review of pharmacoeconomics & outcomes research*, 4(1), 71-7.

Bourbeau, J. (2010). Making pulmonary rehabilitation a success in COPD. *Swiss Medical Weekly*, *140*, w13067. PMID:20809435

Bourbeau, J., Julien, M., Maltais, F., Rouleau, M., Beaupré, A., & Bégin, R. et al. & Chronic Obstructive Pulmonary Disease axis of the Respiratory Network Fonds de la Recherche en Santé du Québec. (. (2003). Reduction of hospital utilization in patients with chronic obstructive pulmonary disease: A disease-specific self-management intervention. *Archives of Internal Medicine*, *163*(5), 585–591. doi:10.1001/archinte.163.5.585 PMID:12622605

Bower, P., & Gilbody, S. (2005). Stepped care in psychological therapies: Access, effectiveness and efficiency. Narrative literature review. *The British Journal of Psychiatry*, *186*(1), 11–17. doi:10.1192/bjp.186.1.11 PMID:15630118

Boyd, C. M., Singh, S., Varadhan, R., Weiss, C. O., Sharma, R., Bass, E. B., & Puhan, M. A. (2012). *Methods for Benefit and Harm Assessment in Systematic Reviews. Methods Research Report. (Prepared by the Johns Hopkins University Evidence-based Practice Center under contract No. 290-2007-10061-I). AHRQ Publication No. 12(13)-EHC150-EF*. Rockville, MD: Agency for Healthcare Research and Quality.

Boyd, R. N., Mitchell, L. E., James, S. T., Ziviani, J., Sakzewski, L., Smith, A., & Scuffham, P. A. et al. (2013). Move it to improve it (Mitii): Study protocol of a randomised controlled trial of a novel web-based multimodal training program for children and adolescents with cerebral palsy. *BMJ Open*, *3*(4), 4. doi:10.1136/bmjopen-2013-002853 PMID:23578686

Braun, L., Sood, V., Hogue, S., Lieberman, B., & Copley-Merriman, C. (2012). High burden and unmet patient needs in chronic kidney disease. *International Journal of Nephrology and Renovascular Disease*, *5*, 151–163. doi:10.2147/IJNRD.S37766 PMID:23293534

Brett, J., Staniszewska, S., Mockford, C., Herron-Marx, S., Hughes, J. R., Tysall, C., & Suleman, R. (2014). Mapping the impact of patient and public involvement on health and social care research: A systematic review. *Health Expectations*, *17*(5), 637–650. doi:10.1111/j.1369-7625.2012.00795.x PMID:22809132

Brimmer, K. (2014, June 2). New technologies, hospital strategies promote patient engagement. *Healthcare Finance News*.

Brink-Muinen, V. D., Van Dulmen, S. M., De Haes, H. C., Visser, A. P., Schellevis, F. G., & Bensing, J. M. (2006). Has patients' involvement in the decision-making process changed over time? *Health Expectations*, *9*(4), 333–342. doi:10.1111/j.1369-7625.2006.00413.x PMID:17083560

Broetz, D., & Birbaumer, N. (2013). Behavioral physiotherapy in post stroke rehabilitation. *NeuroRehabilitation*, *33*, 377–384. PMID:23949069

Brouwers, M., Kho, M., Browman, G., Burgers, J., Cluzeau, F., Feder, G., & Hanna, S. et al. (2010). AGREE II: Advancing guideline development, reporting and evaluation in health care. *Canadian Medical Association Journal*, *182*(18), E839–E842. doi:10.1503/cmaj.090449 PMID:20603348

Brown, G., Brown, M., & Sharma, S. (2000). Health care in the 21st century: Evidence-based medicine, patient preference-based quality, and cost effectiveness. *Quality Management in Health Care*, *9*(1), 23–31. doi:10.1097/00019514-200009010-00004 PMID:11185879

Brown, K. M., Hoye, R., & Nicholson, M. (2012). Self-esteem, self-efficacy, and social connectedness as mediators of the relationship between volunteering and well-being. *Journal of Social Service Research*, *38*(4), 468–483. doi:10.1080/01488376.2012.687706

Brownson, R. C., Fielding, J. E., & Maylahn, C. M. (2009). Evidence-based public health: A fundamental concept for public health practice. *Annual Review of Public Health*, *30*(1), 175–201. doi:10.1146/annurev.publhealth.031308.100134 PMID:19296775

Buffum, M. D., & Brod, M. (1998). Humor and well-being in spouse caregivers of patients with Alzheimer's disease. *Applied Nursing Research*, *11*(1), 12–18. doi:10.1016/S0897-1897(98)80031-1 PMID:9549154

Bujnowska-Fedak, M. M., & Kurpas, D. (2015). The influence of online health information on the attitude and behavior of people Aged 50. *Advances in Experimental Medicine and Biology*, *861*, 1–17. doi:10.1007/5584_2015_130 PMID:26017724

Burg, B., Ingalz, K., Yamashita, M., & Takarada, S. (2009). *U.S. Patent Application 12/415,269*.

Burke, B. L., Arkowitz, H., & Menchola, M. (2003). The efficacy of motivational interviewing: A meta-analysis of controlled clinical trials. *Journal of Consulting and Clinical Psychology*, *71*(5), 843–861. doi:10.1037/0022-006X.71.5.843 PMID:14516234

Burke, L. E., Styn, M. A., Sereika, S. M., Conroy, M. B., Ye, L., Glanz, K., & Ewing, L. J. et al. (2012). Using mHealth technology to enhance self-monitoring for weight loss: A randomized trial. *American Journal of Preventive Medicine*, *43*(1), 20–26. doi:10.1016/j.amepre.2012.03.016 PMID:22704741

Burton, E., Lewin, G., Clemson, L., & Boldy, D. (2013). Effectiveness of a lifestyle exercise program for older people receiving a restorative home care service: Pragmatic randomized controlled trial. *Clinical Interventions in Aging*, *8*, 1591–1601. doi:10.2147/CIA.S44614 PMID:24324331

Buunk, B. P., Gibbons, F. X., & Buunk, A. (1997/2013). *Health, coping, and well-being: Perspectives from social comparison theory*. Mahwah, NJ: Erlbaum.

Byrne, S. M., Cooper, Z., & Fairburn, C. G. (2004). Psychological predictors of weight regain in obesity. *Behaviour Research and Therapy*, *42*(11), 1341–1356. doi:10.1016/j.brat.2003.09.004 PMID:15381442

Cafazzo, J. A., Casselman, M., Hamming, N., Katzman, D. K., & Palmert, M. R. (2012). Design of an mHealth app for the self-management of adolescent type 1 diabetes: A pilot study. *Journal of Medical Internet Research*, *14*(3), e70. doi:10.2196/jmir.2058 PMID:22564332

Cain, J. C., & Wicks, M. N. (2006). Caregivers attributes as correlates of burden in family caregivers coping with chronic obstructive pulmonary disease. *Journal of Family Nursing*, *6*(1), 46–68. doi:10.1177/107484070000600104

Calia, R., Ferrarese, D., Zecchini, J., & Orlandelli, E. (2006). *Vissuti Psicosociali nel Trapianto di rene: Pazienti in lista di attesa, nel post-trapianto e nel ri-trapianto* [Psychosocial Experiences in Kidney Transplant: Patients waiting for transplant, post-transplant and re-transplant]. Roma: Accademia Lancisiana.

Canadian Cancer Society, National Cancer Institute of Canada. Advisory Committee on Records, & Registries. (1987). Canadian cancer statistics. Canadian Cancer Society.

Cancela, J., Moreno, E. M., Arredondo, M. T., & Bonato, P. (2014) Designing auditory cues for Parkinson's disease gait rehabilitation.*Proceedings IEEE Engineering in Medicine and Biology Society* (pp. 5852-5855).

Candy, B., Taylor, S. J., Ramsay, J., Esmond, G., Griffiths, C. J., & Bryar, R. M. (2007). Service implications from a comparison of the evidence on the effectiveness and a survey of provision in England and Wales of COPD specialist nurse services in the community. *International Journal of Nursing Studies*, *44*(4), 601–610. doi:10.1016/j.ijnurstu.2005.12.007 PMID:16504198

Cantisano, N., Rimé, B., & Muñoz-Sastre, M. T. (2013). The social sharing of emotions in HIV/AIDS: A comparative study of HIV/AIDS, diabetic and cancer patients. *Journal of Health Psychology*, *18*(10), 1255–1267. doi:10.1177/1359105312462436 PMID:23129833

Capodaglio, P., Lafortuna, C., Petroni, M. L., Salvadori, A., Gondoni, L., Castelnuovo, G., & Brunani, A. (2013). Rationale for hospital-based rehabilitation in obesity with comorbidities. *European Journal of Physical and Rehabilitation Medicine*, *49*(3), 399–417. PMID:23736902

Carlucci, A., Guerrieri, A., & Nava, S. (2012). Palliative care in COPD patients: Is it only an end-of-life issue? *European Respiratory Review*, *21*(126), 347–354. doi:10.1183/09059180.00001512 PMID:23204123

Carman, K. L., Dardess, P., Maurer, M., Sofaer, S., Adams, K., Bechtel, C., & Sweeney, J. (2013). Patient And Family Engagement: A Framework For Understanding The Elements And Developing Interventions And Policies. *Health Affairs*, *32*(2), 223–231. doi:10.1377/hlthaff.2012.1133 PMID:23381514

Carone, M., Bertolotti, G., Cerveri, I., De Benedetto, F., Fogliani, V., Nardini, S., ... & Edu-Care Working Group. (2002). EDU-CARE, a randomised, multicentre, parallel group study on education and quality of life in COPD. Monaldi archives for chest disease = Archivio Monaldi per le malattie del torace/Fondazione clinica del lavoro, IRCCS [and] Istituto di clinica tisiologica e malattie apparato respiratorio, Università di Napoli. *Secondo ateneo, 57*(1), 25-29.

Carpman, J. R., Grant, M. A., & Simmons, D. A. (1986). *Design that cares: planning health facilities for patients and visitors*. Chicago: American Hospital Pub.

Carter, N., Miller, P., Murphy, B., Payne, V., & Bryant-Lukosius, D. (2014). Healthcare providers' perspectives of the supportive care needs of men with advanced prostate Cancer. *Paper presented at theOncology nursing forum*. doi:10.1188/14.ONF.421-430

Casale, G., & Calvieri, A. (2014). Palliative care in Italy: A historical perspective. *MEDIC*, *22*(1), 21–26.

Casarett, D., Pickard, A., Fishman, J. M., Alexander, S. C., Arnold, R. M., Pollak, K. I., & Tulsky, J. A. (2010). Can metaphors and analogies improve communication with seriously ill patients? *Journal of Palliative Medicine*, *13*(3), 255–260. doi:10.1089/jpm.2009.0221 PMID:19922170

Casas, A., Troosters, T., Garcia-Aymerich, J., Roca, J., Hernández, C., Alonso, A., & Decramer, M. (2006). Integrated care prevents hospitalisations for exacerbations in COPD patients. *The European Respiratory Journal*, *28*(1), 123–130. doi:10.1183/09031936.06.00063205 PMID:16611656

Cassileth, B. R., Zupkis, R. V., Sutton-Smith, K., & March, V. (1980). Information and participation preferences among cancer patients. *Annals of Internal Medicine*, *92*(6), 832–836. doi:10.7326/0003-4819-92-6-832 PMID:7387025

Cass, R., & Sunstein, J. D. (2015). Nudging smokers. *The New England Journal of Medicine*, *372*(22), 2150–2151. doi:10.1056/NEJMe1503200 PMID:25970008

Castelnuovo, G. (2010a). Empirically supported treatments in psychotherapy: Towards an evidence-based or evidence-biased psychology in clinical settings? *Frontiers in Psychology*, *1*, 27. PMID:21833197

Castelnuovo, G. (2010b). No medicine without psychology: The key role of psychological contribution in clinical settings. *Frontiers in Psychology*, *1*, 4. doi:10.3389/fpsyg.2010.00004 PMID:21833187

Castelnuovo, G., Manzoni, G. M., Cuzziol, P., Cesa, G. L., Tuzzi, C., Villa, V., & Molinari, E. et al. (2010). TECNOB: Study design of a randomized controlled trial of a multidisciplinary telecare intervention for obese patients with type-2 diabetes. *BMC Public Health*, *10*(1), 204. doi:10.1186/1471-2458-10-204 PMID:20416042

Castelnuovo, G., Manzoni, G. M., Pietrabissa, G., Corti, S., Giusti, E. M., Molinari, E., & Simpson, S. (2014). Obesity and outpatient rehabilitation using mobile technologies: The potential mHealth approach. *Frontiers in Psychology*, *5*, 559. doi:10.3389/fpsyg.2014.00559 PMID:24959157

Castelnuovo, G., Pietrabissa, G., Manzoni, G. M., Corti, S., Ceccarini, M., Borrello, M., & Molinari, E. et al. (2015a). Chronic care management of globesity: Promoting healthier lifestyles in traditional and mHealth based settings. *Frontiers in Psychology*, October. PMID:26528215

Castelnuovo, G., Zoppis, I., Santoro, E., Ceccarini, M., Pietrabissa, G., Manzoni, G. M., & Sicurello, F. et al. (2015b). Managing chronic pathologies with a stepped mHealth-based approach in clinical psychology and medicine. *Frontiers in Psychology*, *6*, 407. doi:10.3389/fpsyg.2015.00407 PMID:25926801

Cavanaugh, K. L., Wingard, R. M., Hakim, R. M., Eden, S., Shintani, A., Wallston, K. A., & Ikizier, T. A. et al. (2010). Low health literacy associates with increased mortality in ESRD. *Journal of the American Society of Nephrology*, *21*(11), 1979–1985. doi:10.1681/ASN.2009111163 PMID:20671215

Centers for Medicare and Medicaid Services. (2014). *Readmission reduction program*. Retrieved September 29, 2015, from http://www.cms.gov/Medicare/Medicare-Fee-for-Service-payment/AcuteInpatientPPS/Readmissions-Reduction-Program.html

Chan, K. (2013). *Going to the ER? Real-time hospital emergency wait times now online*. Retrieved from http://www.vancitybuzz.com/2013/04/hospital-emergency-room-wait-times-online/

Chan, Y., Wang, T., Chang, C., Chen, L., Chu, H., Lin, S., & Chang, S. (2015). Short-term effects of self-massage combined with home exercise on pain, daily activity, and autonomic function in patients with myofascial pain dysfunction syndrome. *Journal of Physical Therapy Science*, *27*(1), 217–221. doi:10.1589/jpts.27.217 PMID:25642077

Charles, C., Gafni, A., & Whelan, T. (1997). Shared decision-making in the medical encounter: What does it mean? (or it takes at least two to tango). *Social Science & Medicine*, *44*(5), 681–692. doi:10.1016/S0277-9536(96)00221-3 PMID:9032835

Charles, C., Gafni, A., & Whelan, T. (1999). Decision-making in the physician-patient encounter: Revisiting the shared treatment decision-making model. *Social Science & Medicine*, *49*(5), 651–661. doi:10.1016/S0277-9536(99)00145-8 PMID:10452420

Charnock, D., Shepperd, S., Needham, G., & Gann, R. (1999). DISCERN: An instrument for judging the quality of written consumer health information on treatment choices. *Journal of Epidemiology and Community Health*, *53*(2), 105–111. doi:10.1136/jech.53.2.105 PMID:10396471

Chase, D. (2012, September 9). Patient engagement is the blockbuster drug of the century. *Forbes.com.* Retrieved from http://www.forbes.com/sites/davechase/2012/09/09/patient-engagement-is-the-blockbuster-drug-of-the-century/

Chavannes, N. H., Grijsen, M., van den Akker, M., Schepers, H., Nijdam, M., Tiep, B., & Muris, J. (2009). Integrated disease management improves one-year quality of life in primary care COPD patients: A controlled clinical trial. *Primary Care Respiratory Journal, 18*(3), 171–176. doi:10.3132/pcrj.2009.00003 PMID:19142557

Chewning, B., Bylund, C., Shah, B., Arora, N. K., Gueguen, J. A., & Makoul, G. (2012). Patient preferences for shared decisions: A systematic review. *Patient Education and Counseling, 86*(1), 9–18. doi:10.1016/j.pec.2011.02.004 PMID:21474265

Chiarolanza, C., & De Gregorio, E. (2007). *Lavorare con ATLAS.ti. Come analizzare i processi psicosociali* [*Working with ATLAS.ti. How to Analyze Psychosocial Processes*]. Roma: Carocci.

Chien, C. L., Lee, C. M., Wu, Y. W., Chen, T. A., & Wu, Y. T. (2008). Home-based exercise increases capacity but not quality of life in people with chronic heart failure: A systematic review. *The Australian Journal of Physiotherapy, 54*(2), 87–93. doi:10.1016/S0004-9514(08)70041-2 PMID:18491999

Chomutare, T., Fernandez-Luque, L., Arsand, E., & Hartvigsen, G. (2011). Features of mobile diabetes applications: Review of the literature and analysis of current applications compared against evidence-based guidelines. *Journal of Medical Internet Research, 13*(3), e65. doi:10.2196/jmir.1874 PMID:21979293

Chouffani, R. (2013). mHealth clinical apps impacting care, not just with consumers. *TechTarget.* Retrieved from http://searchhealthit.techtarget.com/opinion/MHealth-clinical-apps-impacting-care-not-just-with-consumers?asrc=EM_ERU_27369471&utm_medium=EM&utm_source=ERU&utm_campaign=20140320_ERU%20Transmission%20for%2003/20/2014%20(UserUniverse:%20732731)_myka-reports@techtarget.com&src=5223540

Chow, E., Harth, T., Hruby, G., Finkelstein, J., Wu, J., & Danjoux, C. (2001). How accurate are physicians' clinical predictions of survival and the available prognostic tools in estimating survival times in terminally ill cancer patients? A systematic review. *Clinical Oncology, 13*(3), 209–218. PMID:11527298

Chua, H. F., Ho, S. S., Jasinska, A. J., Polk, T. A., Welsh, R. C., Liberzon, I., & Strecher, V. J. (2011). Self-related neural response to tailored smoking-cessation messages predicts quitting. *Nature, 20*(1), 1. PMID:21358641

Cigoli, V. (2006). *L'albero della discendenza. Clinica dei corpi familiari* [*The Descendents' Tree. A Clinical Approach to Family Bodies*]. Milano: Franco Angeli.

Cinel, C., Poli, R., Citi, L., & Robertson, D. (2013). An exploration of the effects of audio-visual entrainment on Parkinson's disease tremor.*Proceedings IEEE EMBS Conference on Neural Engineering* (pp. 1562-1565).

Cipresso, P., Serino, S., Villani, D., Repetto, C., Selitti, L., Albani, G., & Riva, G. et al. (2012). Is your phone so smart to affect your states? An exploratory study based on psychophysiological measures. *Neurocomputing*, *84*, 23–30. doi:10.1016/j.neucom.2011.12.027

Clark, J., Wray, N., & Ashton, C. (2001). Living with treatment decisions: Regrets and quality of life among men treated for metastatic prostate cancer. *Journal of Clinical Oncology*, *19*(1), 72–80. PMID:11134197

Clark, R., & Mayer, R. (2011). *E-Learning and the Science of Instruction: Proven Guidelines for Consumers and Designers of Multimedia Learning*. New York: Pfeiffer. doi:10.1002/9781118255971

Clayton, J. M., Butow, P. N., Waters, A., Laidsaar-Powell, R. C., O'Brien, A., Boyle, F., & Tattersall, M. H. et al. (2013). Evaluation of a novel individualised communication-skills training intervention to improve doctors' confidence and skills in end-of-life communication. *Palliative Medicine*, *27*(3), 236–243. doi:10.1177/0269216312449683 PMID:22711714

Close, J. C., Wesson, J., Sherrington, C., Hill, K. D., Kurrle, S., Lord, S. R., & Clemson, L. et al. (2014). Can a tailored exercise and home hazard reduction program reduce the rate of falls in community dwelling older people with cognitive impairment: Protocol paper for the i-FOCIS randomised controlled trial. *BMC Geriatrics*, *14*(89), 1–14. PMID:25128411

Cockram, J., Cecins, N., & Jenkins, S. (2006). Maintaining exercise capacity and quality of life following pulmonary rehabilitation. *Respirology (Carlton, Vic.)*, *11*(1), 98–104. doi:10.1111/j.1440-1843.2006.00791.x PMID:16423209

Cohen, D. J., Crabtree, B. F., Etz, R. S., Balasubramanian, B. A., Donahue, K. E., Leviton, L. C., & Green, L. W. et al. (2008). Fidelity versus flexibility. *American Journal of Preventive Medicine*, *35*(5), 381–389. doi:10.1016/j.amepre.2008.08.005 PMID:18929985

Cohen, S. E., & Syme, S. (1985). *Social support and health*. New York: Academic Press.

Cohen, S., & Wills, T. A. (1985). Stress, social support, and the buffering hypothesis. *Psychological Bulletin*, *98*(2), 310–357. doi:10.1037/0033-2909.98.2.310 PMID:3901065

Coleman, K., Austin, B. T., Brach, C., & Wagner, E. H. (2009). Evidence On The Chronic Care Model In The New Millennium. *Health Affairs*, *28*(1), 75–85. doi:10.1377/hlthaff.28.1.75 PMID:19124857

Collaboration, The ADAPTE. (2009). *The ADAPTE Process: Resource Toolkit for Guideline Adaptation. Version 2.0.* Retrieved from http://www.adapte.org

Collier, R. (2011). Federal government unveils patient-oriented research strategy. *Canadian Medical Association Journal*, *183*(13), E993–E994. doi:10.1503/cmaj.109-3978 PMID:21876023

Collin, S. M., Martin, R. M., Metcalfe, C., Gunnell, D., Albertsen, P. C., Neal, D., & Donovan, J. et al. (2008). Prostate-cancer mortality in the USA and UK in 1975-2004: An ecological study. *The Lancet Oncology*, *9*(5), 445–452. doi:10.1016/S1470-2045(08)70104-9 PMID:18424233

Committee on Patient Safety and Quality Improvement. (2005). ACOG Committee Opinion No. 320: Partnering with patients to improve safety. *Obstetrics and Gynecology*, *106*(5), 1123–1128. doi:10.1097/00006250-200511000-00057 PMID:16260544

Commonwealth Fund. (2015). *Mobile health and patient engagement in the safety net: A survey of community health centers and clinics*. Retrieved from http://www.commonwealthfund.org/publications/issue-briefs/2015/may/mobile-health-and-patient-engagement-in-the-safety-net

Coulter, A. (2005). What do patients and the public want from primary care? *BMJ (Clinical Research Ed.)*, *331*(7526), 1199–1201. doi:10.1136/bmj.331.7526.1199 PMID:16293845

Coulter, A. (2011). *Engaging patients in healthcare*. New York: McGraw-Hill Education.

Coulter, A., & Magee, H. (2003). *The European patient of the future*. McGraw Hill Education.

Coulter, C. L., Scarvell, J. M., Neeman, T. M., & Smith, P. N. (2013). Physiotherapist-directed rehabilitation exercises in the outpatient or home setting improve strength, gait speed and cadence after elective total hip replacement: A systematic review. *Journal of Physiotherapy*, *59*(4), 219–226. doi:10.1016/S1836-9553(13)70198-X PMID:24287215

Crawford, M. J., Rutter, D., Manley, C., Weaver, T., & Bhui, K. (2002). Systematic review of involving patients in the planning and development of healthcare. *BMJ (Clinical Research Ed.)*, *325*(7375), 1263. doi:10.1136/bmj.325.7375.1263 PMID:12458240

Crocker, T., Young, J., Forster, A., Brown, L., Ozer, S., & Greenwood, D. C. (2013). The effect of physical rehabilitation on activities of daily living in older residents of long-term care facilities: Systematic review with meta-analysis. *Age and Ageing*, *42*(6), 682–688. doi:10.1093/ageing/aft133 PMID:24004604

Csikszentmihalyi, M. (1975). *Beyond boredom and anxiety*. San Francisco, CA: Jossey-Bass.

Csikszentmihalyi, M. (1997). *Finding flow: The psychology of engagement with everyday life*. New York: Basic Books.

Curtis, D. W., Pino, E. J., Bailey, J. M., Shih, E. I., Waterman, J., Vinterbo, S. A., & Ohno-Machado, L. et al. (2008). SMART—an integrated wireless system for monitoring unattended patients. *Journal of the American Medical Informatics Association*, *15*(1), 44–53. doi:10.1197/jamia.M2016 PMID:17947629

Curtis, J. R. (2008). Palliative and end-of-life care for patients with severe COPD. *The European Respiratory Journal*, *32*(3), 796–803. doi:10.1183/09031936.00126107 PMID:17989116

Curtis, J. R., Engelberg, R. A., Nielsen, E. L., Au, D. H., & Patrick, D. L. (2004). Patient-physician communication about end-of-life care for patients with severe COPD. *The European Respiratory Journal*, *24*(2), 200–205. doi:10.1183/09031936.04.00010104 PMID:15332385

Curtis, J. R., Engelberg, R. A., Wenrich, M. D., Shannon, S. E., Treece, P. D., & Rubenfeld, G. D. (2005). Missed opportunities during family conferences about end-of-life care in the intensive care unit. *American Journal of Respiratory and Critical Care Medicine*, *171*(8), 844–849. doi:10.1164/rccm.200409-1267OC PMID:15640361

Curtis, J. R., Engelberg, R., Young, J. P., Vig, L. K., Reinke, L. F., Wenrich, M. D., & Back, A. L. et al. (2008). An approach to understanding the interaction of hope and desire for explicit prognostic information among individuals with severe chronic obstructive pulmonary disease or advanced cancer. *Journal of Palliative Medicine*, *11*(4), 610–620. doi:10.1089/jpm.2007.0209 PMID:18454614

Dageforde, L. A., & Cavanaugh, K. L. (2013). Health Literacy: Emerging Evidence and Applications in Kidney Disease Care. *Advances in Chronic Kidney Disease*, *20*(4), 311–319. doi:10.1053/j.ackd.2013.04.005 PMID:23809283

Dal Negro, R. W., & Goldberg, A. I. (Eds.). (2005). *Home Long-term oxygen treatment in Italy. The additional value of telemedicine* (pp. 71–85). Springer Publ. doi:10.1007/88-470-0448-9

Dansky, K. H., & Miles, J. (1997). Patient satisfaction with ambulatory healthcare services: Waiting time and filling time. *Hospital & Health Services Administration*, *42*(2), 165–177. PMID:10167452

Darlow, S., & Wen, K. Y. (2015). Development testing of mobile health interventions for cancer patient self-management: A review. *Health Informatics Journal*. PMID:25916831

Dartmouth Atlas Project. (2015). *Understanding of the efficiency and effectiveness of the health care system.* Retrieved from http://www.dartmouthatlas.org/

Davis, K., Schoenbaum, S. C., & Audet, A. M. (2005). A 2020 vision of patient-centered primary care. *Journal of General Internal Medicine*, *20*(10), 953–957. doi:10.1111/j.1525-1497.2005.0178.x PMID:16191145

Davison, B., Szafron, M., Gutwin, C., & Visvanathan, K. (2014). Using a web-based decision support intervention to facilitate patient-physician communication at prostate cancer treatment discussions. *Revue canadienne de soins infirmiers en oncologie [Canadian Oncology Nursing Journal]*, 24(4), 241-247.

Davis, T. C., Crouch, M. A., Wills, G., Miller, S., & Abdehou, D. M. (1990).. . *The Journal of Family Practice*, *31*(5), 533–538. PMID:2230677

Dayer, L., Heldenbrand, S., Anderson, P., Gubbins, P. O., & Martin, B. C. (2013). Smartphone medication adherence apps: Potential benefits to patients and providers. *Journal of the American Pharmacists Association: JAPhA*, *53*(2), 172–181. doi:10.1331/JAPhA.2013.12202 PMID:23571625

De Man, S., Vlerick, P., Gemmel, P., De Bondt, P., Matthys, D., & Dierckx, R. (2005). Impact of waiting on the perception of service quality in nuclear medicine. *Nuclear Medicine Communications*, *26*(6), 541–547. doi:10.1097/00006231-200506000-00010 PMID:15891598 de Ridder, D., Geenen, R., Kuijer, R., & van Middendorp, H. (2008). Psychological adjustment to chronic disease. *Lancet*, *372*(9634), 246–255. doi:10.1016/S0140-6736(08)61078-8 PMID:18640461

de Vos, M. A., Bos, A. P., Plötz, F. B., van Heerde, M., de Graaff, B. M., Tates, K., ... & Willems, D. L. (2015). Talking With Parents About End-of-Life Decisions for Their Children. Pediatrics, peds-2014.

Dean, M., & Street, R. L. Jr. (2014). A 3-stage model of patient-centered communication for addressing cancer patients' emotional distress. *Patient Education and Counseling*, *94*(2), 143–148. doi:10.1016/j.pec.2013.09.025 PMID:24169023

Deci, E. L., & Flaste, R. (1996). *Why We Do What We Do: Understanding Self-Motivation*. New York: Penguin Books.

Deloitte. (2011). *Umfrage 2011 zum Gesundheitswesen in der Schweiz. Wichtigste Ergebnisse, strategische Auswirkungen.*

Denhaerynck, K., Manhaeve, D., Dobbels, F., Garzoni, D., Nolte, C., & De Geest, S. (2007). Prevalence and consequences of nonadherence to hemodialysis regimens. *American Journal of Critical Care*, *16*(3), 222–235. PMID:17460313

Detmar, S. B., Muller, M. J., Wever, L. D., Schornagel, J. H., & Aaronson, N. K. (2001). Patient-physician communication during outpatient palliative treatment visits: An observational study. *Journal of the American Medical Association*, *285*(10), 1351–1357. doi:10.1001/jama.285.10.1351 PMID:11255393

Devlin, A. S. (2008). Judging a Book by Its Cover: Medical Building Facades and Judgments of Care. *Environment and Behavior*, *40*(3), 307–329. doi:10.1177/0013916507302242

Devraj, R., & Gordon, E. J. (2009). Health literacy and kidney disease: Toward a new line of research. *American Journal of Kidney Diseases*, *53*(5), 884–889. doi:10.1053/j.ajkd.2008.12.028 PMID:19324481

Diamantidis, C. J., & Becker, S. (2014). Health information technology (IT) to improve the care of patients with chronic kidney disease (CKD). *BMC Nephrology*, *15*(7). Available at http://www.biomedcentral.com/1471-2369/15/7. doi:10.1186/1471-2369-15-7 PMID:24405907

Doak, C. C., Doak, L. G., & Root, J. H. (1994). Suitability assessment of materials (SAM). *Paper presented at theAmerican Public Health Association Annual Meeting*, Washington, DC.

Doak, C. C., Doak, L. G., & Root, J. H. (1996). Teaching patients with low literacy skills. *AJN The American Journal of Nursing*, *96*(12), 16M. doi:10.1097/00000446-199612000-00022

Dodaro, A., & Recchia, V. (2011). Inappropriateness in ionizing imaging. The central node of the informed consent: From "event" model to "process" model. *Recenti Progressi in Medicina*, *102*, 421–431. PMID:22120778

Dombrowski, S. U., Avenell, A., & Sniehott, F. F. (2011). Behavioural interventions for obese adults with additional risk factors for morbidity: Systematic review of effects on behaviour, weight and disease risk factors. *Obes Facts*, *3*(6), 377–396. doi:10.1159/000323076 PMID:21196792

Dombrowski, S. U., Sniehotta, F. F., Avenell, A., Johnston, M., MacLennan, G., & Ara, Ã. (2012). Identifying active ingredients in complex behavioural interventions for obese adults with obesity-related co-morbidities or additional risk factors for co-morbidities: A systematic review. *Health Psychology Review*, *6*(1), 7–32. doi:10.1080/17437199.2010.513298

Dopson, S., Locock, L., Gabbay, J., Ferlie, E., & Fitzgerald, L. (2003). Evidence-based medicine and the implementation gap. *Health*, *7*(3), 311–330. doi:10.1177/1363459303007003004

Duggan, P. S., Geller, G., Cooper, L. A., & Beach, M. C. (2006). The moral nature of patient-centeredness: Is it "just the right thing to do"? *Patient Education and Counseling*, *62*(2), 271–276. doi:10.1016/j.pec.2005.08.001 PMID:16356677

Dunn, R. A., & Guadagno, R. E. (2012). My avatar and me–Gender and personality predictors of avatar-self discrepancy. *Computers in Human Behavior*, *28*(1), 97–106. doi:10.1016/j.chb.2011.08.015

Eck, E. K., DeBaun, B., & Pugliese, G. (2001). *The Contagious Patient: Identifying, Containing, and Treating Appropriately.* Retrieved http://www.infectioncontroltoday.com/articles/2001/12/the-contagious-patient.aspx

Eggly, S., Penner, L. A., Greene, M., Harper, F. W., Ruckdeschel, J. C., & Albrecht, T. L. (2006). Information seeking during "bad news" oncology interactions: Question asking by patients and their companions. *Social Science & Medicine*, *63*(11), 2974–2985. doi:10.1016/j.socscimed.2006.07.012 PMID:16962218

Ekroos, N., & Jalonen, K. (2007). E-Health and diabetes care. *Journal of Telemedicine and Telecare*, *13*(1), 22–23. doi:10.1258/135763307781645013

El Tantawi, M. M., El Kashlan, M. K., & Saeed, Y. M. (2013). Assessment of the Efficacy of Second Life, a Virtual Learning Environment, in Dental Education. *Journal of Dental Education*, *77*(12), 1639–1652. PMID:24319136

Ellimoottil, C., Polcari, A., Kadlec, A., & Gupta, G. (2012). Readability of websites containing information about prostate cancer treatment options. *The Journal of Urology*, *188*(6), 2171–2176. doi:10.1016/j.juro.2012.07.105 PMID:23083852

Elliot, M. (2006). Stigmergic collaboration: The evolution of group work. *journal of media and culture, 9*(2).

Elwyn, G., Frosch, D., Thomson, R., Joseph-Williams, N., Lloyd, A., Kinnersley, P., & Barry, M. et al. (2012). Shared Decision-making: A Model for Clinical Practice. *Journal of General Internal Medicine*, *27*(10), 1361–1367. doi:10.1007/s11606-012-2077-6 PMID:22618581

Elwyn, G., & Miron-Shatz, T. (2009). Deliberation before determination: The definition and evaluation of good decision-making. *Health Expectations*, *13*(2), 139–147. doi:10.1111/j.1369-7625.2009.00572.x PMID:19740089

Emanuel, E. J., & Emanuel, L. L. (1992). Four models of the physician-patient relationship. *Journal of the American Medical Association*, *267*(16), 2221–2227. doi:10.1001/jama.1992.03480160079038 PMID:1556799

Epstein, R. M., & Street Jr, R. L. Patient-Centered Communication in Cancer Care: Promoting Healing and Reducing Suffering. *National Cancer Institute, NIH Publication* (07-6225).

Epstein, R. M., & Gramling, R. E. (2013). What is shared in shared decision-making? Complex decisions when the evidence is unclear. *Medical Care Research and Review. Supplement to*, *70*(1), 94S–112S.

Epstein, R., & Street, R. L. (2011). Shared Mind: Communication, Decision-making, and Autonomy in Serious Illness. *Annals of Family Medicine*, *9*(5), 454–461. doi:10.1370/afm.1301 PMID:21911765

Erzberger, C. (1998). *Zahlen und Wörter: Die Verbindung quantitativer und qualitativer Daten und Methoden im Forschungsprozeß*. Dt. Studien-Verlag.

Eysenbach, G. (2001). What is e-health? *Journal of Medical Internet Research*, *3*(2), e20. doi:10.2196/jmir.3.2.e20 PMID:11720962

Eysenbach, G. (2011). Can tweets predict citations? Metrics of social impact based on Twitter and correlation with traditional metrics of scientific impact. *Journal of Medical Internet Research*, *13*(4), e123. doi:10.2196/jmir.2012 PMID:22173204

Fadem, S. Z., Walker, D. R., Abbott, G., Friedman, A. L., Goldman, R., Sexton, S., & Peters, T. G. et al. (2011). Satisfaction with renal replacement therapy and education: The American Association of Kidney Patients Survey. *Clinical Journal of the American Society of Nephrology; CJASN*, *6*(3), 605–612. doi:10.2215/CJN.06970810 PMID:21330485

Fagerlin, A., & Schneider, C. E. (2004). Enough: The failure of the living will. *The Hastings Center Report*, *34*(2), 30–42. doi:10.2307/3527683 PMID:15156835

Fagerlin, A., Zikmund-Fisher, B. J., & Ubel, P. A. (2011). Helping patients decide: Ten steps to better risk communication. *Journal of the National Cancer Institute*, *103*(19), 1436–1443. doi:10.1093/jnci/djr318 PMID:21931068

Falk, E. B., O'Donnell, M. B., Tompson, S., Gonzales, R., Chin, S. D., Strecher, V., & An, L. (2014). *Neural systems associated with self-related processing predict population success of health messages*. Mass Commun Health.

Fang, M. C., Panguluri, P., Machtinger, E. L., & Schillinger, D. (2009). Language, literacy, and characterization of stroke among patients taking warfarin for stroke prevention: Implications for health communication. *Patient Education and Counseling*, *75*(3), 403–410. Retrieved from http://www.ajmc.com/journals/supplement/2014/a465_ma14_transitions/a465_mar14_owen_s81t91/P-3#shash.SfblJhR1.dpuf doi:10.1016/j.pec.2008.12.009 PMID:19171448

Farmer, K. C. (1999). Methods for measuring and monitoring medication regimen adherence in clinical trials and clinical practice. *Clinical Therapeutics*, *21*(6), 1074–1090. doi:10.1016/S0149-2918(99)80026-5 PMID:10440628

Faulkner, A. (1998). ABC of palliative care. Communication with patients, families, and other professionals. *BMJ: British Medical Journal*, *316*(7125), 130–132. doi:10.1136/bmj.316.7125.130 PMID:9462321

Fehrman-Ekholm, I., Dunér, F., Brink, B., Tydén, G., & Elinder, C. G. (2001). No Evidence of Accelerated Loss of Kidney Function in Living Kidney Donors: Results from a cross-cultural follow-up. *Transplantation*, *72*(3), 444–449. doi:10.1097/00007890-200108150-00015 PMID:11502974

Ferguson, T. (2007). *E-Patients: How they can help us heal healthcare.* Retrieved from http://e-patients.net/e-Patients_White_Paper.pdf

Ferreira, D., Carreira, H., Silva, S., & Lunet, N. (2013). Assessment of the contents related to screening on Portuguese language websites providing information on breast and prostate cancer. *Cadernos de Saude Publica*, *29*(11), 2163–2176. doi:10.1590/0102-311x00150312 PMID:24233032

Finkelstein, F. O., Story, K., Firanek, C., Barre, P., Takano, T., Soroka, S., & Mendelssohn, D. et al. (2008). Perceived knowledge among patients cared for by Nephrologists about chronic kidney disease and ESRD therapies. *Kidney International*, *74*(9), 1178–1184. doi:10.1038/ki.2008.376 PMID:18668024

Finkelstein, S. M., Speedie, S. M., & Potthoff, S. (2006). Home telehealth improves clinical outcomes at lower cost for home healthcare. *Telemedicine Journal and e-Health*, *12*(2), 128–136. doi:10.1089/tmj.2006.12.128 PMID:16620167

Fiordelli, M., Diviani, N., & Schulz, P. J. (2013). Mapping mHealth research: A decade of evolution. *Journal of Medical Internet Research*, *15*(5), e95. doi:10.2196/jmir.2430 PMID:23697600

Fischer, T. (2009). *Die ärztliche Versorgung im niedergelassenen Bereich aus dem Blickwinkel der Patienten: Schlaglichter auf ein vernachlässigtes Gebiet der Gesundheitspolitik.*

Fischer, G. (2012). Context-Aware Systems -The 'right' information, at the 'right' time, in the 'right' place, in the 'right' way, to the 'right' person. In G. Tortora, S. Levialdi, & M. Tucci (Eds.), *Proceedings of the Conference on Advanced Visual Interfaces (AVI 2012),*Capri, Italy (pp. 287-294). ACM.

Fischhoff, B. (2012). *Communicating Risks and Benefits: An Evidence Based User's Guide.* Government Printing Office.

Fischhoff, B., Brewer, N. T., & Downs, J. S. (2011). *Communicating risks and benefits: an evidence-based user's guide*. Food and Drug Administration.

Fischhoff, B., Watson, S. R., & Hope, C. (1984). Defining risk. *Policy Sciences*, *17*(2), 123–139. doi:10.1007/BF00146924

Fisher, M. S. Sr. (2003). Psychosocial evaluation interview protocol for living related and living unrelated kidney donors. *Social Work in Health Care*, *38*(1), 39–61. doi:10.1300/J010v38n01_03 PMID:14984248

Flegal, K. M., Graubard, B. I., Williamson, D. F., & Gail, M. H. (2005). Excess deaths associated with underweight, overweight, and obesity. *Journal of the American Medical Association*, *293*(15), 1861–1867. doi:10.1001/jama.293.15.1861 PMID:15840860

Fleisher, J. (2013). Hospitals Duel Over Wait Times. *The Wall Street Journal*.

Fong, K., & Mar, R. A. (2015). What Does My Avatar Say About Me? Inferring Personality From Avatars. *Personality and Social Psychology Bulletin*, *41*(2), 237–249. doi:10.1177/0146167214562761 PMID:25576173

Foster, G. D., Makris, A. P., & Bailer, B. A. (2005). Behavioral treatment of obesity. *The American Journal of Clinical Nutrition*, *82*(Suppl. 1), 230S–235S. PMID:16002827

Foster, M., Brice, J. H., Shofer, F., Principe, S., DeWalt, D., Falk, R., & Ferris, M. (2011). Personal disaster preparedness of dialysis patients in North Carolina. *Clinical Journal of the American Society of Nephrology; CJASN*, *6*(10), 2478–2484. doi:10.2215/CJN.03590411 PMID:21852660

Fox, J., & Ahn, S. J. (2013). Avatars: Portraying, Exploring, and Changing Online and Offline Identities. In R. Luppicini (Ed.), *Handbook of Research on Technoself: Identity in a Technological Society* (Vol. 1, pp. 255–271). Hershey: IGI Global. doi:10.4018/978-1-4666-2211-1.ch014

Fox, J., & Bailenson, J. N. (2009). Virtual self-modeling: The effects of vicarious reinforcement and identification on exercise behaviors. *Media Psychology*, *12*(1), 1–25. doi:10.1080/15213260802669474

Fox, J., Bailenson, J. N., & Tricase, L. (2013). The embodiment of sexualized virtual selves: The Proteus effect and experiences of self-objectification via avatars. *Computers in Human Behavior*, *29*(3), 930–938. doi:10.1016/j.chb.2012.12.027

Frank, L., Basch, E., & Selby, J. (2014). The PCORI Perspective on Patient-Centered Outcomes Research. *Journal of the American Medical Association*, *312*(15), 1513–1514. doi:10.1001/jama.2014.11100 PMID:25167382

Fraser, S. D., Roderick, P. J., Casey, M., Taal, M. W., Yuen, H. M., & Nutbeam, D. (2013). Prevalence and associations of limited health literacy in chronic kidney disease: A systematic review. *Nephrology, Dialysis, Transplantation*, *28*(1), 129–137. doi:10.1093/ndt/gfs371 PMID:23222414

Free, C., Phillips, G., Galli, L., Watson, L., Felix, L., Edwards, P., & Haines, A. et al. (2013). The effectiveness of mobile-health technology-based health behaviour change or disease management interventions for health care consumers: A systematic review. *PLoS Medicine*, *10*(1), e1001362. doi:10.1371/journal.pmed.1001362 PMID:23349621

Friberg, F., Lidén, E., Håkanson, C., & Öhlén, J. (2014). Communicating bodily changes: Physicians' ways of enabling patient understanding in gastrointestinal cancer consultations. *Palliative & Supportive Care*, 13(3), 661-671. PMID:24784141

Fried, T. R., & O'Leary, J. R. (2008). Using the experiences of bereaved caregivers to inform patient- and caregiver-centered advance care planning. *Journal of General Internal Medicine*, *23*(10), 1602–1607. doi:10.1007/s11606-008-0748-0 PMID:18665427

Fromer, L. (2011). Implementing chronic care for COPD: Planned visits, care coordination, and patient empowerment for improved outcomes. *International Journal of Chronic Obstructive Pulmonary Disease*, *6*, 605–614. doi:10.2147/COPD.S24692 PMID:22162647

Gaggioli, A., Mazzoni, E., Milani, L., & Riva, G. (2015). The creative link: Investigating the relationship between social network indices, creative performance and flow in blended teams. *Computers in Human Behavior*, *42*, 157–166. doi:10.1016/j.chb.2013.12.003

Gaggioli, A., Riva, G., Milani, L., & Mazzoni, E. (2013). *Networked Flow: Towards an Understanding of Creative Networks*. Heidelberg: Springer. doi:10.1007/978-94-007-5552-9

Gaggioli, A., Scaratti, C., Morganti, L., Stramba-Badiale, M., Agostoni, M., Spatola, C. A., & Riva, G. et al. (2014). Effectiveness of group reminiscence for improving wellbeing of institutionalized elderly adults: Study protocol for a randomized controlled trial. *Trials*, *15*(1), 408. doi:10.1186/1745-6215-15-408 PMID:25344703

Gaikwad, R., & Warren, J. (2009). The role of home-based information and communications technology interventions in chronic disease management: A systematic literature review. *Health Informatics Journal*, *15*(2), 122–146. doi:10.1177/1460458209102973 PMID:19474225

Gance-Cleveland, B. (2005). Family-Centered Care. *Journal for Specialists in Pediatric Nursing*, *10*(3), 151–155. doi:10.1111/j.1744-6155.2005.00028.x PMID:16083436

Garlo, K., O'Leary, J. R., Van Ness, P. H., & Fried, T. R. (2010). Burden in caregivers of older adults with advanced illness. *Journal of the American Geriatrics Society*, *58*(12), 2315–2322. doi:10.1111/j.1532-5415.2010.03177.x PMID:21087225

Gartner Inc. (2015). *Gartner's 2015 hype cycle for emerging technologies identifies the computing innovations that organizations should monitor*. Retrieved from http://www.gartner.com/newsroom/id/3114217

Gaston, C. M., & Mitchell, G. (2005). Information giving and decision-making in patients with advanced cancer: A systematic review. *Social Science & Medicine*, *61*(10), 2252–2264. doi:10.1016/j.socscimed.2005.04.015 PMID:15922501

Gee, J. P. (2003). *What videogames have to teach us about learning and literacy* (2nd ed.). New York: Palgrave Macmillan.

Gee, P. M., Paterniti, D. A., Ward, D., & Soederberg Miller, L. M. (2015). e-Patients Perceptions of Using Personal Health Records for self-management Support of Chronic Illness. *Computers, Informatics, Nursing*, *33*(6), 229–237. doi:10.1097/CIN.0000000000000151 PMID:25899440

General Medical Council. (2013). *Good Medical Practice.* Retrieved from http://www.gmc-uk.org/guidance/news_consultation/20477.asp

Genova, J., Nahon-Serfaty, I., Dansokho, S. C., Gagnon, M. P., Renaud, J. S., & Giguère, A. (2014). The Communication AssessmenT Checklist in Health (CATCH): A Tool for Assessing the Quality of Printed Educational Materials for Clinicians. *The Journal of Continuing Education in the Health Professions*, *34*(4), 232–242. doi:10.1002/chp.21257 PMID:25530293

Gerber, B. S., Brodsky, I. G., Lawless, K. A., Smolen, L. I., Arozullah, A. M., Smith, E. V., & Eiser, A. R. et al. (2005). Implementation and evaluation of a low-literacy diabetes education computer multimedia application. *Diabetes Care*, *28*(7), 1574–1580. doi:10.2337/diacare.28.7.1574 PMID:15983303

Gerbino, G., Dimonte, V., Albasi, C., Lasorsa, C., Vitale, C., & Marangella, M. (2011). Adesione Alla Terapia Del Paziente In Emodialisi[Adherence to Care for the Patient in Dyalisis]. *Giornale Italiano di Nefrologia*, *28*(4), 416–424. PMID:21809311

Gerr, R., Saulsberry, K., Clark, M., & Kerns, C. (2014). *The Shared Accountability Care Model: Keeping Patients Activated, In-Network, and Brand Loyal.* The Advisory Board Company.

Giacomini, M., DeJean, D., Simeonov, D., & Smith, A. (2012). Experiences of living and dying with COPD: A systematic review and synthesis of the qualitative empirical literature. *Archive of. Ontario Health Technology Assessment Series*, *12*(13), 1–47. PMID:23074423

Giangregorio, L. M., Thabane, L., Adachi, J. D., Ashe, M. C., Bleakney, R. R., Braun, E. A., & Papaioannou, A. et al. (2014). Build better bones with exercise: Protocol for a feasibility study of a multicenter randomized controlled trial of 12 months of home exercise in women with a vertebral fracture. *Physical Therapy*, *94*(9), 1337–1352. doi:10.2522/ptj.20130625 PMID:24786946

Giguière, A., Légaré, F., Grad, R., Pluye, R., Haynes, B., Cauchon, M., & Labrecque, M. et al. (2012). Decision boxes for clinicians to support evidence-based practice and shared decision making: The user experience. *Implementation Science; IS*, *7*(72). PMID:22862935

Gillick, M. R. (2004). Advance care planning. *The New England Journal of Medicine*, *350*(1), 7–8. doi:10.1056/NEJMp038202 PMID:14702421

Gillon, R. (1994). Medical ethics: Four principles plus attention to scope. *BMJ (Clinical Research Ed.)*, *309*(6948), 184–188. doi:10.1136/bmj.309.6948.184 PMID:8044100

Girtler, R. (2001). *Methoden der Feldforschung*. Stuttgart: UTB GmbH.(in German)

Glanz, K., Rimer, B. K., & Viswanath, K. (2008). *Health Behavior and Health Education: Theory, Research, and Practice* (4th ed.). San Francisco: Jossey-Bass.

Glaser, B., & Strauss, A. (1967). *The Discovery of Grounded Theory: Strategies for Qualitative Research*. New York: Aldine.

Gläser, J., & Laudel, G. (2009). *Experteninterviews und qualitative Inhaltsanalyse: als Instrumente rekonstruierender Untersuchungen*. Wiesbaden: VS Verlag für Sozialwissenschaften.

Glasgow, R. E. (2013). *Reach, Effectiveness, Adoption, Implementation, and Maintenance (RE-AIM)*. Retrieved from http://www.re-aim.hnfe.vt.edu/presentations/glasgow2013presentation.pdf

Glasgow, R. E., Orleans, C. T., & Wagner, E. H. (2001). Does the chronic care model serve also as a template for improving prevention? *The Milbank Quarterly*, *79*(4), 579–612. doi:10.1111/1468-0009.00222 PMID:11789118

Glasgow, R. E., Toobert, D. J., Riddle, M., Donnelly, J., Mitchell, D. L., & Calder, D. (1989). Diabetes-specific social learning variables and self-care behaviors among persons with type II diabetes. *Health Psychology*, *8*(3), 285–303. doi:10.1037/0278-6133.8.3.285 PMID:2767020

Global Initiative for Chronic Obstructive Lung Disease (GOLD). (2015). *Global Strategy for the Diagnosis, Management, and Prevention of Chronic Obstructive Lung Disease*. Updated 2015. Global Initiative for Chronic Obstructive Lung Disease, Inc. Retrieved from http://www.goldcopd.org/uploads/users/files/GOLD_Report_2015_Sept2.pdf

Global Initiative for Chronic Obstructive Lung Disease (GOLD). (2015). *Strategia globale per la diagnosi, il trattamento e la prevenzione della broncopneumopatia cronica ostruttiva. Updated 2015*. Global Initiative for Chronic Obstructive Lung Disease, Inc. Retrieved from http://www.goldcopd.it/materiale/2015/GOLD_workshop_report_2015.pdf

Go, A. S., Chertow, G. M., Fan, D., McCulloch, C. E., & Hsu, C. Y. (2004). Chronic kidney disease and the risks of death, cardiovascular events, and hospitalization. *The New England Journal of Medicine*, *351*(13), 1296–1305. doi:10.1056/NEJMoa041031 PMID:15385656

Goetzel, R. Z., Anderson, D. R., Whitmer, R. W., Ozminkowski, R. J., Dunn, R. L., & Wasserman, J.Health Enhancement Research Organization (HERO) Research Committee. (1998). The relationship between modifiable health risks and health care expenditures: An analysis of the multi-employer HERO health risk and cost database. *Journal of Occupational and Environmental Medicine*, *40*(10), 843–854. doi:10.1097/00043764-199810000-00003 PMID:9800168

Google (2012). *The Digital Journey to Wellness: Hospital Selection Infographic.*

Gore, J. M., Brophy, C. J., & Greenstone, M. A. (2000). How well do we care for patients with end stage chronic obstructive pulmonary disease (COPD)? A comparison of palliative care and quality of life in COPD and lung cancer. *Thorax*, *55*(12), 1000–1006. doi:10.1136/thorax.55.12.1000 PMID:11083884

Gott, M., Gardiner, C., Small, N., Payne, S., Seamark, D., Barnes, S., & Ruse, C. et al. (2009). Barriers to advance care planning in chronic obstructive pulmonary disease. *Palliative Medicine*, *23*(7), 642–648. doi:10.1177/0269216309106790 PMID:19648222

Graetz, I., Reed, M., Rundall, T., Bellows, J., Brand, R., & Hsu, J. (2009). Care coordination and electronic health records: Connecting clinicians.[). American Medical Informatics Association.]. *AMIA ... Annual Symposium Proceedings / AMIA Symposium. AMIA Symposium*, *2009*, 208. PMID:20351851

Graffigna, G., Barello, S., Riva, G., & Bosio, A. C. (2014). Patient engagement: The key to redesign the exchange between the demand and supply for healthcare in the era of active ageing. In G. Riva, P. Ajmone Marsan, & C. Grassi. (Eds.), Active Ageing and Healthy Living (pp. 85-95). Amsterdam: IOS Press.

Graffigna, G., & Barello, S. (2015). Innovating Healthcare in the Era of Patient Engagement: Challenges, Opportunities & New Trends. In G. Graffigna, S. Barello, & S. Triberti (Eds.), *Patient Engagement: A Consumer-Centered Model to Innovate Healthcare*. Berlin: De Gruyter Open. doi:10.1515/9783110452440-002

Graffigna, G., & Barello, S. (2015). Modelling Patient Engagement in Healthcare: Insight for Research and Practice. In G. Graffigna, S. Barello, & S. Triberti (Eds.), *Patient Engagement: A consumer-centered model to innovate healthcare*. Berlin: DeGruyter Open. doi:10.1515/9783110452440-004

Graffigna, G., Barello, S., Libreri, C., & Bosio, C. A. (2014). How to engage type-2 diabetic patients in their own health management: Implications for clinical practice. *BMC Public Health*, *14*(1), 648. doi:10.1186/1471-2458-14-648 PMID:24966036

Graffigna, G., Barello, S., & Riva, G. (2013). Technologies for patient engagement. *Health Affairs*, *32*(6), 1172–1172. doi:10.1377/hlthaff.2013.0279 PMID:23733998

Graffigna, G., Barello, S., & Riva, G. (2013a). How to make health information technology effective: The challenge of patient engagement. *Archives of Physical Medicine and Rehabilitation*, *94*(10), 2034–2035. doi:10.1016/j.apmr.2013.04.024 PMID:24075414

Graffigna, G., Barello, S., & Triberti, S. (2015). Giving (Back) a Role to Patients in the Delivery of Healthcare Services: Theoretical Roots of Patient Engagement. In G. Graffigna, S. Barello, & S. Triberti (Eds.), *Patient Engagement. A Consumer-Centered Model to Innovate Healthcare* (pp. 13–26). Berlin: De Gruyter Open. doi:10.1515/9783110452440-003

Graffigna, G., Barello, S., & Triberti, S. (2015). *Patient Engagement: A consumer-centered model to innovate healthcare*. Berlin: DeGruyter Open. doi:10.1515/9783110452440

Graffigna, G., Barello, S., Triberti, S., Wiederhold, B. K., Bosio, A. C., & Riva, G. (2014). Enabling eHealth as a pathway for patient engagement: A toolkit for medical practice. *Studies in Health Technology and Informatics*, *199*, 13–21. PMID:24875682

Graffigna, G., Barello, S., Wiederhold, B. K., Bosio, A. C., & Riva, G. (2013a). Positive technology as a driver for health engagement. *Studies in Health Technology and Informatics*, *191*, 9–17. PMID:23792833

Graffigna, G., Vegni, E., Barello, S., Olson, K., & Bosio, C. A. (2011). Studying the social construction of cancer-related fatigue experience: The heuristic value of Ethnoscience. *Patient Education and Counseling*, *82*(3), 402–409. doi:10.1016/j.pec.2010.12.017 PMID:21292426

Gramling, R., Norton, S. A., Ladwig, S., Metzger, M., DeLuca, J., Gramling, D., & Alexander, S. (2013a). Direct observation of prognosis communication in palliative care: A descriptive study. *Journal of Pain and Symptom Management*, *45*(2), 202–212. doi:10.1016/j.jpainsymman.2012.02.004 PMID:22652135

Gramling, R., Norton, S., Ladwig, S., Winters, P., Metzger, M., Quill, T., & Alexander, S. (2013b). Latent Classes of Prognosis Conversations in Palliative Care: A Mixed-Methods Study. *Journal of Palliative Medicine*, *16*(6), 653–660. doi:10.1089/jpm.2012.0381 PMID:23659459

Grant, M., Cavanagh, A., & Yorke, J. (2012). The impact of caring for those with chronic obstructive pulmonary disease (COPD) on carers' psychological well-being: A narrative review. *International Journal of Nursing Studies*, (Mar): 2. PMID:22386988

Grassé, P. P. (1959). La reconstruction du nid et les coordinations interindividuelles chezBellicositermes natalensis et Cubitermes sp. la théorie de la stigmergie: Essai d'interprétation du comportement des termites constructeurs. *Insectes Sociaux*, *6*(1), 41–80. doi:10.1007/BF02223791

Grazie, D., & Wimmer-Puchinger, B. (2014). Rahmen-Gesundheitsziel 3 - Gesundheitskompetenz der Bevölkerung stärken, Bericht der Arbeitsgruppe. Bundesministerium für Gesundheit, Editor (in German).

Greenhalgh, T., & Russell, J. (2010). Why do evaluations of eHealth programs fail? An alternative set of guiding principles. *PLoS Medicine*, *7*(11), 1331. doi:10.1371/journal.pmed.1000360 PMID:21072245

Green, J. A., Mor, M. K., Schields, A. M., Sevick, M. A., Palevsky, P. M., Fine, M. J., & Weisbord, S. D. et al. (2011). Prevalence and demographic and clinical associations of health literacy in patients on maintenance hemodialysis. *Clinical Journal of the American Society of Nephrology; CJASN*, *6*(6), 1354–1360. doi:10.2215/CJN.09761110 PMID:21551025

Green, J. A., Mor, M. K., Shields, A. M., Sevick, M. A., Arnold, R. M., Palevsky, P. M., & Weisbord, S. D. et al. (2013). Associations of health literacy with dialysis adherence and health resource utilization in patients receiving maintenance hemodialysis. *American Journal of Kidney Diseases*, *62*(1), 73–80. doi:10.1053/j.ajkd.2012.12.014 PMID:23352380

Grice, H. P. (1975). Logic and conversation. In P. Cole & J. L. Morgan (Eds.), Syntax and Semantics (Vol. 3, pp. 41-58). New York: Academic Press.

Grimmer, K., Luker, J., Beaton, K., Kumar, S., Crockett, A., & Price, K. (2013). Trialing individualized interventions to prevent functional decline in at-risk older adults (TRIIFL): Study protocol for a randomized controlled trial nested in a longitudinal observational study. *Trials*, *14*(1), 266. doi:10.1186/1745-6215-14-266 PMID:23962259

Grimshaw, J., Eccles, M., Thomas, R., MacLennan, G., Ramsay, C., Fraser, C., & Vale, L. (2006). Toward Evidence-based Quality Improvement. *Journal of General Internal Medicine*, *21*(Suppl. 2), S14–S20. PMID:16637955

Grubbs, V., Gregorich, S. E., Perez-Stable, E. J., & Hsu, C. Y. (2009). Health literacy and access to kidney transplantation. *Clinical Journal of the American Society of Nephrology; CJASN*, *4*(1), 195–200. doi:10.2215/CJN.03290708 PMID:19056617

Gruman, J., Rovner, M. H., French, M. E., Jeffress, D., Sofaer, S., Shaller, D., & Prager, D. J. (2010). From patient education to patient engagement: Implications for the field of patient education. *Patient Education and Counseling*, *78*(3), 350–356. doi:10.1016/j.pec.2010.02.002 PMID:20202780

Gschwind, Y. J., Kressig, R. W., Lacroix, A., Muehlbauer, T., Pfenninger, B., & Granacher, U. (2013). A best practice fall prevention exercise program to improve balance, strength / power, and psychosocial health in older adults: Study protocol for a randomized controlled trial. *BMC Geriatrics*, *13*(1), 105. doi:10.1186/1471-2318-13-105 PMID:24106864

Guadagnoli, E., & Ward, P. (1998). Patient participation in decision-making. *Social Science & Medicine*, *47*(3), 329–339. doi:10.1016/S0277-9536(98)00059-8 PMID:9681902

Gubbi, J., Buyya, R., Marusic, S., & Palaniswami, M. (2013). Internet of Things (IoT): A vision, architectural elements, and future directions. *Future Generation Computer Systems*, *29*(7), 1645–1660. doi:10.1016/j.future.2013.01.010

Gulati, M. (2011). Diagnostic assessment of patients with interstitial lung disease. *Primary Care Respiratory Journal*, *20*(2), 120–127. doi:10.4104/pcrj.2010.00079 PMID:21509417

Gunn, H., Cattaneo, D., Finlayson, M., Freeman, J., & Sosnoff, J. J. (2014). Home or away? Choosing a setting for a falls-prevention program for people with multiple sclerosis. *International Journal of MS Care*, *16*(4), 186–191. doi:10.7224/1537-2073.2014-058 PMID:25694777

Guyatt, G., Oxman, A. D., Sultan, S., Brozek, J., Glasziou, P., Alonso-Coello, P., ... & Jaeschke, R. (2012). GRADE guidelines: 11. Making an overall rating of confidence in effect estimates for a single outcome and for all outcomes. *Journal of clinical epidemiology*.

Guyatt, G., Oxman, A., Akl, E., Kunz, R., Vist, G., Brozek, J., & deBeer, H. et al. (2011). GRADE guidelines: 1. Introduction-GRADE evidence profiles and summary of findings tables. *Journal of Clinical Epidemiology*, *64*(4), 383–394. doi:10.1016/j.jclinepi.2010.04.026 PMID:21195583

Haber, D. (2006). Life review: Implementation, theory, research, and therapy. *International Journal of Aging & Human Development*, *63*(2), 153–171. doi:10.2190/DA9G-RHK5-N9JP-T6CC PMID:17137032

Haff, N., Patel, M. S., Lim, R., Zhu, J., Troxel, A. B., Asch, D. A., & Volpp, K. G. (2015). The role of behavioral economic incentive design and demographic characteristics in financial incentive-based approaches to changing health behaviors: A meta-analysis. *American Journal of Health Promotion*, *29*(5), 314–323. doi:10.4278/ajhp.140714-LIT-333 PMID:25928816

Haggard, L., & Hosking, S. (2003). *Healing the Hospital Environment: Design, Management and Maintenance of Healthcare Premises*. London: Taylor & Francis.

Hagland, M. (2013). CVS Caremark report: Medication non-adherence in U.S. costs up to $290 billion annually. Retrieved from http://www.healthcare-informatics.com/news-item/cvs-caremark-report-medication-non-adherence-us-costs-290-billion-annually

Hall, M. J., Levant, S., & DeFrances, C. J. (2013). Trends in inpatient hospital deaths: National Hospital Discharge Survey, 2000-2010. *NCHS data brief*, (118), 1.

Harms, C., & Biocca, F. (2004). Internal Consistency and Reliability of the Networked Minds - Measure of Social Presence.*Proceedings of the Seventh Annual International Workshop: Presence*. Valencia, CA: Universidad Politecnica de Valencia press.

Harper, D. (2001). *Online Etymology Dictionary*. Retrieved from http://www.etymonline.com/index.php?term=patience&allowed_in_frame=0

Hart, E., & Di Blasi, Z. (2015). Combined flow in musical jam sessions: A pilot qualitative study. *Psychology of Music, 43*(2), 275-290. doi:0305735613502374.

Harter, L. M., Japp, P. M., & Beck, C. S. (2005). *Narratives, health, and healing: Communication theory, research, and practice*. Mahwah, NJ: Lawrence Erlbaum.

Hartmannbund. (2014). *Umfrage „Termintreue" – Datenbasis*. Retrieved from http://www.hartmannbund.de/uploads/Landesverb%C3%A4nde/Niedersachsen/2014-07-09_Handout-Presse.PDF (in German).

Health Insurance Portability and Accountability Act. (1996). *CMS.gov*. Retrieved from https://www.cms.gov/Regulations-and-Guidance/HIPAA-Administrative-Simplification/HIPAAGenInfo/downloads/hipaalaw.pdf

Health On the Net Foundation. (2014). Retrieved from http://www.healthonnet.org/HONcode/Conduct.html

Hebden, L., Balestracci, K., McGeechan, K., Denney-Wilson, E., Harris, M., Bauman, A., & Allman-Farinelli, M. (2013). 'TXT2BFiT' a mobile phone-based healthy lifestyle program for preventing unhealthy weight gain in young adults: Study protocol for a randomized controlled trial. *Trials*, *14*(1), 75. doi:10.1186/1745-6215-14-75 PMID:23506013

Heisler, M., Bouknight, R. R., Hayward, R. A., Smith, D. M., & Kerr, E. A. (2002). The relative importance of physician communication, participatory decision-making, and patient understanding in diabetes self-management. *Journal of General Internal Medicine*, *17*(4), 243–252. doi:10.1046/j.1525-1497.2002.10905.x PMID:11972720

Heisler, M., Vijan, S., Anderson, R. M., Ubel, P. A., Bernstein, S. J., & Hofer, T. P. (2003). When do patients and their physicians agree on diabetes treatment goals and strategies, and what difference does it make? *Journal of General Internal Medicine*, *18*(11), 893–902. doi:10.1046/j.1525-1497.2003.21132.x PMID:14687274

Hellawell, G., Turner, K., Le Monnier, K., & Brewster, S. (2000). Urology and the Internet: An evaluation of Internet use by urology patients and of information available on urological topics. *BJU International*, *86*(3), 191–194. doi:10.1046/j.1464-410x.2000.00831.x PMID:10930912

Hemingway, H., & Marmot, M. (1999a). Clinical Evidence: Psychosocial factors in the etiology and prognosis of coronary heart disease: systematic review of prospective cohort studies. *The Western Journal of Medicine*, *171*(5-6), 342–350. PMID:18751201

Hemingway, H., & Marmot, M. (1999b). Evidence based cardiology: Psychosocial factors in the aetiology and prognosis of coronary heart disease. Systematic review of prospective cohort studies. *BMJ (Clinical Research Ed.)*, *318*(7196), 1460–1467. doi:10.1136/bmj.318.7196.1460 PMID:10346775

Hibbard, J. H., Greene, J., & Overton, V. (2013). Patients with lower activation associated with higher costs; delivery systems should know their patients' 'scores'. *Health Affairs*, *32*(2), 216–222. doi:10.1377/hlthaff.2012.1064 PMID:23381513

Hibbard, J. H., Mahoney, E. R., Stock, R., & Tusler, M. (2007). Do increases in patient activation result in improved self-management behaviors? *Health Services Research*, *42*(4), 1443–1463. doi:10.1111/j.1475-6773.2006.00669.x PMID:17610432

Hibbard, J., & Greene, J. (2013). What the evidence shows about patient activation: Better health outcomes and care experiences; fewer data on costs. *Health Affairs*, *32*(2), 207–214. doi:10.1377/hlthaff.2012.1061 PMID:23381511

Higgins, E. T. (1987). Self-discrepancy: A theory relating self and affect. *Psychological Review*, *94*(3), 319–340. doi:10.1037/0033-295X.94.3.319 PMID:3615707

Himmelstein, D. U., Warren, E., Thorne, D., & Woolhandler, S. (2005, February). MarketWatch: Illness And Injury As Contributors To Bankruptcy. *Health Affairs*. Retrieved from:http://content.healthaffairs.org/content/early/2005/02/02/hlthaff.w5.63/suppl/DC1

Hines, A. L., Barrett, M. S., Jiang, H. J., & Steiner, C. A. (2011). *Conditions with the largest number of adult hospital readmissions by payer*. Retrieved from https://www.hcup-us.ahrq.gov/reports/statbriefs/sb172-Conditions-Readmissions-Payer.jsp

Hoerbst, A., & Ammenwerth, E. (2010). Electronic Health Records. A systematic review on quality requirements. *Methods of Information in Medicine*, *49*(4), 320–336. doi:10.3414/ME10-01-0038 PMID:20603687

Hoffman, A., Volk, R., Saarimaki, A., Stirling, C., Li, L., Härter, M., & Llewellyn-Thomas, H. et al. (2013). Delivering patient decision aids on the Internet: Definitions, theories, current evidence, and emerging research areas. *BMC Medical Informatics and Decision Making*, *13*(Suppl. 2), S13. doi:10.1186/1472-6947-13-S2-S13 PMID:24625064

Holmes-Rovner, M., Stommel, M., Corser, W. D., Olomu, A., Holtrop, J. S., Siddiqi, A., & Dunn, S. L. (2008). Does outpatient telephone coaching add to hospital quality improvement following hospitalization for acute coronary syndrome? *Journal of General Internal Medicine*, *23*(9), 1464–1470. doi:10.1007/s11606-008-0710-1 PMID:18618189

Hood, L. E., & Galas, D. J. (2008). *P4 Medicine: personalized, predictive, preventive, participatory. A change of view that changes everything*. Washington: Computing Community Consortium. Retrieved from http://cra.org/ccc/wp-content/uploads/sites/2/2015/05/P4_Medicine.pdf

Hsieh, H. F., Shannon, S. E., & Curtis, J. R. (2006). Contradictions and communication strategies during end-of-life decision making in the intensive care unit. *Journal of Critical Care*, *21*(4), 294–304. doi:10.1016/j.jcrc.2006.06.003 PMID:17175415

Hudson, B. (2005). Sea change or quick fix? Policy on long term conditions in England. *Health & Social Care in the Community*, *13*(4), 378–385. doi:10.1111/j.1365-2524.2005.00579.x PMID:15969709

Imbeault-Nepton, I., & Otis, M. J. D. (2014). Synchronized walking cadence for TUG in perturbed environments: using Earcon or Tacton cues?*Proceedings of IEEE Internation Symposium on Haptic, Audio and Visual Environments and Games (HAVE)* (pp. 41-46). doi:10.1109/HAVE.2014.6954329

Inghilleri, P., Riva, G., & Riva, E. (2014). *Enabling Positive Change: Flow and Complexity in Daily Experience*. Berlin: De Gruyter Open.

Institute for Healthcare Improvement. (2015). *Triple aim initiative*. Retrieved from http://www.ihi.org/Engage/Initiatives/TripleAim/pages/default.aspx

Institute of Medicine. (2004). *Health literacy: a prescription to end confusion*. Washington, DC: The National Academies.

Institute of Medicine. (2012). *How Can Health Care Organizations Become More Health Literate? Workshop Summary*. Washington, DC: National Academies Press.

International Telecommunication Union. (2015). *The World Telecommunication/ICT Indicators Database*. Retrieved from http://www.itu.int/en/ITU-D/Statistics/Pages/stat/default.aspx

Irizarry, T., DeVito Dabbs, A., & Curran, C. R. (2015). Patient portals and patient engagement: A state of the science review. *Journal of Medical Internet Research*, *17*(6), e148. doi:10.2196/jmir.4255 PMID:26104044

Iuga, A. O., & McGuire, M. J. (2014). Adherence and health care costs. *Risk management and healthcare policy, 7*, 35.

Jacobs, R., Lou, J., Ownby, R., & Caballero, J. (2014). A systematic review of eHealth interventions to improve health literacy. *Health Informatics Journal*. PMID:24916567

Jaggers, J. R., Dudgeon, W., Blair, S. N., Sui, X., Burgess, S., Wilcox, S., & Hand, G. A. (2013). A home-based exercise intervention to increase physical activity among people living with HIV: Study design of a randomized clinical trial. *BMC Public Health*, *13*(1), 502. doi:10.1186/1471-2458-13-502 PMID:23706094

Janssen, D. J., Engelberg, R. A., Wouters, E. F., & Curtis, J. R. (2012). Advance care planning for patients with COPD: Past, present and future. *Patient Education and Counseling*, *86*(1), 19–24. doi:10.1016/j.pec.2011.01.007 PMID:21316899

Janzek-Hawlat, S. (2015). *Impact of waiting times in health care* [Master Thesis]. Faculty of Informatics, Vienna University of Technology.

Javitt, J. (2014). Case study: Using mHealth to manage diabetes. *mHealth News*. Retrieved from http://www.mhealthnews.com/print/24916

Jha, V., Garcia-Garcia, G., Iseki, K., Li, Z., Naicker, S., Plattner, B., & Yang, C. W. et al. (2013). Chronic kidney disease: Global dimension and perspectives. *Lancet*, *382*(9888), 260–272. http://www.ncbi.nlm.nih.gov/pubmed/23727169. doi:10.1016/S0140-6736(13)60687-X PMID:23727169

Jin, S. A. A. (2012). The virtual malleable self and the virtual identity discrepancy model: Investigative frameworks for virtual possible selves and others in avatar-based identity construction and social interaction. *Computers in Human Behavior*, *28*(6), 2160–2168. doi:10.1016/j.chb.2012.06.022

Johnson, M. O. (2011). The shifting landscape of health care: Toward a model of health care empowerment. *American Journal of Public Health*, *101*(2), 265–270. doi:10.2105/AJPH.2009.189829 PMID:21164096

Jolly, K., Taylor, R., Lip, G. Y. H., Greenfield, S., Raftery, J., Mant, J., & Stevens, A. et al. (2007). The Birmingham Rehabilitation Uptake Maximisation Study (BRUM). Homebased compared with hospital-based cardiac rehabilitation in a multi-ethnic population: Cost-effectiveness and patient adherence. *Health Technology Assessment*, *11*(35), 1–118. doi:10.3310/hta11350 PMID:17767899

Jolly, S. E., Navaneethan, S. D., Schold, J. D., Arrigain, S., Koning, V., Burrucker, Y. K., & Nally, J. V. et al. (2015). Development of a chronic kidney disease patient navigator program. *BMC Nephrology*, *16*(1), 69. doi:10.1186/s12882-015-0060-2 PMID:26024966

Jones, V. (2006). The "Diabesity" Epidemic: Let's Rehabilitate America. *Medscape General Medicine*, *8*(2), 34–34. PMID:16926773

Jull, G., & Moore, A. (2013). Manual Therapy. *Manual Therapy*, *18*(6), 447–448. doi:10.1016/j.math.2013.09.006 PMID:24188381

Katz, E. (1999). Theorizing diffusion: Tarde and Sorokin revisited. *The Annals of the American Academy of Political and Social Science*, *566*(1), 144–155. doi:10.1177/0002716299566001012

Katz, M. G., Jacobson, T. A., Veldar, E., & Kripalani, S. (2007). Patient Literacy and Question-asking Behavior During the Medical Encounter: A Mixed-metholds Analysis. *Journal of General Internal Medicine*, *22*(6), 782–786. doi:10.1007/s11606-007-0184-6 PMID:17431697

Kaye, R., Kokia, E., Shalev, V., Idar, D., & Chinitz, D. (2010). Barriers and success factors in health information technology: A practitioner's perspective. *Journal of Management & Marketing in Healthcare*, *3*(2), 163–175. doi:10.1179/175330310X12736577732764

Kayser, K., Watson, E., & Andrade, J. T. (2007). Cancer as a we-disease: Examining the process of coping from a relational perspective. *Families, Systems & Health*, *25*(4), 404–418. doi:10.1037/1091-7527.25.4.404

Kennedy, J. F. (1962). *Special message to Congress on protecting consumer interest.* Presidential Papers. President's Office Files.

Kent, P., Laird, R., & Haines, T. (2015). The effect of changing movement and posture using motion-sensor biofeedback, versus guidelines-based care, on the clinical outcomes of people with sub-acute or chronic low back pain-a multicentre, cluster-randomised, placebo-controlled, pilot trial. *BMC Musculoskeletal Disorders*, *16*(1), 131. doi:10.1186/s12891-015-0591-5 PMID:26022102

Keogh, E., Rosser, B. A., & Eccleston, C. (2010). e-Health and chronic pain management: Current status and developments. *Pain*, (151): 18–21.

Kernis, M. H. (2013). *Self-esteem issues and answers: A sourcebook of current perspectives.* New York: Psychology Press.

Kessels, R. P. (2003). Patients' Memory for Medical Information. *Journal of the Royal Society of Medicine*, *96*(5), 219–222. doi:10.1258/jrsm.96.5.219 PMID:12724430

Khaylis, A., Yiaslas, T., Bergstrom, J., & Gore-Felton, C. (2010). A review of efficacious technology-based weight-loss interventions: Five key components. *Telemedicine Journal and e-Health*, *16*(9), 931–938. doi:10.1089/tmj.2010.0065 PMID:21091286

Kim, Y., & Sundar, S. S. (2012). Visualizing ideal self vs. actual self through avatars: Impact on preventive health outcomes. *Computers in Human Behavior*, *28*(4), 1356–1364. doi:10.1016/j.chb.2012.02.021

Kizer, K. W. (2001). Establishing healthcare performance standards in an era of consumerism. *The New England Journal of Medicine*, *286*(10), 1213–1217. PMID:11559267

Klazinga, N. (2003). Development and validation of an international appraisal instrument for assessing the quality of clinical practice guidelines: The AGREE project. *Quality & Safety in Health Care*, *12*(1), 18–23. doi:10.1136/qhc.12.1.18 PMID:12571340

Kleinpeter, M. A. (2003). Health literacy affects peritoneal dialysis performance and outcomes. *Advances in Peritoneal Dialysis. Conference on Peritoneal Dialysis*, *19*, 115–119. PMID:14763046

Knauft, E., Nielsen, E. L., Engelberg, R. A., Patrick, D. L., & Curtis, J. R. (2005). Barriers and facilitators to end-of-life care communication for patients with COPD. *Chest*, *127*(6), 2188–2196. doi:10.1378/chest.127.6.2188 PMID:15947336

Kobayashi, L. C., Wardle, J., & von Wagner, C. (2014). Limited health literacy is a barrier to colorectal cancer screening in England: Evidence from the English Longitudinal Study of Ageing. *Preventive Medicine*, *61*, 100–105. doi:10.1016/j.ypmed.2013.11.012 PMID:24287122

Koedoot, C. G., Oort, F. J., De Haan, R. J., Bakker, P. J. M., De Graeff, A., & de Haes, J. C. J. M. (2004). The content and amount of information given by medical oncologists when telling patients with advanced cancer what their treatment options are: Palliative chemotherapy and watchful-waiting. *European Journal of Cancer*, *40*(2), 225–235. doi:10.1016/j.ejca.2003.10.008 PMID:14728937

Kolko, B. E. (1998). Representing bodies in virtual space: The rhetoric of avatar design. *The Information Society*, *15*(3), 177–186. doi:10.1080/019722499128484

Kraal, J. J., Peek, N., van den Akker-Van Marle, M. E., & Kemps, H. M. (2013). Effects and costs of home-based training with telemonitoring guidance in low to moderate risk patients entering cardiac rehabilitation: The FIT@Home study. *BMC Cardiovascular Disorders*, *13*(1), 82. doi:10.1186/1471-2261-13-82 PMID:24103384

Kresser, C. (2014a). Diabesity Retrieved from http://chriskresser.com/diabesity#

Kresser, C. (2014b). Diabesity: the #1 cause of death and disease? Retrieved from http://chriskresser.com/diabesity-the-1-cause-of-death-and-disease

Krueger, R. A. (1994). *Focus groups. A practical Guide for Applied Research*. Thousand Oaks, CA: Sage Publications.

Kruis, A. L., & Chavannes, N. H. (2010). Potential benefits of integrated COPD management in primary care. *Monaldi Archives for Chest Disease*, *73*(3), 130–134. PMID:21214043

Krumholz, H. M., Amatruda, J., Smith, G. L., Mattera, J. A., Roumanis, S. A., Radford, M. J., & Vaccarino, V. et al. (2002). Randomized trial of an education and support intervention to prevent readmission of patients with heart failure. *Journal of the American College of Cardiology*, *39*(1), 83–89. doi:10.1016/S0735-1097(01)01699-0 PMID:11755291

Kugler, C., Vlaminck, H., Haverich, A., & Maes, B. (2005). Nonadherence with diet and fluid restrictions among adults having hemodialysis. *Journal of Nursing Scholarship*, *37*(1), 25–29. doi:10.1111/j.1547-5069.2005.00009.x PMID:15813583

Lacasse, Y., Brosseau, L., Milne, S., Martin, S., Wong, E., Guyatt, G. H., & Goldstein, R. S. (2002). Pulmonary rehabilitation for chronic obstructive pulmonary disease. *Cochrane Database of Systematic Reviews*, (3): CD003793. PMID:12137716

Lafata, J. E., Morris, H. L., Dobie, E., Heisler, M., Werner, R. M., & Dumenci, L. (2013). Patient-reported use of collaborative goal setting and glycemic control among patients with diabetes. *Patient Education and Counseling*, *92*(1), 94–99. doi:10.1016/j.pec.2013.01.016 PMID:23433777

Lai, J. (2006). *U.S. Patent No. 7081807*. Washington, DC: U.S. Patent and Trademark Office.

Lamiani, G., Barello, S., Browning, D. M., Vegni, E., & Meyer, E. C. (2012). Uncovering and validating clinicians' experiential knowledge when facing difficult conversations: A cross-cultural perspective. *Patient Education and Counseling*, *87*(3), 307–312. doi:10.1016/j.pec.2011.11.012 PMID:22196987

Lamiani, G., Strada, I., Mancuso, M. E., Coppola, A., Vegni, E., & Moja, E. A. (2015). Factors influencing illness representations and perceived adherence in haemophilic patients: A pilot study. *Haemophilia*, *21*(5), 598–604. doi:10.1111/hae.12654 PMID:25684356

Lammers, W. M. (2014). *So lässt sich die Wartezeit in der Praxis reduzieren*. ÄrzteZeitung. (in German)

Lancet, T.The Lancet. (2005). Will consumerism lead to better health? *Lancet*, *366*(9483), 343. doi:10.1016/S0140-6736(05)66999-1 PMID:16060053

Lancia, F. (2012). T-LAB 8.0 – User's Manual. Available at http://tlab.it/it/bibliography.php

Lancia, F. (2004). *Strumenti per l'analisi dei testi. Introduzione all'uso di T-LAB* [*Instruments for Textual Analysis. An Introduction to the Use of T-LAB*]. Milano: Franco Angeli.

Lang, E., Wyer, P., & Haynes, R. (2007). Knowledge translation: Closing the evidence-to-practice gap. *Annals of Emergency Medicine*, *49*(3), 355–363. doi:10.1016/j.annemergmed.2006.08.022 PMID:17084943

LaPointe Rudow, D., Hays, R., Baliga, P., Cohen, DJ, Cooper, M., & Danovitch, G, M., ... & Rodrigue, J. R. (2015). Consensus conference on best practices in live kidney donation: Recommendations to optimize education, access, and care. *American Journal of Transplantation*, *15*(4), 914–922. doi:10.1111/ajt.13173 PMID:25648884

Laschet, H. (2014). *Kommentar zur Wartezeit-Umfrage: Säumige Patienten?* ÄrzteZeitung. (in German)

Lau, D. T., Berman, R., Halpern, L., Pickard, A. S., Schrauf, R., & Witt, W. (2010). Exploring factors that influence informal caregiving in medication management for home hospice patients. *Journal of Palliative Medicine*, *13*(9), 1085–1090. doi:10.1089/jpm.2010.0082 PMID:20836633

Lavorini, F., Levy, M. L., Corrigan, C., & Crompton, G.ADMIT Working Group. (2010). The ADMIT series–Issues in Inhalation Therapy. 6) Training tools for inhalation devices. *Primary Care Respiratory Journal*, *19*(4), 335–341. doi:10.4104/pcrj.2010.00065 PMID:21049263

Laws, M. B., Beach, M. C., Lee, Y., Rogers, W. H., Saha, S., Korthuis, P. T., & Wilson, I. B. et al. (2013). Provider-patient adherence dialogue in HIV care: Results of a multisite study. *AIDS and Behavior*, *17*(1), 148–159. doi:10.1007/s10461-012-0143-z PMID:22290609

Laws, M. B., Lee, Y., Rogers, W. H., Beach, M. C., Saha, S., Korthuis, P. T., & Wilson, I. B. et al. (2014). Provider–Patient Communication About Adherence to Anti-retroviral Regimens Differs by Patient Race and Ethnicity. *AIDS and Behavior*, *18*(7), 1279–1287. doi:10.1007/s10461-014-0697-z PMID:24464408

Lazzarato, M. (2002). *Puissances de l'invention: la psychologie Économique de Gabriel Tarde contre l'Économie politique.* Paris: Empêcheurs de penser en rond.

Leary, M. R., & Kowalski, R. M. (1990). Impression management: A literature review and two-component model. *Psychological Bulletin*, *107*(1), 34–47. doi:10.1037/0033-2909.107.1.34

Leary, M. R., Tchividijian, L. R., & Kraxberger, B. E. (1994). Self-presentation can be hazardous to your health: Impression management and health risk. *Health Psychology*, *13*(6), 461–470. doi:10.1037/0278-6133.13.6.461 PMID:7889900

Lee, H. N., Lee, S. Y., Lee, Y. S., Han, J. Y., Choo, M. S., & Lee, K. S. (2013). Pelvic floor muscle training using an extracorporeal biofeedback device for female stress urinary incontinence. *International Urogenicology Journal*, *24*(5), 831–838. doi:10.1007/s00192-012-1943-4 PMID:23052631

Leiter, E. H., Strobel, M., O'Neill, A., Schultz, D., Schile, A., & Reifsnyder, P. C. (2013). Comparison of Two New Mouse Models of Polygenic Type 2 Diabetes at the Jackson Laboratory, NONcNZO10Lt/J and TALLYHO/JngJ. *J Diabetes Res*, *2013*, 165327. doi:10.1155/2013/165327 PMID:23671854

Lennerling, A., & Nyberg, G. (2004). Written information for potential living kidney donors. *Transplant International*, *17*(8), 449–452. doi:10.1111/j.1432-2277.2004.tb00468.x PMID:15322746

Levey, A. S., Schoolwerth, A. C., Burrows, N. R., Williams, D. E., Stith, K. R., & McClellan, W. (2009). Comprehensive public health strategies for preventing the development, progression, and complications of CKD: Report of an expert panel convened by the Centers for Disease Control and Prevention. *American Journal of Kidney Diseases*, *53*(3), 522–535. doi:10.1053/j.ajkd.2008.11.019 PMID:19231739

Levinson, W., Kao, A., Kuby, A., & Thisted, R. A. (2005). Not all patients want to participate in decision making. A national study of public preferences. *Journal of General Internal Medicine*, *20*(6), 531–535. doi:10.1111/j.1525-1497.2005.04101.x PMID:15987329

Levinson, W., Roter, D. L., Mullooly, J. P., Dull, V. T., & Frankel, R. M. (1997). Physician-patient communication. The relationship with malpractice claims among primary care physicians and surgeons. *Journal of the American Medical Association*, *277*(7), 553–559. doi:10.1001/jama.1997.03540310051034 PMID:9032162

Levit, K., Smith, C., Cowan, C., Lazenby, H., Sensenig, A., & Catlin, A. (2003). Trends in US health care spending, 2001. *Health Affairs*, *22*(1), 154–164. doi:10.1377/hlthaff.22.1.154 PMID:12528847

Levy, P., Nocerini, R., & Grazier, K. (2007). Paying for disease management. *Disease Management, 10*(4), 235–244. doi:10.1089/dis.2007.104646 PMID:17718662

Lidén, E., Öhlén, J., Hydén, L. C., & Friberg, F. (2010). Ways of talking about illness and prognosis in palliative cancer care consultations—two interactional frames. *Supportive Care in Cancer, 18*(4), 399–408. doi:10.1007/s00520-009-0673-8 PMID:19504353

Linder, S. M., Rosenfeldt, A. B., Reiss, A., Buchanan, S., Sahu, K., Bay, C. R., & Alberts, J. L. et al. (2013). The home stroke rehabilitation and monitoring system trial: A randomized controlled trial. *International Journal of Stroke, 8*(1), 46–53. doi:10.1111/j.1747-4949.2012.00971.x PMID:23280269

Lin, N., Dean, A., & Ensel, W. M. (2013). *Social support, life events, and depression.* New York: Academic Press.

Little, P., Everitt, H., Williamson, I., Warner, G., Moore, M., Gould, C., & Payne, S. et al. (2001). Preferences of patients for patient centred approach to consultation in primary care: Observational study. *BMJ (Clinical Research Ed.), 322*(7284), 468–540. doi:10.1136/bmj.322.7284.468 PMID:11222423

Loblaw, D., Virgo, K., Nam, R., Somerfield, M., Ben-Josef, E., Mendelson, D., & Talcott, J. et al. (2007). Initial hormonal management of androgen-sensitive metastatic, recurrent, or progressive prostate cancer: 2007 update of an American Society of Clinical Oncology practice guideline. *Journal of Clinical Oncology, 25*(12), 1596–1605. doi:10.1200/JCO.2006.10.1949 PMID:17404365

Locke, E. A., & Latham, G. P. (2002). Building a practically useful theory of goal setting and task motivation. *The American Psychologist, 57*(9), 705–717. doi:10.1037/0003-066X.57.9.705 PMID:12237980

Loke, S.-K. (2015). How do virtual world experiences bring about learning? A critical review of theories. *Australasian Journal of Educational Technology, 31*(1), 112–122.

Lomanowska, A. M., & Guitton, M. J. (2014). My avatar is pregnant! Representation of pregnancy, birth, and maternity in a virtual world. *Computers in Human Behavior, 31*, 322–331. doi:10.1016/j.chb.2013.10.058

Lommi, M., Matarese, M., Alvaro, R., Piredda, M., & De Marinis, M. G. (2015). The experiences of self-care in community-dwelling older people: A meta-synthesis. *International Journal of Nursing Studies, 52*(12), 1854–1867. doi:10.1016/j.ijnurstu.2015.06.012 PMID:26296653

Longtin, Y., Sax, H., Leape, L. L., Sheridan, S. E., Donaldson, L., & Pittet, D. (2010). Patient Participation: Current Knowledge and Applicability to Patient Safety. *Mayo Clinic Proceedings, 85*(1), 53–62. doi:10.4065/mcp.2009.0248 PMID:20042562

Lopez, A. D., & Murray, C. C. (1998). The global burden of disease, 1990–2020. *Nature Medicine, 4*(11), 1241–1243. doi:10.1038/3218 PMID:9809543

Lovera, G., Basile, A., Bertolotti, M., Comazzi, A. M., Clerici, C. A., Gandione, M., & Ponton, P. et al. (2000). L'assistenza psicologica nei trapianti d'organo.[Psychological Care in Organ Transplants]. *Annali dell'Istituto Superiore di Sanita*, *36*(2), 225–246. PMID:11213654

Lozano, R., Naghavi, M., Foreman, K., Lim, S., Shibuya, K., Aboyans, V., & AlMazroa, M. A. et al. (2013). Global and regional mortality from 235 causes of death for 20 age groups in 1990 and 2010: A systematic analysis for the Global Burden of Disease Study. *Lancet*, *380*(9859), 2095–2128. doi:10.1016/S0140-6736(12)61728-0 PMID:23245604

Lucas, G. M., Gratch, J., King, A., & Morency, L. (2014). It's only a computer: Virtual humans increase willingness to disclose. *Computers in Human Behavior*, *37*, 94–100. doi:10.1016/j.chb.2014.04.043

Lusuardi, M., De Benedetto, F., Paggiaro, P., Sanguinetti, C. M., Brazzola, G., Ferri, P., & Donner, C. F. (2006). A Randomized Controlled Trial on Office Spirometry in Asthma and COPD in Standard General Practice. *Chest*, *129*(4), 844–852. doi:10.1378/chest.129.4.844 PMID:16608929

Luxton, D. D., Kayl, R. A., & Mishkind, M. C. (2012). mHealth data security: The need for HIPAA-compliant standardization. *Telemedicine Journal and e-Health*, *18*(4), 284–288. doi:10.1089/tmj.2011.0180 PMID:22400974

Maglie, R. (in press). Can you read this leaflet? User-friendliness of Patient Information Leaflets in the UK and in Italy.*Proceedings of the International Conference hosted by CERLIS, The language of Medicine: Science, Practice and Academia*, University of Bergamo.

Majani, G., & Cavallini, L. (2010). Il ruolo del paziente nella gestione di una terapia a lungo termine. Dalla compliance all'adherence.[Patient's role in the management of a long term treatment. From compliance to adherence]. *Giornale Italiano di Nefrologia*, *27*(3), 316–318. PMID:20540027

Makoul, G., & Clayman, M. L. (2006). An integrative model of shared decision making in medical encounters. *Patient Education and Counseling*, *60*(3), 301–312. doi:10.1016/j.pec.2005.06.010 PMID:16051459

Malkin, R. A. (2007). Design of health care technologies for the developing world. *Annual Review of Biomedical Engineering*, *9*(1), 567–587. doi:10.1146/annurev.bioeng.9.060906.151913 PMID:17430083

Mallampalli, A. (2004). Nutritional management of the patient with chronic obstructive pulmonary disease. *Nutrition in Clinical Practice*, *19*(6), 550–556. doi:10.1177/0115426504019006550 PMID:16215153

Malvey, D., & Slovensky, D. J. (2014). mHealth. Transforming Healthcare. New York: Springer.

Mangold, M., Peintinger, M, & Kopetzki, C. (2010). Behandlungsablehnung trotz vitaler Indikation. RdM - Recht der Medizin 2010/4. (in German)

Manns, B., Hemmelgarn, B., Lillie, E., Crowe, S., Cyr, A., Gladish, M., & Laupacis, A. et al. (2014). Setting research priorities for patients on or nearing dialysis. *Clinical Journal of the American Society of Nephrology; CJASN*, *9*(10), 1813–1821. doi:10.2215/CJN.01610214 PMID:24832095

Mansell, D., Poses, R. M., Kazis, L., & Duefield, C. A. (2000). Clinical factors that influence patients' desire for participation in decisions about illness. *Archives of Internal Medicine*, *160*(19), 2991–2996. doi:10.1001/archinte.160.19.2991 PMID:11041908

Manzoni, G. M., Castelnuovo, G., & Molinari, E. (2008). Weight loss with a low-carbohydrate, Mediterranean, or low-fat diet. *The New England Journal of Medicine*, *359*(20), 2170, author reply 2171–2172. PMID:19009669

Manzoni, G. M., Castelnuovo, G., & Proietti, R. (2011). Assessment of psychosocial risk factors is missing in the 2010 ACCF/AHA guideline for assessment of cardiovascular risk in asymptomatic adults. *Journal of the American College of Cardiology*, *57*(14), 1569–1570. doi:10.1016/j.jacc.2010.12.015 PMID:21453841

Manzoni, G. M., Cribbie, R. A., Villa, V., Arpin-Cribbie, C. A., Gondoni, L., & Castelnuovo, G. (2010). Psychological well-being in obese inpatients with ischemic heart disease at entry and at discharge from a four-week cardiac rehabilitation program. *Frontiers in Psychology*, *1*, 38. PMID:21833207

Manzoni, G. M., Pagnini, F., Corti, S., Molinari, E., & Castelnuovo, G. (2011a). Internet-based behavioral interventions for obesity: An updated systematic review. *Clinical Practice and Epidemiology in Mental Health*, *7*(1), 19–28. doi:10.2174/1745017901107010019 PMID:21552423

Manzoni, G. M., Villa, V., Compare, A., Castelnuovo, G., Nibbio, F., Titon, A. M., & Gondoni, L. A. et al. (2011b). Short-term effects of a multi-disciplinary cardiac rehabilitation programme on psychological well-being, exercise capacity and weight in a sample of obese in-patients with coronary heart disease: A practice-level study. *Psychology Health and Medicine*, *16*(2), 178–189. doi:10.1080/13548506.2010.542167 PMID:21328146

Marberry, S. O. (2006). *Improving Healthcare with Better Building Design*. Chicago, IL: Health Administration Press.

Marcus, M. D., & Wildes, J. E. (2009). Obesity: Is it a mental disorder? *International Journal of Eating Disorders*, *42*(8), 739–753. doi:10.1002/eat.20725 PMID:19610015

Marek, K. D., & Antle, L. (2008). Patient safety and quality: An evidence-based handbook for nurses. In R. G. Hughes (Ed.), *Medication management of the community-dwelling older adult*. Rockville, MD: Agency for Healthcare Research and Quality.

Marsh, G. E. Jr. (1993). Hospital Interior Architecture: Creating Healing Environments for Special Patient Populations. *The New England Journal of Medicine*, *328*(12), 894–895. doi:10.1056/NEJM199303253281224

Martey, R. M., Stromer-Galley, J., Consalvo, M., Wu, J., Banks, J., & Strzalkowski, T. (2015). Communicating age in Second Life: The contributions of textual and visual factors. *New Media & Society*, *17*(1), 41–61. doi:10.1177/1461444813504270

Martinez-Perez, B., de la Torre-Diez, I., & Lopez-Coronado, M. (2013). Mobile health applications for the most prevalent conditions by the World Health Organization: Review and analysis. *Journal of Medical Internet Research*, *15*(6), e120. doi:10.2196/jmir.2600 PMID:23770578

Maurer, J., Rebbapragada, V., Borson, S., Goldstein, R., Kunik, M. E., Yohannes, A. M., & Hanania, N. A. (2008). Anxiety and depression in COPD: current understanding, unanswered questions, and research needs. *Chest Journal, 134(4_suppl)*, 43S-56S.

Maurer, M., Dardess, P., Carman, K. L., Frazier, K., & Smeeding, L. (2012). *Guide to patient and family engagement: environmental scan report*. Rockville, MD: Agency for Healthcare Research and Quality.

Mayer, R., & Moreno, R. (2003). Nine Ways to Reduce Cognitive Load in Multimedia Learning. *Educational Psychologist*, *38*(1), 43–52. doi:10.1207/S15326985EP3801_6

Mayring, P. (2002). *Einführung in die qualitative Sozialforschung*. Weinheim: Beltz. (in German)

Mazzoni, D., Laghi, M., & Cicognani, E. (2013). Qualità della vita e fattori psicosociali nei pazienti con insufficienza renale[Quality of life and psychosocial factors in patients with Renal Insufficiency]. *Psicologia della Salute*, *3*, 5–27. doi:10.3280/PDS2013-003001

McAuley, E., Wójcicki, T. R., Gothe, N. P., Mailey, E. L., Szabo, A. N., Fanning, J., & Mullen, S. P. et al. (2013). Effects of a DVD-delivered exercise intervention on physical function in older adults. *The Journals of Gerontology. Series A, Biological Sciences and Medical Sciences*, *68*(9), 1076–1082. doi:10.1093/gerona/glt014 PMID:23401566

McCarley, P. (2009). Patient empowerment and motivational interviewing: Engaging patients to self-manage their own care. *Nephrology Nursing Journal*, *36*(4), 409–413. PMID:19715108

McCormick, B., & Stone, I. (2007). Economic costs of obesity and the case for government intervention. *Obesity Reviews*, *8*(Suppl. 1), 161–164. doi:10.1111/j.1467-789X.2007.00337.x PMID:17316321

McGrady, E., Conger, S., Blanke, S., & Landry, B. J. (2010). Emerging technologies in healthcare: Navigating risks, evaluating rewards. *Journal of Healthcare Management*, *55*(5), 353. PMID:21077584

McKinstry, B. (2000). Do patients wish to be involved in decision making in the consultation? A cross sectional survey with video vignettes. *BMJ (Clinical Research Ed.)*, *321*(7265), 867–871. doi:10.1136/bmj.321.7265.867 PMID:11021866

McWhorter, J. (2012). Gosh, Golly, Gee. *New Republic*. Retrieved from htttp://www.newrepublic.com/article/politics/magazine/103945/romney-language-mcwhorter

McWhorter, J. (2013, February). Txting is killing language. JK!!! *TED2013*. Retrieved from http://www.ted.com/talks/john_mcwhorter_txtng_is_killing_language_jk#t-126831

Mehta, S. P., & Roy, J. S. (2011). Systematic revie of home physiotherapy after hip fracture surgery. *Journal of Rehabilitation Medicine*, *43*(6), 477–480. doi:10.2340/16501977-0808 PMID:21491074

Menichetti, J., Libreri, C., Lozza, E., & Graffigna, G. (2014). Giving patients a starring role in their own care: A bibliometric analysis of the on-going literature debate.[Epubaheadof print]. *Health Expectations*, n/a. doi:10.1111/hex.12299 PMID:25369557

Menichetti, J., Libreri, C., Lozza, E., & Graffigna, G. (2014). Giving patients a starring role in their own care: A bibliometric analysis of the on-going literature debate. *Health Expectations*, November, 1–11. PMID:25369557

Meppelink, C., van Weert, J., Haven, C. J., & Smit, E. G. (2015). The Effectiveness of Health Animations in Audiences with Different Health Literacy Levels: An Experimental Study. *Journal of Medical Internet Research*, *17*(1), e11. doi:10.2196/jmir.3979 PMID:25586711

Mercer, V. (2011). Chronic Disease Management. In W. T. O'Donohue & C. Draper (Eds.), *Stepped Care and e-Health: Practical Applications to Behavioral Disorders* (pp. 151–179). New York: Springer. doi:10.1007/978-1-4419-6510-3_9

Messano, G. A., Spaziani, E., Turchetta, F., Ceci, F., Corelli, S., Casciaro, G., & Stagnitti, F. et al. (2013). Risk management in surgery. *Il Giornale di Chirurgia -. The Journal of Surgery*, *34*(7-8), 231–237.

Mhatre, P. V., Vilares, I., Stibb, S. M., Albert, M. V., Pickering, L., Marciniak, C. M., & Toledo, S. et al. (2013). Wii Fit balance board playing improves balance and gait in Parkinson disease. *PM & R*, *5*(9), 769–777. doi:10.1016/j.pmrj.2013.05.019 PMID:23770422

Miceli, J., & Wolosin, R. J. (2004). *You're running late - now what? Patient satisfaction, wait time and physician behavior.* Orlando, Florida: World organization of national colleges, academies and academic associations of General Practitioners/Family Physicians.

Michie, S., & Abraham, C. (2008). Advancing the science of behaviour change: A plea for scientific reporting. *Addiction (Abingdon, England)*, *103*(9), 1409–1410. doi:10.1111/j.1360-0443.2008.02291.x PMID:18783495

Michie, S., Johnston, M., Abraham, C., & Walker, A. (2005). Making psychological theory useful for implementing evidence based practice: A consensus approach. *Quality & Safety in Health Care*, *14*(1), 26–33. doi:10.1136/qshc.2004.011155 PMID:15692000

Michie, S., van Stralen, M. M., & West, R. (2011). The behaviour change wheel: A new method for characterising and designing behaviour change interventions. *Implementation Science; IS*, *6*(1), 42. doi:10.1186/1748-5908-6-42 PMID:21513547

Miller, W., & Rollinck, S. (2002). *Motivational interviewing: preparing people to change*. New York: Guilford Press.

Minetti, E., Zanini, S., & Saita, E. (2011). Evaluation of Effectiveness of Information for the Candidate to Kidney Donation. In W. Weimar, M. Bos, & J. van Buschbach (Eds.), Organ Transplantation: Ethical, Legal and Psychological Aspects (pp. 322-328), Vol II, Pabst Science Publisher.

Minetti, E., Zanini, S., & Civati, G. (2004). *Scheda informativa per il potenziale donatore vivente di rene* [[*Fact Sheet for the Potential Kidney Donor]*]. Ancona: Riunione Scientifica Nord Italia Transplant Program.

Ministero della Salute. (2010). *Piano nazionale della prevenzione 2010–2012*.

Misono, A. S., Cutrona, S. L., Choudhry, N. K., Fischer, M. A., Stedman, M. R., Liberman, J. N., & Shrank, W. H. et al. (2010). Healthcare information technology interventions to improve cardiovascular and diabetes medication adherence. *The American Journal of Managed Care*, *16*(12), 82–92. PMID:21314228

Monninkhof, E., van der Valk, P., van der Palen, J., van Herwaarden, C., & Zielhuis, G. (2003). Effects of a comprehensive self-management programme in patients with chronic obstructive pulmonary disease. *The European Respiratory Journal*, *22*(5), 815–820. doi:10.1183/09031936.03.00047003 PMID:14621090

Montgomery, A. A., Emmett, C. L., Fahey, T., Jones, C., Ricketts, I., Patel, R. R., & Murphy, D. J. et al. (2007). Two decision aids for mode of delivery among women with previous caesarean section: Randomised controlled trial. *BMJ (Clinical Research Ed.)*, *334*(7607), 1305. doi:10.1136/bmj.39217.671019.55 PMID:17540908

Moore, J. O., Marshall, M. A., Inch, B. C., Judge, D. C., Moss, F. H., Gilroy, S. J., & Zusman, R. M. et al. (2014). Technology-supported apprenticeship in the management of hypertension: A randomized control trial. *Journal of Clinical Outcomes Management*, *21*(3), 110–122.

Moore, P. J., Adler, N. E., & Robertson, P. A. (2000). Medical malpractice: The effect of doctor-patient relations on medical patient perceptions and malpractice intentions. *The Western Journal of Medicine*, *173*(4), 244–250. doi:10.1136/ewjm.173.4.244 PMID:11017984

Morie, J. F., & Chance, E. (2011). Extending the reach of health care for obesity and diabetes using virtual worlds. *Journal of Diabetes Science and Technology*, *5*(2), 272–276. doi:10.1177/193229681100500211 PMID:21527093

Morris, D. B. (2001). Narrative, ethics, and pain: Thinking with stories. *Narrative*, 55-77.

Morrison, R. S., & Meier, D. E. (2004). Palliative care. *The New England Journal of Medicine*, *350*(25), 2582–2590. doi:10.1056/NEJMcp035232 PMID:15201415

Mortazavi, B., Nyamathi, S., Lee, S. I., Wilkerson, T., Ghasemzadeh, H., & Sarrafzadeh, M. (2014). Near-realistic mobile exergames with wireless wearable sensors. *Biomedical and Health Informatics. IEEE Journal of*, *18*(2), 449–456.

Moss Richins, S. (2015). *Emerging Technologies in Healthcare*. London: CRC Press, Taylor & Francis Group. doi:10.1201/b18431

Mundi Index. (2012). *Land Vergleich > Krankenhausbetten pro Einwohner*. Retrieved from http://www.indexmundi.com/g/r.aspx?v=2227&l=de

Murphy, K., Casey, D., Devane, D., Cooney, A., McCarthy, B., Mee, L., & O'Shea, E. et al. (2011). A cluster randomised controlled trial evaluating the effectiveness of a structured pulmonary rehabilitation education programme for improving the health status of people with chronic obstructive pulmonary disease (COPD): The PRINCE study protocol. *BMC Pulmonary Medicine*, *11*(1), 4. doi:10.1186/1471-2466-11-4 PMID:21244668

Murphy, M., Black, N., Lamping, D., McKee, C., Sanderson, C., Askham, J., & Marteau, T. (1998). Consensus development methods, and their use in clinical guideline development. *Health Technology Assessment (Winchester, England)*, *2*(3), i. PMID:9561895

Murray, S. A., Kendall, M., Boyd, K., & Sheikh, A. (2005). Illness trajectories and palliative care. *BMJ (Clinical Research Ed.)*, *330*(7498), 1007–1011. doi:10.1136/bmj.330.7498.1007 PMID:15860828

Murray, T., Hardy, D., Spruijt-Metz, D., Hekler, E., & Raij, A. (2013). Avatar interfaces for biobehavioral feedback. In A. Marcus (Ed.), *Design, User Experience, and Usability. Health, Learning, Playing, Cultural, and Cross-Cultural User Experience* (pp. 424–434). Heidelberg: Springer. doi:10.1007/978-3-642-39241-2_47

National Committee for Quality Assurance. (2012). Insights for Improvement. Reducing Readmission: Measuring Health Plan Performance. Retrieved from http://www.ncqa.org/portals/0/Publications/2012%20BI_NCQA%20ReAdMi%20_Pub.pdf

Naylor, C., Parsonage, M., McDaid, D., Knap, M., Fossey, M., & Galea, A. (2012). *Long-term conditions and mental health. The cost of co-morbidities.* The Kings Fund Report. Retrieved from http://www.kingsfund.org.uk/sites/files/kf/field/field_publication_file/long-term-conditions-mental-health-cost-comorbidities-naylor-feb12.pdf

Neuhauser, L. (2011). Readability, Comprehension and Usability. In B. Fischhoff, N. Brewer, & J. S. Downs (Eds.), *Communicating Risks and Benefits: An Evidence-Based User's Guide. US Department of Health and Human Services Food and Drug Administration. Risk Communication Advisory Committee and consultants.*

Neumeyer-Gromen, A., Lampert, T., Stark, K., & Kallischnigg, G. (2004). Disease management programs for depression: A systematic review and meta-analysis of randomized controlled trials. *Medical Care*, *42*(12), 1211–1221. doi:10.1097/00005650-200412000-00008 PMID:15550801

Newman, M. G., Szkodny, L. E., Llera, S. J., & Przeworski, A. (2011). A review of technology-assisted self-help and minimal contact therapies for anxiety and depression: Is human contact necessary for therapeutic efðcacy? *Clinical Psychology Review*, *31*(1), 89–103. doi:10.1016/j.cpr.2010.09.008 PMID:21130939

Nguyen, T., & Lau, D. C. (2012). The obesity epidemic and its impact on hypertension. *The Canadian Journal of Cardiology*, *28*(3), 326–333. doi:10.1016/j.cjca.2012.01.001 PMID:22595448

Nhavoto, J. A., & Gronlund, A. (2014). Mobile technologies and geographic information systems to improve health care systems: A literature review. *JMIR Mhealth and Uhealth*, *2*(2), e21. doi:10.2196/mhealth.3216 PMID:25099368

Nielsen-Bohlman, L., Panzer, A. M., & Kindig, D. A. (2004). *Health literacy: A prescription to end confusion*. Washington, D.C.: National Academies Press.

Nielsen, J. (1999). *Designing web usability: The practice of simplicity*. New Riders Publishing.

Nielsen, J. (2004). *Designing web usability*. Pearson Deutschland GmbH.

Norman, C. D., & Skinner, H. A. (2006a). eHEALS: The eHealth literacy scale. *Journal of Medical Internet Research*, *8*(4), e27. doi:10.2196/jmir.8.4.e27 PMID:17213046

Norman, C. D., & Skinner, H. A. (2006b). eHealth literacy: Essential skills for consumer health in a networked world. *Journal of Medical Internet Research*, *8*(2), e9. doi:10.2196/jmir.8.2.e9 PMID:16867972

Norton, S. A., Metzger, M., DeLuca, J., Alexander, S. C., Quill, T. E., & Gramling, R. (2013). Palliative Care Communication: Linking Patients' Prognoses, Values, and Goals of Care. *Research in Nursing & Health*, *36*(6), 582–590. doi:10.1002/nur.21563 PMID:24114740

Novak, I. (2011). Effective home programme intervention for adults: A systematic review. *Clinical Rehabilitation*, *25*(12), 1066–1085. doi:10.1177/0269215511410727 PMID:21831927

Nuño, R., Coleman, K., Bengoa, R., & Sauto, R. (2012). Integrated care for chronic conditions: The contribution of the ICCC Framework. *Health Policy (Amsterdam)*, *105*(1), 55–64. doi:10.1016/j.healthpol.2011.10.006 PMID:22071454

Nursing & Midwifery Council. (2015). *The code - Professional standards of practice and behaviour for nurses and midwives*. Retrieved from http://www.nmc.org.uk/standards/code/

O'Donnell, R. R. (2011). Stepped Care and E-Health in Behavioral Managed Care. In W. T. O'Donohue & C. Draper (Eds.), *Stepped Care and e-Health: Practical Applications to Behavioral Disorders* (pp. 263–282). New York: Springer. doi:10.1007/978-1-4419-6510-3_14

O'Donohue, W. T., & Draper, C. (2011a). The Case for Evidence-Based Stepped Care as Part of a Reformed Delivery System. In W. T. O'Donohue & C. Draper (Eds.), *Stepped Care and e-Health: Practical Applications to Behavioral Disorders* (pp. 1–16). New York: Springer. doi:10.1007/978-1-4419-6510-3_1

O'Donohue, W. T., & Draper, C. (Eds.). (2011b). *Stepped Care and e-Health: Practical Applications to Behavioral Disorders*. New York: Springer.

Ocloo, J. E., & Fulop, N. J. (2012). Developing a 'Critical' approach to patient and public involvement in patient safety in the NHS: Learning lessons from other parts of the public sector? *Health Expectations*, *15*(4), 424–432. doi:10.1111/j.1369-7625.2011.00695.x PMID:21711471

Ofman, J. J., Badamgarav, E., Henning, J. M., Knight, K., Gano, A. D. Jr, Levan, R. K., & Weingarten, S. R. et al. (2004). Does disease management improve clinical and economic outcomes in patients with chronic diseases? A systematic review. *The American Journal of Medicine*, *117*(3), 182–192. doi:10.1016/j.amjmed.2004.03.018 PMID:15300966

Ogah, I., & Wassersug, R. (2013). How reliable are "reputable sources" for medical information on the Internet? The case of hormonal therapy to treat prostate cancer. *Paper presented at the Urologic Oncology: Seminars and Original Investigations.*

Oh, H., Rizo, C., & Enkin, M. et al.. (2005). What Is e-health (3): A systematic review of published definitions. *Journal of Medical Internet Research*, (7): e1.

Omran, A. R. (2005). First published 1971). The epidemiological transition: A theory of the epidemiology of population change. *The Milbank Quarterly*, *83*(4), 731–757. doi:10.1111/j.1468-0009.2005.00398.x PMID:16279965

Ong, L. M. L., Visser, M. R. M., Kruyver, I. P. M., Bensing, J. M., Van Den Brink-Muinen, A., Stouthard, J. M. L., & De Haes, J. C. J. M. et al. (1998). The Roter Interaction Analysis System (RIAS) in oncological consultations: Psychometric properties. *Psycho-Oncology*, *7*(5), 387–401. doi:10.1002/(SICI)1099-1611(1998090)7:5<387::AID-PON316>3.0.CO;2-G PMID:9809330

Ontario, H. Q. (2013). In-home care for optimizing chronic disease management in the community: An evidence-based analysis. *Ontario Health Technology Assessment Series*, *13*(5), 1–65. PMID:24167539

Organization, W. H. (2011). mHealth: New horizons for health through mobile technologies: Second global survey on eHealth. Global observatory for eHealth series (Vol. 3). Retrieved from http://www.who.int/goe/publications/goe_mhealth_web.pdf

Osborn, C. Y., Cavanaugh, K., Wallston, K. A., White, R. O., & Rothman, R. L. (2009). Diabetes numeracy: An overlooked factor in understanding racial disparities in glycemic control. *Diabetes Care*, *32*(9), 1614–1619. doi:10.2337/dc09-0425 PMID:19401443

Osterlund Efraimsson, E., Klang, B., Larsson, K., Ehrenberg, A., & Fossum, B. (2009). Communication and self-management education at nurse-led COPD clinics in primary health care. *Patient Education and Counseling*, *77*(2), 209–217. doi:10.1016/j.pec.2009.03.033 PMID:19414234

Outpatient Service Trialists. (2004). Rehabilitation therapy services for stroke patients living at home: Systematic review of randomized trials. *Lancet*, *363*(9406), 352–356. doi:10.1016/S0140-6736(04)15434-2 PMID:15070563

Oxman, A.GRADE Working Group. (2004). Grading quality of evidence and strength of recommendations. *BMJ (Clinical Research Ed.)*, *328*(19), 1490–1494. PMID:15205295

Pagnini, F., Banfi, P., Lunetta, C., Rossi, G., Castelnuovo, G., Marconi, A., & Molinari, E. et al. (2012). Respiratory function of people with amyotrophic lateral sclerosis and caregiver distress level: A correlational study. *BioPsychoSocial Medicine*, *6*(1), 14. doi:10.1186/1751-0759-6-14 PMID:22721255

Pagnini, F., Lunetta, C., Rossi, G., Banfi, P., Gorni, K., Cellotto, N., & Corbo, M. et al. (2011). Existential well-being and spirituality of individuals with amyotrophic lateral sclerosis is related to psychological well-being of their caregivers. *Amyotrophic Lateral Sclerosis; Official Publication of the World Federation of Neurology Research Group on Motor Neuron Diseases*, *12*(2), 105–108. doi:10.3109/17482968.2010.502941 PMID:20653520

Pagnini, F., Rossi, G., Lunetta, C., Banfi, P., Castelnuovo, G., Corbo, M., & Molinari, E. (2010). Burden, depression, and anxiety in caregivers of people with amyotrophic lateral sclerosis. *Psychology Health and Medicine*, *15*(6), 685–693. doi:10.1080/13548506.2010.507773 PMID:21154021

Pander Maat, H., & Lentz, L. (2010). Improving the Usability of Patient Information Leaflets. *Patient Education and Counseling*, *80*(1), 113–119. doi:10.1016/j.pec.2009.09.030 PMID:19854022

Papalia, R., Vasta, S., Tecame, A., D'Adamio, S., Maffulli, N., & Denaro, V. (2013). Home-based vs supervised rehabilitation programs following knee surgery: A systematic review. *British Medical Bulletin*, *108*(1), 55–72. doi:10.1093/bmb/ldt014 PMID:23690452

Parker, S., Zipurksy, J., Ma, H., & Siegel, C. (2013, October). Randomized controlled trial demonstrates a web-based multimedia program used prior to first-time colonoscopy decreased patient anxiety, sedation requirement and procedure time while increasing knowledge. Dartmouth-Hitchcock Medical Center, Geisel School of Medicine at Dartmouth. *Poster presented at theMeeting of the American College of Gastroenterology*, San Diego, CA.

Park, L. G., Howie-Esquivel, J., Chung, M. L., & Dracup, K. (2014). A text messaging intervention to promote medication adherence for patients with coronary heart disease: A randomized controlled trial. *Patient Education and Counseling*, *94*(2), 261–268. doi:10.1016/j.pec.2013.10.027 PMID:24321403

Park, M. J., & Kim, H. S. (2012). Evaluation of mobile phone and Internet intervention on waist circumference and blood pressure in post-menopausal women with abdominal obesity. *International Journal of Medical Informatics*, *81*(6), 388–394. doi:10.1016/j.ijmedinf.2011.12.011 PMID:22265810

Pasqua, F., Biscione, G. L., Crigna, G., Gargano, R., Cardaci, V., Ferri, L., & Clini, E. et al. (2009). Use of functional independence measure in rehabilitation of inpatients with respiratory failure. *Respiratory Medicine*, *103*(3), 471–476. doi:10.1016/j.rmed.2008.09.007 PMID:18977645

Passamante, A. P. (1998). *U.S. Patent No. 5752621*. Washington, DC: U.S. Patent and Trademark Office.

Patel, K., Janssen, D. J., & Curtis, J. R. (2012). Advance care planning in COPD. *Respirology (Carlton, Vic.)*, *17*(1), 72–78. doi:10.1111/j.1440-1843.2011.02087.x PMID:22008225

Pauwels, R. A., Buist, A. S., Calverley, P. M. A., Jenkins, C. R., & Hurd, S. S.NHLBI/WHO. (2001). NHLBI/WHO global strategy for the diagnosis, management, and prevention of chronic obstructive pulmonary disease. *American Journal of Respiratory and Critical Care Medicine*, *163*(5), 1256–1276. doi:10.1164/ajrccm.163.5.2101039 PMID:11316667

Payne, S., Smith, P., & Dean, S. (1999). Identifying the concerns of informal carers in palliative care. *Palliative Medicine, 13*(1), 37–44. doi:10.1191/026921699666872524 PMID:10320874

Pellas, N., & Kazanidis, I. (2013). On the value of Second Life for students' engagement in blended and online courses: A comparative study from the Higher Education in Greece. *Education and Information Technologies.*

Pellas, N., & Kazanidis, I. (2014). Engaging students in blended and online collaborative courses at university level through Second Life: Comparative perspectives and instructional affordances. *New Review of Hypermedia and Multimedia, 20*(2), 123–144. doi:10.1080/13614568.2013.856958

Pellegrini, C. A., Duncan, J. M., Moller, A. C., Buscemi, J., Sularz, A., DeMott, A., & Spring, B. et al. (2012). A smartphone-supported weight loss program: Design of the ENGAGED randomized controlled trial. *BMC Public Health, 12*, 1041. PMID:23194256

Pepa, L., Ciabattoni, L., Verdini, F., Capecci, M., & Ceravolo, M. G. (2014). Smartphone based fuzzy logic freezing of gait detection in Parkinson's disease.*Proceeding IEEE/ASME Conference on Mechatronic and Embedded Systems and Applications (MESA)* (pp. 1-6).

Perednia, D. A., & Allen, A. (1995). Telemedicine technology and clinical applications. *Journal of the American Medical Association, 273*(6), 483–488. doi:10.1001/jama.1995.03520300057037 PMID:7837367

Peters, E. (2012a). Affect and emotion. Communicating Risks and Benefits: An Evidence Based User's Guide, 89.

Peters, E. (2012b). Quantitative information. In B. B Fischhoff, N. Brewer, & J. S. Downs (Ed.), Communicating Risks and Benefits: An Evidence Based User's Guide: An Evidence Based User's Guide (pp. 53). US Department of Health and Human Services Food and Drug Administration. Risk Communication Advisory Committee and consultants.

Peters, E., Dieckmann, N., Dixon, A., Hibbard, J. H., & Mertz, C. K. (2007). Less is more in presenting quality information to consumers. *Medical Care Research and Review, 64*(2), 169–190. doi:10.1177/10775587070640020301 PMID:17406019

Petkova, V. I., & Ehrsson, H. H. (2008). If I were you: Perceptual illusion of body swapping. *PLoS ONE, 3*(12), e3832. PMID:19050755

Pew Internet and American Life Project Health Fact Sheet. (2012). *Pew Internet.* Retrieved from http://www.pewinternet.org/fact-sheets/health-fact-sheet/

Phalen, J. M., & Eaton, C. B. (2008). *The role of e-health in patient engagement and quality improvement. e-health solutions for healthcare disparities.* New York: Springer.

Pham, K., Thornton, J. D., Engelberg, R. A., Jackson, J. C., & Curtis, J. R. (2008). Alterations during medical interpretation of ICU family conferences that interfere with or enhance communication. *CHEST Journal, 134*(1), 109–116. doi:10.1378/chest.07-2852 PMID:18347204

Pharmaceutical Research and Manufacturers of America. (2011). *Improving prescription medicine adherence is key to better health care*. Retrieved from http://www.phrma.org/sites/default/files/pdf/PhRMA_Improving%20Medication%20Adherence_Issue%20Brief.pdf

Pierratos, A. (2013). Patient Education in Chronic Kidney Disease and Dialysis. *Seminars in Dialysis*, *26*(2), 135–137. doi:10.1111/sdi.12081 PMID:23520986

Pietrabissa, G., Manzoni, G. M., Corti, S., Vegliante, N., Molinari, E., & Castelnuovo, G. (2012). Addressing motivation in globesity treatment: A new challenge for clinical psychology. *Frontiers in Psychology*, *3*, 317. doi:10.3389/fpsyg.2012.00317 PMID:22969744

Piette, J. D., Striplin, D., Marinec, N., Chen, J., Trivedi, R. B., Aron, D. C., & Aikens, J. E. et al. (2015). A Mobile Health Intervention Supporting Heart Failure Patients and Their Informal Caregivers: A Randomized Comparative Effectiveness Trial. *Journal of Medical Internet Research*, *17*(6), e142. doi:10.2196/jmir.4550 PMID:26063161

Piette, J., Rosland, A., Marinec, N., Striplin, D., Bernstein, S., & Silveira, M. (2013). Engagement With Automated Patient Monitoring and Self-Management Support Calls. *Medical Care*, *51*(3), 216–223. doi:10.1097/MLR.0b013e318277ebf8 PMID:23222527

Pignone, M., DeWalt, D. A., Sheridan, S., Berkman, N., & Lohr, K. N. (2005). Interventions to improve health outcomes for patients with low literacy. *Journal of General Internal Medicine*, *20*(2), 185–192. doi:10.1111/j.1525-1497.2005.40208.x PMID:15836553

Pittet, D., Allegranzi, B., Storr, J., & Donaldson, L. (2005). 'Clean Care is Safer Care': The Global Patient Safety Challenge 2005–2006. *International Journal of Infectious Diseases*, *10*(6), 419–424. doi:10.1016/j.ijid.2006.06.001 PMID:16914344

Plastina, A. F. (in press). Patient (Mis)understanding of Prescription Drug Ads in Social Media: Multimodal Discourse Analysis of eDTCA. *Proceedings of the International Conference hosted by CERLIS, The language of Medicine: Science, Practice and Academia*, University of Bergamo.

Polaschek, N. (2003). Negotiated care: A model for nursing work in the renal setting. *Journal of Advanced Nursing*, *42*(4), 355–363. doi:10.1046/j.1365-2648.2003.02627.x PMID:12752880

Pollock, J. B., & Jaffery, J. B. (2007). Knowledge of phosphorus compared with other nutrients in maintenance dialysis patients. *Journal of Renal Nutrition*, *17*(5), 323–328. doi:10.1053/j.jrn.2007.05.009 PMID:17720101

Postolache, G., Girao, P. S., & Postolache, O. (2013). Requirements and barriers to pervasive health adoption. In S. C. Mukhopadhyay & O. A. Postolache (Eds.), *Pervasive and Mobile Sensing and Computing for Health Care. Technological and Social Issues* (pp. 315–352). Springer Verlag. doi:10.1007/978-3-642-32538-0_15

Potomac, M., & Doak, C. C. (2002). Pfizer Principles for Clear Health Communication.

Prochaska, J. O., Di Clemente, C. C., & Norcross, J. C. (1992). In search of how people change. Applications to addictive behaviors. *The American Psychologist*, *47*(9), 1102–1114. doi:10.1037/0003-066X.47.9.1102 PMID:1329589

Provenzi, L., Borgatti, R., Menozzi, G., & Montirosso, R. (2015). A dynamic system analysis of dyadic flexibility and stability across the Face-to-Face Still-Face procedure: Application of the State Space Grid. *Infant Behavior and Development*, *38*, 1–10. doi:10.1016/j.infbeh.2014.10.001 PMID:25463152

Pruthi, R., Belsante, J., Kurpad, R., Nielsen, M., & Wallen, E. (2011). Robotic cystectomy and the Internet: Separating fact from fiction. *Paper presented at the Urologic Oncology: Seminars and Original Investigations*. doi:10.1016/j.urolonc.2009.04.010

Przyborski, A., & Wohlrab-Sahr, M. (2010). *Qualitative Sozialforschung: Ein Arbeitsbuch*. München: Oldenbourg Wissenschaftsverlag. (in German)

Randall, J., Singh, B., Warren, B., Travis, S., Mortensen, N., & George, B. (2010). Delayed surgery for acute severe colitis is associated with increased risk of postoperative complications. *British Journal of Surgery*, *97*(3), 404–409. doi:10.1002/bjs.6874 PMID:20101648

Rao, G., Burke, L. E., Spring, B. J., Ewing, L. J., Turk, M., Lichtenstein, A. H., & Coons, M. et al. (2011). New and emerging weight management strategies for busy ambulatory settings: A scientific statement from the American Heart Association endorsed by the Society of Behavioral Medicine. *Circulation*, *124*(10), 1182–1203. doi:10.1161/CIR.0b013e31822b9543 PMID:21824925

Rau, J. (2014). *Medicare fines 2,610 hospitals in third round of readmission penalties*. Retrieved from http://khn.org/news/medicare-readmissions-penalties-2015

Raynor, D. K. (2007). The Importance of Medicines Information for Patients. *Prescriber*, *18*(2), 60–62. doi:10.1002/psb.15

Recchia, V., Dodaro, A., & Braga, L. (2013). Event-based versus process-based informed consent to address scientific evidence and uncertainties in ionising medical imaging. *Insights into Imaging*, *4*(5), 647–653. doi:10.1007/s13244-013-0272-6 PMID:23904249

Rechel, B., Doyle, Y., Grundy, E., & McKee, M. (2009). *Policy brief. 10 Health system and policy analysis. How can health system respond to population ageing?* WHO Report. Retrieved from http://www.euro.who.int/__data/assets/pdf_file/0004/64966/E92560.pdf

Ricciardi, L., Mostashari, F., & Murphy, J. et al.. (2013). A national action plan to support consumer engagement via e-health. *Health Affairs (Project Hope)*, (32): 376–384.

Ricciardi, L., Mostashari, F., Murphy, J., Daniel, J. G., & Siminerio, E. P. (2013). A national action plan to support consumer engagement via e-health. *Health Affairs*, *32*(2), 376–384. doi:10.1377/hlthaff.2012.1216 PMID:23381531

Rich, M. W., Beckham, V., Wittenberg, C., Leven, C. L., Freedland, K. E., & Carney, R. M. (1995). A multidisciplinary intervention to prevent the readmission of elderly patients with congestive heart failure. *The New England Journal of Medicine*, *333*(18), 1190–1195. doi:10.1056/NEJM199511023331806 PMID:7565975

Richmond, C. A., Ross, N. A., & Egeland, G. M. (2007). Social support and thriving health: A new approach to understanding the health of indigenous Canadians. *American Journal of Public Health, 97*(10), 1827–1833. doi:10.2105/AJPH.2006.096917 PMID:17761564

Riper, H., Andersson, G., Christensen, H., Cuijpers, P., Lange, A., & Eysenbach, G. (2010). Theme issue on e-mental health: A growing field in internet research. *Journal of Medical Internet Research, 12*(5), e74. doi:10.2196/jmir.1713 PMID:21169177

Riva, G. (in press) Embodied Medicine: What Human-Computer Confluence Can Offer to Health Care. In A. Gaggioli, A. Ferscha, G. Riva, S. Dunne, and I. Viaud-Delmon (Eds.), Human Computer Confluence: Transforming Human Experience Through Symbiotic Technologies, Berlin: De Gruyter Open

Riva, G., Milani, L., & Gaggioli, A. (Eds.). (2010). Networked Flow: comprendere e sviluppare la creatività di rete. Milano, IT: LED.

Riva, G. (2008). *Psicologia dei nuovi media*. Bologna: Il Mulino.

Riva, G., Banos, R. M., Botella, C., Wiederhold, B. K., & Gaggioli, A. (2012). Positive technology: Using interactive technologies to promote positive functioning. *Cyberpsychology, Behavior, and Social Networking, 15*(2), 69–77. doi:10.1089/cyber.2011.0139 PMID:22149077

Riva, G., Castelnuovo, G., & Mantovani, F. (2006). Transformation of flow in rehabilitation: The role of advanced communication technologies. *Behavior Research Methods, 38*(2), 237–244. doi:10.3758/BF03192775 PMID:16956100

Roberts, S., Williams, J., Yeates, D., & Goldacre, M. (2007). Mortality in patients with and without colectomy admitted to hospital for ulcerative colitis and Crohn's disease: Record linkage studies. *British Medical Journal, 17*(7628), 1033–3. doi:10.1136/bmj.39345.714039.55 PMID:17977817

Rodger, M. W., Young, W. R., & Craig, C. M. (2014). Synthesis of walking sounds for alleviating gait disturbances in Parkinson's. *IEEE Transactions on Neural Systems and Rehabilitation Engineering, 22*(3), 543–548. doi:10.1109/TNSRE.2013.2285410 PMID:24235275

Rodrigues, J. J., Lopes, I. M., Silva, B. M., & Torre Ide, L. (2013). A new mobile ubiquitous computing application to control obesity: SapoFit. *Informatics for Health & Social Care, 38*(1), 37–53. doi:10.3109/17538157.2012.674586 PMID:22657250

Rodriguez, K. L., Bayliss, N., Alexander, S. C., Jeffreys, A. S., Olsen, M. K., Pollak, K. I., & Arnold, R. M. (2010). How oncologists and their patients with advanced cancer communicate about health-related quality of life. *Psycho-Oncology, 19*(5), 490–499. doi:10.1002/pon.1579 PMID:19449348

Rodriguez, K. L., Gambino, F. J., Butow, P., Hagerty, R., & Arnold, R. M. (2007). Pushing up daisies: Implicit and explicit language in oncologist–patient communication about death. *Supportive Care in Cancer, 15*(2), 153–161. doi:10.1007/s00520-006-0108-8 PMID:16969631

Rodriguez, K. M. (2013). Intrinsic and extrinsic factors affecting patient engagement in diabetes self-management: Perspectives of a certified diabetes educator. *Clinical Therapeutics*, *35*(2), 170–178. doi:10.1016/j.clinthera.2013.01.002 PMID:23411000

Rosen, P., Anell, A., & Hjortsberg, C. (2001). Patient views on choice and participation in primary health care. *Health Policy (Amsterdam)*, *55*(2), 121–128. doi:10.1016/S0168-8510(00)00122-6 PMID:11163651

Rossi Ferrario, S., Zotti, A. M., Pasetti, C., Comazzi, F., Giorgi, I., Negri, M., & Omarini, P. et al. (2009). Communicating medical information: A little lesson from italian patients. *Giornale Italiano di Medicina del Lavoro Ed Ergonomia*, *31*(3Suppl B), b12–b16. PMID:20518222

Roter, D. L. (2002). *The Roter Method for Interaction Process Analysis*. RIAS Manual.

Roter, D. L., & Larson, S. (2002). The Roter interaction analysis system (RIAS): Utility and flexibility for analysis of medical interactions. *Patient Education and Counseling*, *46*(4), 243–251. doi:10.1016/S0738-3991(02)00012-5 PMID:11932123

Rothberg, A. E., Peeters, A., & Herman, W. H. (2014). Cost-Effectiveness of Obesity Prevention and Treatment. In A. G. Bray & C. Bouchard (Eds.), *Handbook of Obesity. Clinical Applications* (pp. 453–470). London: CRC Press, Taylor & Francis Group.

Rothenbacher, D., Lutz, M. P., & Porzsolt, F. (1997). Treatment decisions in palliative cancer care: Patients' preferences for involvement and doctors' knowledge about it. *European Journal of Cancer*, *33*(8), 1184–1189. doi:10.1016/S0959-8049(97)00034-8 PMID:9301440

Rot, I., Ogah, I., & Wassersug, R. (2012). The language of prostate cancer treatments and implications for informed decision making by patients. *European Journal of Cancer Care*, *21*(6), 766–775. doi:10.1111/j.1365-2354.2012.01359.x PMID:22574619

Routh, J. C., Gong, E. M., Cannon, G. M. Jr, & Nelson, C. P. (2011). Does a controversial topic affect the quality of urologic information on the Internet? *Urology*, *78*(5), 1051–1056. doi:10.1016/j.urology.2011.06.050 PMID:21945281

Rozanski, A., Blumenthal, J. A., & Kaplan, J. (1999). Impact of psychological factors on the pathogenesis of cardiovascular disease and implications for therapy. *Circulation*, *99*(16), 2192–2217. doi:10.1161/01.CIR.99.16.2192 PMID:10217662

Rubinelli, S. (2013). Rational versus unreasonable persuasion in doctor-patient communication: A normative account. *Patient Education and Counseling*, *92*(3), 296–301. doi:10.1016/j.pec.2013.06.005 PMID:23830240

Ruiter, R. A. C., & Kok, G. (2011). Planning to frighten people? Think again! In *Writing Health Communication: An Evidence-Based Guide for professionals.*

Rupolo, G., & Poznanzki, C. (1999). *Psicologia e psichiatria del trapianto d'organi* [*Psychology and Psychiatry on Organ Tranplants*]. Milano: Masson.

Ryff, C. D., & Singer, B. (2000). Interpersonal flourishing: A positive health agenda for the new millennium. *Personality and Social Psychology Review*, *4*(1), 30–44. doi:10.1207/S15327957PSPR0401_4

Saba, G. W., Saita, E., & Novelli, M. (2011). Pearls Toolbox: l'equipaggiamento psicologico per il medico [Pearls Toolbox: Psychological tools for the medical doctor]. In E. Saita (a cura di) Pensare alla salute e alla malattia [Thinking of Health and Illness] (pp. 53-67). Milano: EDUcatt.

Sabato, E., Leo, C. G., & Sabina, S. (2009). Continuity of health care in patients with chronic respiratory insufficiency: A macro-model of care integration between hospital and home. *Multidisciplinary Respiratory Medicine*, *4*, 112–120.

Sabato, E., Sabina, S., & Leo, C. G. (2014). Standard Care. In R. W. Dal Negro & R. V. Hodder (Eds.), *Long-Term Oxygen Therapy New Insights and perspectives* (pp. 161–170). Springer-Verlag Italia Srl.

Safeer, R. S., Cooke, C. E., & Keenan, J. (2006). The impact of health literacy on cardiovascular disease. *Vascular Health and Risk Management*, *2*(4), 457–464. doi:10.2147/vhrm.2006.2.4.457 PMID:17323600

Safran, C. (2004). *United States House Ways and Means Health Subcommittee testimony*. Washington, D.C.

Saita, E. (2012). Il corpo condiviso. La motivazione a donare parti di sé.[The Shared Body. The motivation to donate a part of him/herSelf]. *Ricerche di Psicologia*, *4*, 639–641.

Saita, E., & Zanini, S. (2011). Donare un rene: le determinanti di una scelta. (Donating a Kidney: determinants of the choice). In G. Castelnuovo, R. Menici, & M. Fedi (Eds.), *La donazione in Italia. Situazione e prospettive della donazione di sangue, organi, tessuti, cellule e midollo osseo* [Donation in Italy. Current Status and Prospectives in Blood, Organs, Tissues, Cells and Bone-Marrow]. (pp. 195–205). Milano: Springer-Verlag.

Saita, E., Zanini, S., & Fenaroli, V. (2012). Il trapianto di rene da vivente: Le motivazioni a donare e a ricevere un rene.[Kidney Transplant from Living Donor: Motivations to Give and Receive a Kidney]. *Ricerche di Psicologia*, *4*, 693–711. doi:10.3280/RIP2012-004008

Salmon, C. T., & Atkin, C. (2003). Using media campaigns for health promotion. Handbook of health communication, 285-313.

Salonen, A., Ryhänen, A., & Leino-Kilpi, H. (2014). Educational benefits of Internet and computer-based programmes for prostate cancer patients: A systematic review. *Patient Education and Counseling*, *94*(1), 10–19. PMID:24021418

Santoro, E. (2013). [Social media and medical apps: how they can change health communication, education and care]. *Recenti Progressi in Medicina*, *104*(5), 179–180. PMID:23748682

Santoro, E., Caldarola, P., & Villella, A. (2011). [Using Web 2.0 technologies and social media for the cardiologist's education and update]. *Giornale Italiano di Cardiologia*, *12*(3), 174–181. PMID:21560473

Santoro, E., Castelnuovo, G., Zoppis, I., Mauri, G., & Sicurello, F. (2015). Social media and mobile applications in chronic disease prevention and management. *Frontiers in Psychology*, *6*, 567. doi:10.3389/fpsyg.2015.00567 PMID:25999884

Santoro, E., & Quintaliani, G. (2013). [Using web 2.0 technologies and social media for the nephrologist]. *Giornale Italiano di Nefrologia*, *30*(1). PMID:23832442

Santus, P., Picciolo, S., Proietto, A., Falcone, F., Mangiacavallo, A., Pellegrino, G., & Centanni, S. et al. (2012). Doctor-patient relationship: A resource to improve respiratory diseases management. *European Journal of Internal Medicine*, *23*(5), 442–446. doi:10.1016/j.ejim.2012.04.004 PMID:22726373

Sawyer, R. K. (2003). *Group creativity: Music, theater, collaboration*. Mahwah, NJ: LEA.

Sawyer, R. K. (2006). Group creativity: Musical performance and collaboration. *Psychology of Music*, *34*(2), 148–165. doi:10.1177/0305735606061850

Sawyer, R. K. (2007). *Group genius: The creative power of collaboration*. New York: Basic Books.

Say, R., Murtagh, M., & Thomson, R. (2006). Patients' preference for involvement in medical decision making: A narrative review. *Patient Education and Counseling*, *60*(2), 102–114. doi:10.1016/j.pec.2005.02.003 PMID:16442453

Schell, J. O., Green, J. A., Tulsky, J. A., & Arnold, R. M. (2013). Communication Skills Training for Dialysis Decision-Making and End-of-Life Care in Nephrology. *Clinical Journal of American Society of Nephrology*, *8*(4), 675–680. doi:10.2215/CJN.05220512 PMID:23143502

Schell, J. O., Patel, U. D., Steinhauser, K. E., Ammarell, N., & Tulsky, J. A. (2012). Discussion of kidney disease trajectory by elderly patients and Nephrologists: A qualitative study. *American Journal of Kidney Diseases*, *59*(4), 495–503. doi:10.1053/j.ajkd.2011.11.023 PMID:22221483

Schiel, R., Kaps, A., & Bieber, G. (2012). Electronic health technology for the assessment of physical activity and eating habits in children and adolescents with overweight and obesity IDA. *Appetite*, *58*(2), 432–437. doi:10.1016/j.appet.2011.11.021 PMID:22155072

Schieppati, A., & Remuzzi, G. (2005). Chronic renal disease as a public health problem: Epidemiology, social, and economic implications. *Kidney International*, *68*(Suppl. 98), S7–S10. doi:10.1111/j.1523-1755.2005.09801.x PMID:16108976

Schneiderman, N., Antoni, M. H., Saab, P. G., & Ironson, G. (2001). Health psychology: Psychosocial and biobehavioral aspects of chronic disease management. *Annual Review of Psychology*, *52*(1), 555–580. doi:10.1146/annurev.psych.52.1.555 PMID:11148317

Schocker, L. (2013). Young People Are Sleeping With Their Phones. Their Parents Are Sleeping With People. Retrieved from http://www.huffingtonpost.com/2013/09/16/sleep-phone-tablet-bed_n_3924161.html

Schoffman, D. E., Turner-McGrievy, G., Jones, S. J., & Wilcox, S. (2013). Mobile apps for pediatric obesity prevention and treatment, healthy eating, and physical activity promotion: Just fun and games? *Translational Behavioral Medicine*, *3*(3), 320–325. doi:10.1007/s13142-013-0206-3 PMID:24073184

Schopler, J., & Galinsky, M. (2014). Expanding our view of support groups as open systems. In M. Galinsky & J. Schopler (Eds.), *Support groups: Current perspectives on theory and practice* (pp. 3–10). New York: The Haworth Press, Inc.

Schunk, D. H., Pintrich, P. R., & Meece, J. L. (2008). *Motivation in education: Theory, research, and applications*. Upper Saddle River, New Jersey: Pearson/Merrill Prentice Hall.

Seamark, D., Blake, S., Seamark, C., Hyland, M. E., Greaves, C., Pinnuck, M., ... & East Devon Respiratory Research Group. (2012). Is hospitalisation for COPD an opportunity for advance care planning? A qualitative study. *Primary care respiratory journal: journal of the General Practice Airways Group*, 21(3), 261-266.

Seligman, H. K., Wang, F. F., Palacios, J. L., Wilson, C. C., Daher, C., Piette, J. D., & Schillinger, D. (2005). Physician notification of their diabetes patients' limited health literacy. A randomized, controlled trial. *Journal of General Internal Medicine*, *20*(11), 1001–1007. doi:10.1111/j.1525-1497.2005.00189.x PMID:16307624

Serino, S., Pedroli, E., Keizer, A., Triberti, S., Dakanalis, A., Pallavicini, F., & Riva, G. et al. (2015). Virtual Reality Body Swapping: A Tool for Modifying the Allocentric Memory of the Body. *Cyberpsychology, Behavior, and Social Networking*. doi:10.1089/cyber.2015.0229 PMID:26506136

Sexton, D. L., & Munro, B. H. (1985). Impact of a husband's chronic illness (COPD) on the spouse's life. *Research in Nursing & Health*, *8*(1), 83–90. doi:10.1002/nur.4770080115 PMID:3846320

Shaheen, S., Mohammed, A., & Grbic, N. (2015). Mobile Services for Diabetic Patients' Sustainable Lifestyle. In S. Adibi (Ed.), *mHealth Multidisciplinary Verticals* (pp. 51–61). London: CRC Press, Taylor & Francis Group.

Sharifi, M., Dryden, E. M., Horan, C. M., Price, S., Marshall, R., Hacker, K., & Taveras, E. M. et al. (2013). Leveraging text messaging and mobile technology to support pediatric obesity-related behavior change: A qualitative study using parent focus groups and interviews. *Journal of Medical Internet Research*, *15*(12), e272. doi:10.2196/jmir.2780 PMID:24317406

Sharma, G., Kuo, Y. F., Freeman, J. L., Zhang, D. D., & Goodwin, J. S. (2010). Outpatient follow-up visit and 30-day emergency department visit and readmission in patients hospitalized for chronic obstructive pulmonary disease. *Archives of Internal Medicine*, *170*(18), 1664–1670. doi:10.1001/archinternmed.2010.345 PMID:20937926

Shaw, R. J., Bosworth, H. B., Silva, S. S., Lipkus, I. M., Davis, L. L., Sha, R. S., & Johnson, C. M. (2013). Mobile health messages help sustain recent weight loss. *The American Journal of Medicine*, *126*(11), 1002–1009. doi:10.1016/j.amjmed.2013.07.001 PMID:24050486

Shea, J., Guerra, C., Weiner, J., Aguirre, A., Ravenell, K., & Asch, D. (2008). Adapting a patient satisfaction instrument for low literate and Spanish-speaking populations: Comparison of three formats. *Patient Education and Counseling*, *73*(1), 132–140. doi:10.1016/j.pec.2008.03.026 PMID:18486414

Sheridan, S. L., Draeger, L. B., Pignone, M. P., Keyserling, T. C., Simpson, R. J., Rimer, B., & Gizlice, Z. et al. (2011). A randomized trial of an intervention to improve use and adherence to effective coronary heart disease prevention strategies. *BMC Health Services Research*, *11*(1), 331. doi:10.1186/1472-6963-11-331 PMID:22141447

Shiffman, R., Dixon, J., Brandt, C., Essalhi, A., Hsiao, A., Michel, G., & O'Connell, R. (2005). The GuideLine Implementability Appraisal (GLIA): Development of an instrument to identify obstacles to guideline implementation. *BMC Medical Informatics and Decision Making*, *5*(23). doi:10.1186/1472-6947-5-23 PMID:16048653

Shipman, C., White, S., Gysels, M., & White, P. (2009). Access to care in advanced COPD: Factors that influence contact with general practice services. *Primary Care Respiratory Journal*, *18*(4), 273–278. doi:10.4104/pcrj.2009.00013 PMID:19333517

Siegel, C., Lofland, J., Naim, A., Gollins, J., Walls, D., Rudder, L., & Reynolds, C. (2015). Gastroenterologists' Views of Shared Decision Making for Patients with Inflammatory Bowel Disease. *Digestive Diseases and Sciences*, *60*(9), 2636–2645. doi:10.1007/s10620-015-3675-z PMID:25939543

Siemonsma, P., Döpp, C., Alpay, L., Tak, E., van Meeteren, N., & Chorus, A. (2014). Determinants influencing the implementation of home-based stroke rehabilitation: A systematic review. *Disability and Rehabilitation*, *36*(24), 2019–2030. doi:10.3109/09638288.2014.885091 PMID:24520957

Simbula, S., Guglielmi, D., & Schaufeli, W. B. (2011). A three-wave study of job resources, self-efficacy, and work engagement among Italian schoolteachers. *European Journal of Work and Organizational Psychology*, *20*(3), 285–304. doi:10.1080/13594320903513916

Simpson, D. D. (2004). A conceptual framework for drug treatment process and outcomes. *Journal of Substance Abuse Treatment*, *27*(2), 99–121. doi:10.1016/j.jsat.2004.06.001 PMID:15450644

Simpson, S. G., & Slowey, L. (2011). Video therapy for atypical eating disorder and obesity: A case study. *Clinical Practice and Epidemiology in Mental Health*, *7*(1), 38–43. doi:10.2174/1745017901107010038 PMID:21559235

Sinclair, J., Hingston, P., & Masek, M. (2007). Considerations for the design of exergames. *Proceeding GRAPHITE'07 International Conference on Computer Graphics and Interactive Techniques in Australia and Southeast Asia* (pp. 289-295). doi:10.1145/1321261.1321313

Smith, S. C., O'Conor, R., Curtis, L., Waite, K., Deary, I., Paasche-Orlow, M., & Wolf, M. S. (2015). Low health literacy predicts decline in physical function among older adults: findings from the LitCog cohort study. *Journal of epidemiology and community health*, jech-2014-204915.

Smith, D. M., Lowenstein, G., Rozin, P., Sherriff, R. L., & Ubel, P. A. (2007). Sensitivity to disgust, stigma, and adjustment to life with a colostomy. *Journal of Research in Personality*, *41*(4), 787–803. doi:10.1016/j.jrp.2006.09.006 PMID:17940585

Smith, S. G., Curtis, L. M., Wardle, J., von Wagner, C., & Wolf, M. S. (2013). Skill set or mind set? Associations between health literacy, patient activation and health. *PLoS ONE*, *8*(9), e74373. doi:10.1371/journal.pone.0074373 PMID:24023942

Sokol, M. C., McGuigan, K. A., Verbrugge, R. R., & Epstein, R. S. (2005). Impact of medication adherence on hospitalization risk and healthcare cost. *Medical Care*, *43*(6), 521–530. doi:10.1097/01.mlr.0000163641.86870.af PMID:15908846

Soobrah, R., & Clark, S. K. (2012). Your patient information website: How good is it? *Colorectal Disease*, *14*(3), e90–e94. doi:10.1111/j.1463-1318.2011.02792.x PMID:21883807

Sørensen, K., Van den Broucke, S., Fullam, J., Doyle, G., Pelikan, J., Slonska, Z., & Brand, H. (2012). Health literacy and public health: A systematic review and integration of definitions and models. *BMC Public Health*, *12*(1), 80. doi:10.1186/1471-2458-12-80 PMID:22276600

Spence, A., Hasson, F., Waldron, M., Kernohan, G., McLaughlin, D., Cochrane, B., & Watson, B. (2008). Active carers: Living with chronic obstructive pulmonary disease. *International Journal of Palliative Nursing*, *14*(8), 368–372. doi:10.12968/ijpn.2008.14.8.30771 PMID:19023952

Spoth, R., & Redmond, C. (2000). Research on family engagement in preventive interventions: Toward improved use of scientific findings in primary prevention practice. *The Journal of Primary Prevention*, *21*(2), 267–284. doi:10.1023/A:1007039421026

Spruit, M. A., Singh, S. J., Garvey, C., ZuWallack, R., Nici, L., Rochester, C., & Wouters, E. F. et al. (2013). An official American Thoracic Society/European Respiratory Society statement: Key concepts and advances in pulmonary rehabilitation. *American Journal of Respiratory and Critical Care Medicine*, *188*(8), e13–e64. doi:10.1164/rccm.201309-1634ST PMID:24127811

Srikesavan, C. S., Shay, B., Robinson, D. B., & Szturm, T. (2013). Task-oriented training with computer gaming in people with rheumatoid arthritisor osteoarthritis of the hand: Study protocol of a randomized controlled pilot trial. *Trials*, *14*(1), 69. doi:10.1186/1745-6215-14-69 PMID:23497529

Stacey, D., Légaré, F., Col, N. F., Bennett, C. L., Barry, M. J., Eden, K. B., & Wu, J. H. C. et al. (2014). Decision aids for people facing health treatment or screening decisions. *Cochrane Database of Systematic Reviews*, *January*. doi:10.1002/14651858.CD001431.pub4 PMID:24470076

Staeck, F. (2014). *Wartezeiten-Debatte: Regierung gegen Vergleich von PKV mit GKV*. ÄrzteZeitung. (in German)

Stamey, T. A., McNeal, J. E., Yemoto, C. M., Sigal, B. M., & Johnstone, I. M. (1999). Biological determinants of cancer progression in men with prostate cancer. *Journal of the American Medical Association*, *281*(15), 1395–1400. doi:10.1001/jama.281.15.1395 PMID:10217055

Stange, K. C., Nutting, P. A., Miller, W. L., Jaén, C. R., Crabtree, B. F., Flocke, S. A., & Gill, J. M. (2010). Defining and measuring the patient-centered medical home. *Journal of General Internal Medicine*, *25*(6), 601–612. doi:10.1007/s11606-010-1291-3 PMID:20467909

Statistik Austria. (2015a). *Demographie*. Retrieved from http://www.statistik.at/web_de/statistiken/soziales/gender-statistik/demographie/

Statistik Austria. (2015b). *Stationäre Aufenthalte*. Retrieved from http://www.statistik.at/web_de/statistiken/gesundheit/stationaere_aufenthalte/index.html

Stewart, M. (2003). *Patient-centered medicine: transforming the clinical method.* Radcliffe Publishing.

Stewart, M. A. (1995). Effective physician–patient communication and health outcomes: A review. *Canadian Medical Association Journal*, *152*, 1423–1433. PMID:7728691

Stockie, S. (2012). *Making patient-centred care a reality for Ontario Hospitals* [Unpublished MBA Thesis]. York University, Toronto.

Stoilkova, A., Janssen, D. J., & Wouters, E. F. (2013). Educational programmes in COPD management interventions: A systematic review. *Respiratory Medicine*, *107*(11), 1637–1650. doi:10.1016/j.rmed.2013.08.006 PMID:24012387

Strauss, A. L. (1998). *Grundlagen qualitativer Sozialforschung: Datenanalyse und Theoriebildung in der empirischen soziologischen Forschung*. Fink. (in German)

Street, R. L., Elwyn, G., & Epstein, R. (2012). Patient preferences and health care outcomes: An ecological perspective. *Expert Review of Pharmacoeconomics & Outcomes Research*, *12*(2), 167–180. doi:10.1586/erp.12.3 PMID:22458618

Street, R. L. Jr. (1991). Information-giving in medical consultations: The influence of patients' communicative styles and personal characteristics. *Social Science & Medicine*, *32*(5), 541–548. doi:10.1016/0277-9536(91)90288-N PMID:2017721

Street, R. L. Jr. (2013). How clinician-patient communication contributes to health improvement: Modeling pathways from talk to outcome. *Patient Education and Counseling*, *92*(3), 286–291. doi:10.1016/j.pec.2013.05.004 PMID:23746769

Street, R. L. Jr, Gordon, H. S., Ward, M. M., Krupat, E., & Kravitz, R. L. (2005). Patient participation in medical consultations: Why some patients are more involved than others. *Medical Care*, *43*(10), 960–969. doi:10.1097/01.mlr.0000178172.40344.70 PMID:16166865

Street, R. L. Jr, Makoul, G., Arora, N. K., & Epstein, R. M. (2009). How does communication heal? Pathways linking clinician–patient communication to health outcomes. *Patient Education and Counseling*, *74*(3), 295–301. doi:10.1016/j.pec.2008.11.015 PMID:19150199

Street, R. L., Piziak, V. K., Carpentier, W. S., Herzog, J., Hejl, J., Skinner, G., & McLellan, L. (1993). Provider-patient communication and metabolic control. *Diabetes Care*, *16*(5), 714–721. doi:10.2337/diacare.16.5.714 PMID:8495610

Strull, W. M., Lo, B., & Charles, G. (1984). Do patients want to participate in medical decision making? *Journal of the American Medical Association*, *252*(21), 2990–2994. doi:10.1001/jama.1984.03350210038026 PMID:6502860

Sullivan, G. M. (2011). A primer on the validity of assessment instruments. *Journal of graduate medical education, 3*(2), 119-120.

Sullivan, M. (2003). The new subjective medicine: Taking the patient's point of view on health care and health. *Social Science & Medicine*, *56*(7), 1595–1604. doi:10.1016/S0277-9536(02)00159-4 PMID:12614708

Suls, J., & Wheeler, L. (Eds.). (2000). *Handbook of social comparison*. New York: Kluwer Academic/Plenum. doi:10.1007/978-1-4615-4237-7

Suomi, R., Mäntymäki, M., & Söderlund, S. (2014). Promoting Health in Virtual Worlds: Lessons From Second Life. *Journal of Medical Internet Research*, *16*(10), e229. doi:10.2196/jmir.3177 PMID:25313009

Sutton, S. R., & Eiser, J. R. (1984). The effect of fear-arousing communications on cigarette smoking: An expectancy-value approach. *Journal of Behavioral Medicine*, *7*(1), 13–33. doi:10.1007/BF00845345 PMID:6716470

Swan, M. (2009). Emerging patient-driven health care models: An examination of health social networks, consumer personalized medicine and quantified self-tracking. *International Journal of Environmental Research and Public Health*, *6*(2), 492–525. doi:10.3390/ijerph6020492 PMID:19440396

Sweigart, L., Burden, M., Carlton, K. H., & Fillwalk, J. (2014). Virtual simulations across curriculum prepare nursing students for patient interviews. *Clinical Simulation in Nursing*, *10*(3), e139–e145. doi:10.1016/j.ecns.2013.10.003

Sweigart, L., & Hodson-Carlton, K. (2013). Improving student interview skills: The virtual avatar as client. *Nurse Educator*, *38*(1), 11–15. doi:10.1097/NNE.0b013e318276df2d PMID:23222623

Swencionis, C., & Rendell, S. L. (2012). The psychology of obesity. *Abdominal Imaging*, *37*(5), 733–737. doi:10.1007/s00261-012-9863-9 PMID:22392131

Tajfel, H., & Turner, J. C. (2004). The Social Identity Theory of Intergroup Behavior. In J. T. Jost, & J. Sidanius (Eds.), Political Psychology: Key Readings (pp. 276–293). New York: Psychology Press.

Takekawa, T., Abo, M., Ebihara, K., Taguchi, K., Sase, Y., & Kakuda, W. (2013). Long-term effects of injection of botulinum toxin type A combined with home-based functional training for post-stroke patients with spastic upper limb hemiparesis. *Acta Neurologica Belgica*, *113*(4), 469–475. doi:10.1007/s13760-013-0208-4 PMID:23716062

Tang, S. T., Liu, T. W., Liu, L. N., Chiu, C. F., Hsieh, R. K., & Tsai, C. M. (2014). Physician–patient end-of-life care discussions: Correlates and associations with end-of-life care preferences of cancer patients—a cross-sectional survey study. *Palliative Medicine*, *28*(10), 1222–1230. doi:10.1177/0269216314540974 PMID:24965755

Tarde, G. (1890). *Les lois de l'imitation*. Paris: Kimé éditeur.

Tarde, G. (1902). *Pstchologie économique. Tome second.* Paris.

Tarde, G. (1902). *Psychologie économique. Tome premier.* Paris.

Tarozzi, M. (2008). *Che cos'è la grounded theory* [*What Grounded Theory is*]. Roma: Carocci.

Taylor, S. J. (1994). Waiting for Service: The Relationship between Delays and Evaluations of Service. *Journal of Marketing*, *58*(2), 56–69. doi:10.2307/1252269

Techniker Krankenkasse. (2014). *TK-Meinungspuls Gesundheit 2014*. Retrieved from http://www.tk.de/tk/themen/meinungspuls-gesundheit-oktober-2014/meinungspuls-gesundheit-oktober-2014-studienband/660168

Temel, J. S., Greer, J. A., Muzikansky, A., Gallagher, E. R., Admane, S., Jackson, V. A., & Lynch, T. J. et al. (2010). Early palliative care for patients with metastatic non–small-cell lung cancer. *The New England Journal of Medicine*, *363*(8), 733–742. doi:10.1056/NEJMoa1000678 PMID:20818875

Tennant, B., Stellefson, M., Dodd, V., Chaney, B., Chaney, D., Paige, S., & Alber, J. (2015). eHealth Literacy and Web 2.0 Health Information Seeking Behaviors Among Baby Boomers and Older Adults. *Journal of Medical Internet Research*, *17*(3), e70. doi:10.2196/jmir.3992 PMID:25783036

Terranova, G., Ferro, M., Carpeggiani, C., Recchia, V., Braga, L., Semelka, R. C., & Picano, E. (2012). Low quality and lack of clarity of current informed consent forms in cardiology: How to improve them. *JACC: Cardiovascular Imaging*, *5*(6), 649–655. doi:10.1016/j.jcmg.2012.03.007 PMID:22698536

The SUPPORT Principal Investigators. (1995). A controlled trial to improve care for seriously ill hospitalized patients: The study to understand prognoses and preferences for outcomes and risks of treatments (SUPPORT). *Journal of the American Medical Association*, *274*, 1591–1598. doi:10.1001/jama.1995.03530200027032 PMID:7474243

The U. S. Affordable Care Act of March 2010. (2011). U.S. Federal Register, *76*(108), 32331. Retrieved from http://www.gpo.gov/fdsys/pkg/FR-2011-06-06/pdf/2011-13801.pdf

The World Bank Group. (2015). Retrieved from http://Worldbank.org

Thoits, P. A. (2013). Self, identity, stress, and mental health. In C. S. Aneshensel, J. C. Phelan, & A. Bierman (Eds.), *Handbook of the sociology of mental health*. New York: Springer. doi:10.1007/978-94-007-4276-5_18

Thomas T., Kedia, P. & Cohen, R. D. (2007). Impact of an Internet-based educational program on colonoscopy attendance and quality (abstract). *American Journal of Gastroenterology* Supplement S454.

Thomas, C. (2014). The role of the social worker. *Nephrology News & Issues*, *28*(2), 23–24. PMID:24649752

Thomas, M. J., Simpson, J., Riley, R., & Grant, E. (2010). The impact of home-based physiotherapy interventions on breathlesness during activities of daily living in severe COPD: A systematic review. *Physiotherapy*, *96*(2), 108–119. doi:10.1016/j.physio.2009.09.006 PMID:20420957

Thomas, S., Fazakarley, L., Thomas, P. W., Brenton, S., Collyer, S., Perring, S., & Hillier, C. et al. (2014). Testing the feasibility and acceptability of using the Nintendo Wii in the home to increase activity levels, vitality and well-being in people with multiple sclerosis (Mii-vitaliSe): Protocol for a pilot randomised controlled study. *BMJ Open*, *4*(5), e005172. doi:10.1136/bmjopen-2014-005172 PMID:24812193

Thompson, K. D., Connor, S. J., Walls, D., Gollins, J., Stewart, S. K., Bewtra, M., … & Siegel, C. A. (2016). Patients with ulcerative colitis are more concerned about complications of their disease than side effects of medications. *Inflamm. Bowel Dis.*, 22(4), 940-947.

Thompson, A. G. H. (2007). The meaning of patient involvement and participation in health care consultations: A taxonomy. *Social Science & Medicine*, *64*(6), 1297–1310. doi:10.1016/j.socscimed.2006.11.002 PMID:17174016

Tiep, B., & Carter, R. (2008). Oxygen conserving devices and methodologies. *Chronic Respiratory Disease*, *5*(2), 109–114. doi:10.1177/1479972308090691 PMID:18539725

Tiffany, J. M., & Hoglund, B. A. (2014). Facilitating Learning Through Virtual Reality Simulation: Welcome to Nightingale Isle. In Virtual, Augmented Reality and Serious Games for Healthcare 1 (pp. 159-174). Springer Berlin Heidelberg.

Timmermans, L. M., van der Maazen, R. W., Verhaak, C. M., van Roosmalen, M. S., van Daal, W. A., & Kraaimaat, F. W. (2005). Patient participation in discussing palliative radiotherapy. *Patient Education and Counseling*, *57*(1), 53–61. doi:10.1016/j.pec.2004.03.016 PMID:15797153

Tokel, S. T., & İsler, V. (2013). Acceptance of virtual worlds as learning space. *Innovations in Education and Teaching International*.

Torres-Huitzil, C., & Alvarez-Landero, A. (2015). Accelerometer-Based Human Activity Recognition in Smartphones for Healthcare Services. In S. Adibi (Ed.), *Mobile Health: A Technology Road Map* (pp. 147–170). Berlin: Springer. doi:10.1007/978-3-319-12817-7_7

Tousignant, M., Corriveau, H., Kairy, D., Berg, K., Dubois, M. F., Gosselin, S., & Danells, C. et al. (2014). Tai Chi-based exercise program provided via telerehabilitation compared to home visits in a post-stroke population who have returned home without intensive rehabilitation: Study protocol for a randomized, non-inferiority clinical trial. *Trials*, *15*(1), 42. doi:10.1186/1745-6215-15-42 PMID:24479760

Tout, D. S., Davis, E., Velasquez, A., Banerjee, T., & Powe, N. R. (2013). Assessment of Printed Patient-Educational Materials for Chronic Kidney Disease. *American Journal of Nephrology*, *38*(3), 184–194. doi:10.1159/000354314 PMID:23970127

Tractica. (2015). *Home health technologies, medical monitoring and management, remote consultations, eldercare, and health and wellness applications: Global market analysis andforecast.* Retrieved August, 2015, from https://www.tractica.com/research/home-health-technologies/

Trepte, S., & Reinecke, L. (2010). Avatar creation and video game enjoyment: Effects of life-satisfaction, game competitiveness, and identification with the avatar. *Journal of Media Psychology: Theories, Methods, and Applications*, *22*(4), 171–184. doi:10.1027/1864-1105/a000022

Trepte, S., Reinecke, L., & Behr, K.-M. (2009). Creating virtual alter egos or superheroines? Gamers' strategies of avatar creation in terms of gender and sex. *International Journal of Gaming and Computer-Mediated Simulations*, *1*(2), 52–76. doi:10.4018/jgcms.2009040104

Triberti, S., & Argenton, L. (2013). *Psicologia dei videogiochi.* Milano: Apogeo.

Triberti, S., Barello, S., Graffigna, G., Riva, G., Candelieri, A., & Archetti, F. (2014). Evaluating patient engagement and user experience of a positive technology intervention: the H-CIM case. In G. Graffigna, S. Barello, & S. Triberti (Eds.), *Patient Engagement. A consumer Centered Model to Innovate Healthcare* (pp. 66–77). De Gruyter Open.

Triberti, S., & Liberati, E. G. (2014). Patient centered virtual reality: an opportunity to improve the quality of patient's experience. In P. Cipresso & S. Serino (Eds.), *Virtual Reality Technologies, Medical Applications and Challenges* (pp. 1–30). New York: Nova Science.

Triberti, S., & Riva, G. (2014a). Positive technology for enhancing the patient engagement experiences. In G. Graffigna, S. Barello, & S. Triberti (Eds.), *Patient Engagement. A consumer Centered Model to Innovate Healthcare* (pp. 44–55). De Gruyter Open.

Triberti, S., & Riva, G. (2014b). Engaging users to design positive technologies for patient engagement: the perfect interaction model. In G. Graffigna, S. Barello, & S. Triberti (Eds.), *Patient Engagement. A consumer Centered Model to Innovate Healthcare* (pp. 56–65). De Gruyter Open.

Triberti, S., & Riva, G. (2015a). Positive Technology for Enhancing the Patient Engagement Experiences. In S. Barello, G. Graffigna, & S. Triberti (Eds.), *Patient Engagement: a comsumer-centered model to innovate healthcare*. Berlin: De Gruyter Open. doi:10.1515/9783110452440-005

Triberti, S., & Riva, G. (2015b). Engaging Users to Design Positive Technologies for Patient Engagement: the Perfect Interaction Model. In S. Barello, G. Graffigna, & S. Triberti (Eds.), *Patient Engagement: a comsumer- centered model to innovate healthcare*. Berlin: De Gruyter Open. doi:10.1515/9783110452440-006

Truog, R. D., Brown, S. D., Browning, D., Hundert, E. M., Rider, E. A., Bell, S. K., & Meyer, E. C. (2015). Microethics: The ethics of everyday clinical practice. *The Hastings Center Report*, *45*(1), 11–17. doi:10.1002/hast.413 PMID:25600383

Tulsky, J. A., Fischer, G. S., Rose, M. R., & Arnold, R. M. (1998). Opening the black box: How do physicians communicate about advance directives? *Annals of Internal Medicine*, *129*(6), 441–449. doi:10.7326/0003-4819-129-6-199809150-00003 PMID:9735081

Tunsäter, A., Moutakis, M., Borg, S., Persson, U., Strömberg, L., & Nielsen, A. L. (2007). Retrospective incremental cost analysis of a hospital-based COPD Disease Management Programme in Sweden. *Health Policy (Amsterdam)*, *81*(2-3), 309–319. doi:10.1016/j.healthpol.2006.05.013 PMID:16904788

Turner, B. J., Weiner, M., Berry, S. D., Lillie, K., Fosnocht, K., & Hollenbeak, C. S. (2008). Overcoming poor attendance to first scheduled colonoscopy: A randomized trial of peer coach or brochure support. *Journal of General Internal Medicine*, *23*(1), 58–63. doi:10.1007/s11606-007-0445-4 PMID:18030540

Turner-McGrievy, G. M., Beets, M. W., Moore, J. B., Kaczynski, A. T., Barr-Anderson, D. J., & Tate, D. F. (2013). Comparison of traditional versus mobile app self-monitoring of physical activity and dietary intake among overweight adults participating in an mHealth weight loss program. *Journal of the American Medical Informatics Association*, *20*(3), 513–518. doi:10.1136/amiajnl-2012-001510 PMID:23429637

Tzallas, A. T., Tsipouras, M. G., Rigas, G., Tsalikakis, D. G., Karvounis, E. C., Chondrogiorgi, M., & Fotiadis, D. I. et al. (2014). PERFORM: A system for monitoring, assessment and management of patients with Parkinson's disease. *Sensors (Basel)*, *14*(11), 21329–21357. doi:10.3390/s141121329 PMID:25393786

US Department of Health and Human Services. (2010). *CfMMS*. Toolkit for Making Written Material Clear and Effective.

US Federal Plain Language Guidelines. (2010). Retrieved from http://www.plainlanguage.gov/howto/guidelines/bigdoc/fullbigdoc.pdf

User-Centered Design Basics. (2015). Retrieved from http://www.usability.gov/what-and-why/user-centered-design.html

Valdes, K., Naughton, N., & Michlovitz, S. (2014). Therapist supervised clinic-based therapy versus instruction in a home program following distal radius fracture: A systematic review. *Journal of Hand Therapy*, *27*(3), 165–174. doi:10.1016/j.jht.2013.12.010 PMID:24508093

Vale, M. J., Jelinek, M. V., Best, J. D., Dart, A. M., Grigg, L. E., Hare, D. L., & McNeil, J. J. et al. (2003). Coaching patients On Achieving Cardiovascular Health (COACH): A multicenter randomized trial in patients with coronary heart disease. *Archives of Internal Medicine*, *163*(22), 2775–2783. doi:10.1001/archinte.163.22.2775 PMID:14662633

Van Boven, J. F. M., Vegter, S., Van Der Molen, T., & Postma, M. J. (2013). COPD in the working age population: The economic impact on both patients and government. *COPD: Journal of Chronic Obstructive Pulmonary Disease*, *10*(6), 629–639. doi:10.3109/15412555.2013.813446 PMID:23845002

Van der Vaart, R., van Deursen, A., Drossaert, C., Taal, E., van Dijk, J., & van de Laar, M. (2011). Does the eHealth Literacy Scale (eHEALS) measure what it intends to measure? Validation of a Dutch version of the eHEALS in two adult populations. *Journal of Medical Internet Research, 13*(4), e86. doi:10.2196/jmir.1840 PMID:22071338

van Eemeren, F. H., & Grootendorst, R. (2004). *A systematic theory of argumentation*. Cambridge, MA: Cambridge University Press.

Vasalou, A., & Joinson, A. N. (2009). Me, myself and I: The role of interactional context on self-presentation through avatars. *Computers in Human Behavior, 25*(2), 510–520. doi:10.1016/j.chb.2008.11.007

Vera, M., Le Blanc, P. M., Taris, T. W., & Salanova, M. (2014). Patterns of engagement: The relationship between efficacy beliefs and task engagement at the individual versus collective level. *Journal of Applied Social Psychology, 44*(2), 133–144. doi:10.1111/jasp.12219

Vermylen, J. H., Szmuiowicz, E., & Kalhan, R. (2015). Palliative care in COPD: An unmet area for quality improvement. *International Journal of Chronic Obstructive Pulmonary Disease, 10*, 1543–1551. doi:10.2147/COPD.S74641 PMID:26345486

Vervloet, M., Linn, A. J., van Weert, J. C., De Bakker, D. H., Bouvy, M. L., & Van Dijk, L. (2012). The effectiveness of interventions using electronic reminders to improve adherence to chronic medication: A systematic review of the literature. *Journal of the American Medical Informatics Association, 19*(5), 696–704. doi:10.1136/amiajnl-2011-000748 PMID:22534082

Villagra, V. G. (2004). Integrating disease management into the outpatient delivery system during and after managed care. *Health Affairs (Project Hope)*, (Suppl. Web Exclusives), W4-281–283. PMID:15451998

Villagra, V. G., & Ahmed, T. (2004). Effectiveness of a disease management program for patients with diabetes. *Health Affairs (Project Hope), 23*(4), 255–266. doi:10.1377/hlthaff.23.4.255 PMID:15318587

Villani, D., Gatti, E., Confalonieri, E., & Riva, G. (2012). Am I my avatar? A tool to investigate virtual body image representation in adolescence. *Cyberpsychology, Behavior, and Social Networking, 15*(8), 435–440. doi:10.1089/cyber.2012.0057 PMID:22823468

Vin-Raviv, N., Hillyer, G. C., Hershman, D. L., Galea, S., Leoce, N., Bovbjerg, D. H., & Neugut, A. I. et al. (2013). Racial Disparities in Posttraumatic Stress After Diagnosis of Localized Breast Cancer: The BQUAL Study. *Journal of the National Cancer Institute, 107*(7). doi:10.1093/jnci/djt024 PMID:23434900

Visse, M. A., Teunissen, T., Peters, A., Widdershoven, G. A., & Abma, T. A. (2010). Dialogue for air, air for dialogue: Towards shared responsibilities in COPD practice. *Health Care Analysis, 18*(4), 358–373. doi:10.1007/s10728-009-0139-7 PMID:20063199

Visser, A. (2000). Chronic diseases, aging, and dementia: Implications for patient education and counseling. *Patient Education and Counseling*, *39*(2-3), 293–309. doi:10.1016/S0738-3991(99)00002-6

Vissers, J., & Beech, R. (2005). *Health operations management: Patient flow logistics in health care. Routledge health management series*. London, NY: Routledge.

Vitacca, M., & Comini, L. (2012). How do patients die in a rehabilitative unit dedicated to advanced respiratory diseases? *Multidisciplinary Respiratory Medicine*, *7*(1), 18. doi:10.1186/2049-6958-7-18 PMID:22958591

Voelkel, N. F. (2000). Raising awareness of COPD in primary care. *Chest*, *117*(5), 372s–375s. doi:10.1378/chest.117.5_suppl_2.372S PMID:10843979

Volandes, A. E. (2015). *The conversation: a revolutionary plan for end-of-life care*. Bloomsbury Publishing USA.

Von Korff, M., & Tiemans, B. (2000). Individualized stepped care of chronic illness. *The Western Journal of Medicine*, *172*(2), 133–137. doi:10.1136/ewjm.172.2.133 PMID:10693379

Wadden, T. A., Brownell, K. D., & Foster, G. D. (2002). Obesity: Responding to the global epidemic. *Journal of Consulting and Clinical Psychology*, *70*(3), 510–525. doi:10.1037/0022-006X.70.3.510 PMID:12090366

Wagner, E. H. (2000). The role of patient care teams in chronic disease management. *British Medical Journal*, *320*(7234), 569–572. doi:10.1136/bmj.320.7234.569 PMID:10688568

Wagner, E. H., Austin, B. T., Davis, C., Hindmarsh, M., Schaefer, J., & Bonomi, A. (2001a). Improving chronic illness care: Translating evidence into action. *Health Affairs (Project Hope)*, *20*(6), 64–78. doi:10.1377/hlthaff.20.6.64 PMID:11816692

Wagner, E. H., Glasgow, R. E., Davis, C., Bonomi, A. E., Provost, L., McCulloch, D., & Sixta, C. et al. (2001b). Quality improvement in chronic illness care: A collaborative approach. *The Joint Commission Journal on Quality Improvement*, *27*(2), 63–80. PMID:11221012

Wagner, S., Hansen, F. O., Pedersen, C. F., Memon, M., Aysha, F. H., Mathissen, M., & Wesby, O. L. et al. (2013). CareStore Platform for seamless deployment of ambient assited living applications and devices. *Proceedings of International Conference on Pervasive Computing Technologies for Healthcare and Workshops* (pp. 240-243).

Waller, G., Stringer, H., & Meyer, C. (2012). What cognitive behavioral techniques do therapists report using when delivering cognitive behavioral therapy for the eating disorders? *Journal of Consulting and Clinical Psychology*, *80*(1), 171–175. doi:10.1037/a0026559 PMID:22141595

Wallner, J. (2013). Rechtsethischer Anspruch und faktische Grenzen von Patientenaufklärung und Informed Consent.[in German]. *Zeitschrift für Gesundheitspolitik*, *2013*(4).

Walters, J. (2010). COPD - Diagnosis, management and the role of the GP. *Australian Family Physician*, *39*(3), 100–103. PMID:20369108

Walters, J. A., Turnock, A. C., Walters, E. H., & Wood-Baker, R. (2010). Action plans with limited patient education only for exacerbations of chronic obstructive pulmonary disease. *Cochrane Database of Systematic Reviews*, *5*, CD005074. PMID:20464737

Walton, D. (2010). Types of dialogues and burdens of proof. In P. Baroni, F. Cerutti, M. Giacomin, & G. R. Simari (Eds.). *Computational Models of Argument:Proceedings of COMMA 2010* (13-24). Amsterdam: IOS Press.

Walton, D., Atkinson, K., Bench-Capon, T., Wyner, A., & Cartwright, D. (2010). Argumentation in the framework of deliberation dialogue. In C. Bjola, & M. Kornprobst (Eds.), Arguing Global Governance (pp. 201-230). London: Routledge.

Walton, D. (1999). Profiles of Dialogue for Evaluating Arguments from Ignorance. *Argumentation, 13*(1), 53–71. doi:10.1023/A:1007738812877

Walton, D. (2006). How to make and defend a proposal in a deliberation dialogue. *Artificial Intelligence and Law, 14*(3), 177–239. doi:10.1007/s10506-006-9025-x

Walton, D., & Krabbe, E. (1995). *Commitment in Dialogue: Basic Concepts of Interpersonal Reasoning*. Albany, NY: State University of New York Press.

Walton, D., Reed, C., & Macagno, F. (2008). *Argumentation Schemes*. Cambridge, MA: Cambridge University Press. doi:10.1017/CBO9780511802034

Walton, D., Toniolo, A., & Norman, T. (2014). Missing phases of deliberation dialogue for real applications.*Proceedings of the 11th International Workshop on Argumentation in Multi-Agent Systems,* 1-20.

Wang, T. (2015). Digital health funding tops $4.1B: 2014 year in review. Retrieved September 15, 2015, from: http://rockhealth.com/2015/01/digital-health-funding-tops-4-1b-2014-year-review/

Warburton, S. (2009). Second Life in higher education: Assessing the potential for and the barriers to deploying virtual worlds in learning and teaching. *British Journal of Educational Technology, 40*(3), 414–426. doi:10.1111/j.1467-8535.2009.00952.x

Warren, E., Footman, K., Tinelli, M., McKee, M., & Knai, C. (2014). Do cancer-specific websites meet patient's information needs? *Patient Education and Counseling*, *95*(1), 126–136. doi:10.1016/j.pec.2013.12.013 PMID:24447523

Weaver, J. L., Bradley, C. T., & Brasel, K. J. (2012). Family engagement regarding the critically ill patient. *The Surgical Clinics of North America*, *92*(6), 1637–1647. doi:10.1016/j.suc.2012.08.004 PMID:23153887

Weeks, J. C., Catalano, P. J., Cronin, A., Finkelman, M. D., Mack, J. W., Keating, N. L., & Schrag, D. (2012). Patients' expectations about effects of chemotherapy for advanced cancer. *The New England Journal of Medicine*, *367*(17), 1616–1625. doi:10.1056/NEJMoa1204410 PMID:23094723

Weingarten, S. R., Henning, J. M., Badamgarav, E., Knight, K., Hasselblad, V., Gano, A. Jr, & Ofman, J. J. (2002). Interventions used in disease management programmes for patients with chronic illness-which ones work? Meta-analysis of published reports. *BMJ (Clinical Research Ed.), 325*(7370), 925. doi:10.1136/bmj.325.7370.925 PMID:12399340

Weisband, S., & Kiesler, S. (1996, April). Self disclosure on computer forms: Meta-analysis and implications. Proceedings of the SIGCHI conference on human factors in computing systems (pp. 3-10). ACM.

Weissman, J. S., Stern, R. S., & Epstein, A. M. (1994). The impact of patient socioeconomic status and other social factors on readmission: A prospective study in four Massachusetts hospitals. *Inquiry*, 31(2), 163–172. PMID:8021022

West, D. (2012). How mobile devices are transforming healthcare. *Issues in technology innovation*, 18(1), 1-11.

White, D. B., Braddock, C. H., Bereknyei, S., & Curtis, J. R. (2007a). Toward shared decision making at the end of life in intensive care units: Opportunities for improvement. *Archives of Internal Medicine, 167*(5), 461–467. doi:10.1001/archinte.167.5.461 PMID:17353493

White, D. B., Engelberg, R. A., Wenrich, M. D., Lo, B., & Curtis, J. R. (2007b). Prognostication during physician-family discussions about limiting life support in intensive care units*. *Critical Care Medicine, 35*(2), 442–448. doi:10.1097/01.CCM.0000254723.28270.14 PMID:17205000

Whitlock, G., Lewington, S., Sherliker, P., Clarke, R., Emberson, J., Halsey, J., & Peto, R. et al. Prospective Studies Collaboration. (2009). Body-mass index and cause-specific mortality in 900 000 adults: Collaborative analyses of 57 prospective studies. *Lancet, 373*(9669), 1083–1096. doi:10.1016/S0140-6736(09)60318-4 PMID:19299006

Whittaker, R. (2012). Issues in mHealth: Findings from key informant interviews. *Journal of Medical Internet Research, 14*(5), e129. doi:10.2196/jmir.1989 PMID:23032424

WHO World Health Organization. (2008a). *World Health Statistics*. Switzerland: World Health Organization.

WHO World Health Organization. (2008b). The global burden of disease: 2004 update. Geneva.

Wijayasinghe, D. S. (2013). *I arrive on time but end up waiting to see my doctor. Why?* The Globe and Mail.

Williams, T., & Samarth, A. (2011). *Electronic Health Records for Dummies*. Hobokem, NJ: Wiley Publishing, Inc.

Wilson, S. R., Strub, P., Buist, A. S., Knowles, S. B., Lavori, P. W., Lapidus, J., & Vollmer, W. M. (2010). Shared treatment decision making improves adherence and outcomes in poorly controlled asthma. *American Journal of Respiratory and Critical Care Medicine, 181*(6), 566–577. doi:10.1164/rccm.200906-0907OC PMID:20019345

Wing, R. R. (2002). Behavioral weight control. In T. A. Wadden & A. J. Stunkard (Eds.), *Handbook of obesity treatment* (pp. 301–316). New York: Guilford Press.

Winzelberg, G. S., Hanson, L. C., & Tulsky, J. A. (2005). Beyond autonomy: Diversifying end-of-life decision-making approaches to serve patients and families. *Journal of the American Geriatrics Society*, *53*(6), 1046–1050. doi:10.1111/j.1532-5415.2005.53317.x PMID:15935032

Witte, K., & Allen, M. (2000). A meta-analysis of fear appeals: Implications for effective public health campaigns. *Health Education & Behavior*, *27*(5), 591–615. doi:10.1177/109019810002700506 PMID:11009129

Witteman, H. O., Scherer, L. D., Angott, A. M., Ubel, P. A., Dickson, M., Holtzman, L. G., . . . Zikmund-Fisher, B. J. (2012). Hold My Hand: Explicitly Showing Tradeoffs and Fit Between Values and Options Helps People Make Choices Concordant With Their Stated Values. Proceedings of 34th. Chicago: Annual Meeting of The Society for Medical Decision Making. Retrieved from https://smdm.confex.com/smdm/2012az/webprogram/Paper7417.html

Wittenberg-Lyles, E., Oliver, D. P., Demiris, G., Burt, S., & Regehr, K. (2009). Inviting the absent members: Examining how caregivers' participation affects hospice team communication. *Palliative Medicine*. PMID:20007820

Wittenberg-Lyles, E., Oliver, D. P., Kruse, R. L., Demiris, G., Gage, L. A., & Wagner, K. (2013). Family caregiver participation in hospice interdisciplinary team meetings: How does it affect the nature and content of communication? *Health Communication*, *28*(2), 110–118. doi:10.1080/10410236.2011.652935 PMID:22435889

Wolff, J. L., & Roter, D. L. (2011). Family presence in routine medical visits: A meta-analytical review. *Social Science & Medicine*, *72*(6), 823–831. doi:10.1016/j.socscimed.2011.01.015 PMID:21353358

Wong, F., Stewart, D., Dancey, J., Meana, M., McAndrews, M., Bunston, T., & Cheung, A. (2000). Men with prostate cancer: Influence of psychological factors on informational needs and decision making. *Journal of Psychosomatic Research*, *49*(1), 13–19. doi:10.1016/S0022-3999(99)00109-9 PMID:11053599

Woolf, S. H., Grol, R., Hutchinson, A., Eccles, M., & Grimshaw, J. (1999). Clinical guidelines: Potential benefits, limitations, and harms of clinical guidelines. *BMJ: British Medical Journal*, *318*(7182), 527–530. doi:10.1136/bmj.318.7182.527 PMID:10024268

World Health Organization. (1997). The Vienna Recommendations on Health Promoting Hospitals.

World Health Organization. (2015). *Health expenditure, total (% of GDP)*. Retrieved from http://www.who.int/gho/health_financing/total_expenditure/en/

Wright, J. A., Wallston, K. A., Elasy, T. A., Ikizler, T. A., & Cavanaugh, K. L. (2011). Development and results of a kidney disease knowledge survey given to patients with CKD. *American Journal of Kidney Diseases*, *57*(3), 387–395. doi:10.1053/j.ajkd.2010.09.018 PMID:21168943

Wright, S. M. (2001). Contribution of a lecturer-practitioner in implementing evidence-based health care. *Clinical Effectiveness in Nursing*, *5*(1), 30–34. doi:10.1054/cein.2000.0170 PMID:11761876

Wu, L. M., Austin, J., Hamilton, J. G., Valdimarsdottir, H., Isola, L., Rowley, S., & Rini, C. et al. (2012). Self-efficacy beliefs mediate the relationship between subjective cognitive functioning and physical and mental well-being after hematopoietic stem cell transplant. *Psycho-Oncology*, *21*(11), 1175–1184. doi:10.1002/pon.2012 PMID:21739524

Yang, Y. T., & Silverman, R. D. (2014). Mobile health applications: The patchwork of legal and liability issues suggests strategies to improve oversight. *Health Affairs*, *33*(2), 222–227. doi:10.1377/hlthaff.2013.0958 PMID:24493764

Yawn, B. P., & Kaplan, A. (2008). Co-morbidities in people with COPD: A result of multiple diseases, or multiple manifestations of smoking and reactive inflammation? *Primary Care Respiratory Journal*, *17*(4), 199–205. doi:10.3132/pcrj.2008.00021 PMID:18338090

Yee, N., & Bailenson, J. (2007). The Proteus effect: The effect of transformed self-representation on behavior. *Human Communication Research*, *33*(3), 271–290. doi:10.1111/j.1468-2958.2007.00299.x

Yee, N., Bailenson, J., & Ducheneaut, N. (2009). The proteus effect: Implications of transformed digital self-sepresentation on online and offline behavior. *Communication Research*, *36*(2), 285–312. doi:10.1177/0093650208330254

Yin, H. S., Dreyer, B. P., Foltin, G., van Schaick, L., & Mendelsohn, A. L. (2007). Association of low caregiver health literacy with reported use of non-standardized dosing instruments and lack of knowledge of weight-based dosing. *Ambulatory Pediatrics*, *7*(4), 292–298. doi:10.1016/j.ambp.2007.04.004 PMID:17660100

Young, B. A. (2013). Health Literacy in Nephrology: Why is it Important? *American Journal of Kidney Diseases*, *62*(1), 3–6. doi:10.1053/j.ajkd.2013.04.003 PMID:23773837

Zan, S., Agboola, S., Moore, S. A., Parks, K. A., Kvedar, J. C., & Jethwani, K. (2015). Patient Engagement With a Mobile Web-Based Telemonitoring System for Heart Failure Self Management: A Pilot Study. *Journal of Medical Internet Research*, *3*(2), e33. doi:10.2196/mhealth.3789 PMID:25842282

Zhao, Y., Anhalt, F., Fietzek, U. M., & D'Angelo, L. T. (2013). Multi-cue unit: An independent device and actuator of a wearable system for gait-support in Parkinson patients.*Proceedings of IEEE International Conference on Microwaves, Communications, Antennas and Electronics Systems (COMCAS)* (pp. 1-5). doi:10.1109/COMCAS.2013.6685287

Zikmund-Fisher, B. J., Windschitl, P. D., Exe, N., & Ubel, P. A. (2011). 'I'll do what they did": Social norm information and cancer treatment decisions. *Patient Education and Counseling*, *85*(2), 225–229. doi:10.1016/j.pec.2011.01.031 PMID:21367557

Zimmet, P. Z., Magliano, D. J., Herman, W. H., & Shaw, J. E. (2014). Diabetes: A 21st century challenge. *The Lancet Diabetes & Endocrinology*, *2*(1), 56–64. doi:10.1016/S2213-8587(13)70112-8 PMID:24622669

Zolfaghari, M., Asgari, P., & Bahramnezhad, F., AhmadiRad, S., & Haghani, H. (2015). Comparison of two educational methods (family-centered and patient-centered) on hemodialysis: Related complications. *Iranian Journal Of Nursing & Midwifery Research*, *20*(1), 87–92. PMID:25709696

Zwerink, M., Brusse-Keizer, M., van der Valk, P. D., Zielhuis, G. A., Monninkhof, E. M., van der Palen, J., & Effing, T. et al. (2014). Self management for patients with chronic obstructive pulmonary disease. *Cochrane Database of Systematic Reviews*, *3*, CD002990. PMID:24665053

About the Contributors

Guendalina Graffigna received a PhD in Social Psychology at Catholic University of the Sacred Hearth of Milan (Italy) where she actually is Associate Professor. At the same University, she teaches "Qualitative Methodology," she is the Associate Director for the level II Master Degree in "Qualitative Methods applied to Social and Marketing Research" and she is member of the Scientific Committee for the PhD School in Psychology. Guendalina is also the editorial manager for the Journal "Micro & Macro Marketing". Before her actual appointments, Guendalina has been a Post Doc fellow (A.A. 2007-2008) and a visiting professor in Qualitative Methods (A.A. 2008-2009) at the International Institute for Qualitative Methodology, University of Alberta, with which she still collaborates for several research and teaching initiatives. Beside her academic achievements, Guendalina acts as qualitative scientific advisor at GfK-Eurisko in Milan, where she is an online qualitative research specialist and is Director of the Study and Training Centre of ASSIRM (Italian Association of Marketing Research Institutes). In July 2012, Guendalina was awarded with the prize of Qualitative Health Research Leadership 2012 from the Global Congress for Qualitative Health Research Committee. Her research and scientific activities are mainly devoted to patient engagement in health and wellbeing, healthcare organization innovation and digital health. She has spent the last 10 years of activity in constructing bridges between scientific/academic knowledge and professional practice, particularly in the sectors of consumer and health research. At present, she is coordinating and intra- and inter-university reflection for contributing to priorities and policy discussions at the European Level on patient health engagement.

***

Chiara Acquati is an assistant professor at the Graduate College of Social Work, University of Houston. She has received her doctoral degree from the University of Louisville, a Master of Social Work from Boston College, and a Master in Clinical Psychology from the Catholic University of the Sacred Heart, Milan. Her research interests include couples coping with cancer, distress screening, adolescent and young adult (AYA) cancer patients' sexuality and reproductive issues, and psychosocial interventions. Her work has been presented at national and international conferences.

Geri Lynn Baumblatt, MA, is the Executive Director of Patient Engagement at Emmi Solutions, where she has worked with a team of writers, medical illustrators, animators, clinicians, and patients to create a large library of multimedia patient engagement programs and IVR phone calls. She regularly speaks and writes about patient engagement, health literacy, the patient experience, and shared decision making for organizations like AHRQ, the Institute for Healthcare Advancement, Health Literacy Missouri, and the Center for Plain Language, Stanford Medicine X, The Brookings Institute, The Beryl Institute, and the Society for Medical Decision Making. She also serves as an Editorial Board member for the Journal of Patient Experience.

Jacqueline (Jackie) Bender, PhD is a Scientist at ELLICSR Health, Wellness and Cancer Survivorship Centre, and the Centre for Global eHealth Innovation at the University Health Network, and an Assistant Professor in the Dalla Lana School of Public Health at the University of Toronto. Her research focuses on designing and evaluating ways to improve the health and health care experience of people with cancer through the use of social support and information and communication technologies.

Sarah Bigi received her PhD in Linguistics from Università Cattolica del Sacro Cuore in Milan (Italy), where she currently holds a grant from the Italian Ministry of Research (FIRB 2013) for a project on "Strategies and mechanisms of persuasion in chronic care." Her research interests include the study of argumentative practices and decision-making in chronic care encounters.

Maria Borrello is a clinical psychologist and a PhD student in Clinical Psychology at University of Bergamo. She holds a MSc degree in Clinical Psychology at University of Roma "La Sapienza," and also a Master in Scholastic Psychology. Her research activity is carried out in cooperation with Catholic University of Milan. Her research focus is mainly on obesity, the use of motivational interviewing in obesity treatments and mHealth.

Gianluca Castelnuovo PhD and PsyD is Researcher in Clinical Psychology and Associate Professor of Clinical Psychology, Rehabilitation Psychology and Psychopathology at the Faculty of Psychology in the Catholic University of Milan. He is also Senior Researcher in the Clinical Psychology Lab, Saint Joseph Hospital, IRCCS Istituto Auxologico Italiano, Verbania, Italy. He has conducted several research projects and published many papers about clinical psychology and psychotherapy, overall about the use of Virtual Reality, Telepsychology, eHealth and mHealth in medicine and clinical psychology, particularly in the eating disorders, obesity and diabetes fields.

Roberto Cattivelli, Ph.D. and Psy.D., is a researcher in the Clinical Psychology Lab, Saint Joseph Hospital, IRCCS Istituto Auxologico Italiano, Verbania, Italy. He received his Ph.D. in Behavior Analysis and Psychology from the University of Parma and his Psy.D. in Cognitive Behavioral Therapy, focused in third-generation behavioral intervention, at IESCUM, Parma, Italy. He conducted several research projects and published papers about psychotherapy, clinical and health psychology, education and behavior modification.

Alice Chirico has a M.S. degree in Psychology from Catholic University of the Sacred Heart, with a dissertation focused on Networked Flow models in musical contexts. She is a PhD Student at Catholic University of Sacred Heart. Her main research interests concern Flow experience, group flow and Networked Flow modeling in various contexts.

Stefania Corti is Psychologist and Ericksonian Psychotherapist with a PhD in Clinical Psychology.

Antonio Dodaro is currently a legal expert on patients' rights, a professional trainer, mediator and an independent researcher. His education includes: a Master's Degree in Law (University of Ferrara, 1991); a Post-graduate Specialization in Tax Law and Tax Accounting for Companies at the School of Management LUISS (University of Rome, 1993); a Post-graduate of an Advanced course in Tax Law at the University of Lecce (2000); an Enabling Legal Advocacy in front of the Courts (1993-1997). His professional qualifications include: Conciliator, Chamber Referee and Ombudsman at the Chambers of Commerce of Brindisi, Lecce and Ferrara. From 2008 to 2014, he collaborated with the IFC-CNR Institute of Clinical Physiology in research and training activities: Post-graduate Interactive Master in Social Communication - organization, class tutoring, administrative and legal support, lectures (negotiation, facilitation, tax and non-profit legislation); research on patients' rights protection and informed consent in ionizing radiation; Strategic Planning Wide Area; use of the methodology OST Open Space Technology; CME courses SUIT ASL Lecce (2010) and SUIT ASL Brindisi (2013 and 2014) entitled: "The good use of medical radiation. SUIT Stop Useless Imaging Testing". He has worked in the past as: legal, tax, and fundraising consultant for companies and research institutes; Head of Public Relations for the Regional Coordination ACLI Consumers League; Head at the office of Maglie for the Movement of Defense of the Citizen; professional trainer in Tax Law for the Chamber of Commerce of Lecce; forensic practitioner and collaborator in Tax, Administrative and Health Law for Sideri and Cioffi Attorneys (Lecce); responsible for Management and Personnel Training for Prod.AC (Lecce). He is the author of several national and international peer-reviewed research articles.

Jennifer Freytag is a PhD candidate at Texas A&M University. She is a licensed Texas attorney who has practiced elder law and probate.

Federica Galli is a Clinical Psychologist, PhD and Researcher at the Department of Health Sciences of the University of Milan. She graduated at "Sapienza" from the University of Rome, where afterwards, she completed a PhD in Neuroscience and a post-graduation in Clinical Psychology and Psychotherapy. She is an assistant professor of Clinical Psychology at the University of Milan and Developmental Psychopathology at the University of Pavia. Her research area has been primarily focused on the psychological components of chronic pain disorders (mainly headaches) both at pediatric age and adulthood, and is now shifting towards the relational and communicative skills of the medical encounter. She is the author of many national and international papers on psychological and psychopathological components of headaches and other pain disorders.

Juliana Genova obtained her PHD in French Literature, followed by a MA in Health Communication. She is currently a communication adviser with the Department of Foreign Affairs, International Trade and Development. Her research interests focus on the use of scientific evidence, and best practices in knowledge translation and application.

Emanuele Maria Giusti has an MS in Clinical Psychology from the Catholic University of Milan.

Stefan Janzek-Hawlat has a Master degree in Business Informatics and Medical Informatics. Currently he is a business analyst at the Main Association of Austrian Social Security Institutions.

Giulia Lamiani is Research Fellow in Clinical Psychology at the University of Milan where she is involved in teaching communication skills to medical students and healthcare professionals. She graduated in Education from the Catholic University of Milan and in Psychology at the University of Turin. Within the Fulbright Program, she received her Master's in Health Education from Boston University in

2006. She worked at the Children's Hospital Harvard Medical School as a visiting fellow and as a psychologist. Her research interests focus on clinician-patient communication, end-of-life care, patient education and patient safety.

Carlo Giacomo Leo (PhD) is an Economist with a background in health economics (HE) and health technology assessment (HTA). Since 09/2013, he has been a Lecturer at the School of Medicine, Tufts University, Boston. From 06/2012 to 07/2013, he was a research fellow at Tufts Medical Center, Division of Clinical Decision Making, Boston. Since 2005, he has been a Researcher at the Institute of Clinical Physiology of the Italian National Research Council (CNR-IFC) and since 02/2014 he has been the Head of the Lecce section of CNR-IFC. His interests in the fields of HE and HTA are focused on the economic evaluation of health care programs, analysis, modelling, representation and implementation of healthcare pathways.

Rosita B. Maglie is a researcher and lecturer in English Language and Translation at the University of Bari. Her main research interests are in Specialized Discourse, Corpus-based Translation Studies, and Applied Linguistics. Her PhD dissertation, along with other publications, focuses on the use of domain-specific parallel and comparable corpora specially collected in order to investigate English and Italian Medical Purposes (2004, 2005, 2007, 2009, 2011). Another area of interest includes cross-cultural communication in fashion advertising, a topic on which she has published different papers (2010, 2011 and 2012). Her past publications exemplify her main areas of study: Understanding the Language of Medicine (2009) Aracne, and English4Fashion (2010) Wip Edizioni. Additionally, she is interested in area of study, examining the approaches of teaching English to young learners by engaging with cross-cultural differences and gender variance. Two of her recent articles are on this research field (2012, 2014).

Julia Menichetti is a psychologist and a PhD student at Catholic University. Her themes of interest are: active ageing, health promoting interventions, and health psychology.

Enrico E. Minetti has been Chief of the Nephrology Unit - University Hospital Careggi, Firenze, Italy from 2012 to the present. From 2007 - 2012 Enrico was Chief of the Transplantation Nephrology Sub-Unit Ospedale Niguarda-Cà Granda, Milano, Italy and 2004 – 2007 Chief of the Renal Haemodynamic Laboratory Ospedale Niguarda-Cà Granda, Milano, Italy. From 1989 – 2004 Enrico was an Assistant in Nephrology Ospedale Niguarda-Cà Granda, Milano, Italy. In 1985, Enrico received a Master Degree in Medicine and Surgery from the University of Milano, Italy.

Isabel Moreira is a clinical and health psychologist specializing in working with children, adolescents and adults. She divides her time between clinical practice and academic research as a PhD student in the Public Health at the University of Porto Medical School. She actively collaborates in various research projects with teams from the University of Porto Medical School, the EPIUnit - Institute of Public Health of University of Porto, and the Instituto de Telecomunicações, Lisboa.

Margherita Novelli is a Psychologist with a Ph.D in Clinical Psychology.

Raul Oliveira is a Physiotherapist and professor in the Faculdade de Motricidade Humana, Universidade de Lisboa and a researcher at the Laboratory of Motor Behavior in some faculty. He specializes in physiotherapy science, and has obtained a PhD degree in the Human Movement/Sciences of Physiotherapy. He participates in research projects at the Laboratory of Motor Behavior and the Instituto de Telecomunicações da Universidade de Lisboa.

Curtis A. Olson, PhD, is an Assistant Professor in the Department of Medicine at the Geisel School of Medicine at Dartmouth. He has a doctorate in adult and continuing education from the University of Wisconsin-Madison and has been involved in health care professional education for more than 20 years. Dr Olson also serves as Editor-in-Chief of the Journal of Continuing Education in the Health Professions. As Editor, he contributes to the continuing professional development of researchers and authors in the field and to shaping the research agenda in continuing education. He is also Principal and Owner of Clear Creek Research Services, LLC, a consulting firm specializing in evaluations of continuing education programs for health care professionals.

Giada Pietrabissa earned a master's degree in 2009 after graduating from the University of the Sacred Heart in Milan, where she also entered the psychology PhD programs in 2012. Since 2010, she has been providing psychological support to patients undergoing an intensive hospital-based and medically-managed programs for weight reduction and rehabilitation at the Istituto Auxologico Italiano, IRCCS, Saint Joseph Hospital, Verbania, Italy. During her clinical experience she has gained extensive knowledge working with people suffering from obesity and eating disorders, in particular, studying how to prevent relapses by enhancing their motivation to change unhealthy habits. As part of a research team, she is currently investigating factors and beliefs predicting reluctance to seek treatment among heart patients, developing new approaches to improve individuals' compliance to treatment. She has also completed several investigations on methods and assessment tools in clinical psychology and psychotherapy, and she is strongly interested in services using information and communication technologies (ICTs) for improving prevention, diagnosis, treatment, monitoring and health management. In 2015, she received the qualification of brief strategic psychotherapist after studying for 4 years at the Brief Strategic Therapy center, Arezzo, Italy. Moreover, the experience gained during periods of research abroad (Family Therapy Institute, San Diego, CA, United States - 2011 and University of South Australia, Adelaide, SA, Australia - 2015) also gave her the opportunity to expand her knowledge in different areas of psychology.

Gabriela Postolache is with the Unidade de Fisiologia e Clinica Translacional, Instituto de Medicina Molecular, Universidade de Lisboa. She obtained her PhD degree in Life Sciences. Her expertise is in electrophysiology, biomedical instruments, non-invasive and unobtrusive measurements of body signals. She collaborates in research projects related with autonomic nervous system assessment and monitoring, cardiac arrhythmia, electronic health records for wheelchair users, electronic health records for physiotherapy.

Octavian Postolache is a professor at Instituto Universitario de Lisboa, and researcher at Instituto de Telecomunicações, Lisbon. He obtained a PhD degree in Electrical Engineering. His fields of interests are smart sensors for biomedical and environmental applications, pervasive sensing and computing, wireless sensor networks, signal processing with applications in biomedical and telecommunications, non-destructive testing and diagnosis based on smart eddy currents, smart sensors, computational intelligence with application in automated measurement systems. He is currently the leader of a research project regarding the implementation of electronic health records for physiotherapy.

Virginia Recchia is a research scientist in health communication and knowledge management at the Institute of Clinical Physiology of the Italian National Research Council (CNR-IFC). Her education includes a Ph.D. in e-Business Management and Engineering at the eBMS eBusiness Management School of ISUFI (University of Salento, 2006), a Post-graduate European Master in Environmental Management with honors and prize (Erasmus University of Rotterdam, 1998), a M.Sc. degree in Communication Sciences with honors (University of Torino, 1997). Journalist as occasional contributor since 1997, she worked in the past as: research scientist at ISBEM Euro Mediterranean Scientific Biomedical Institute (Brindisi, 2001-2006), web content manager at Global Database Services – Bizmatica Group (Milano, 2000-2001), project manager at Ecomag - American Appraisal Italia Group (Agrate Brianza, 1999-2000), and research fellow at FEEM Fondazione ENI Enrico Mattei (Milano, 1998-1999). Her scientific activities regard patient-physician communication, health literacy/numeracy, process-based informed consent, risk communication, and shared decision-making in ionizing radiation exams. Further research lines involve health knowledge management, interactive CME Continuous Medical Education and eLearning, OST Open Space Technology and other participatory research methods in public health.

Emanuela Saita, PhD, is an Associate Professor at the Catholic University of Milan (IT) where she teaches Health Psychology and Methods and Techniques of the Clinical Interview. For many years, she has been studying psychological reactions to chronic disease diagnoses, focusing on coping and caregiving. Currently, she is interested in different kinds of intervention addressed to chronic patients and in the transition to parenthood and perinatal grief. She coordinates both European and National research projects.

Richard L. Street, Jr., is a professor in the Department of Communication at Texas A&M University. He is also a professor of medicine at Baylor College of Medicine and chief of the Health Decision-Making and Communication Program at the Center for Innovations in Quality, Effectiveness and Safety at the Michael E. DeBakey VA Medical Center.

Hilda Tellioglu is an associate professor at the Institute of Design and Assessment of Technology of Vienna, University of Technology and Dean of Studies of Business Informatics. Besides more than 140 peer-reviewed publications she was the principle investigator of several (inter)national research projects (kommTUi, TOPIC) and has participated in several others (like DESARTE, MAPPER, TRICE, FETCH). Her research focuses on: modeling and knowledge management in manufacturing, automobile industries, software design and development, healthcare, and architecture; tangible interaction design; design thinking; computer-supported cooperative worlds; and gender and diversity in computer science.

Stefano Triberti obtained his PhD in Psychology at Università Cattolica del Sacro Cuore, Milan, Italy in 2016. Currently, his research interests regard User Experience of new technologies for healthcare and well-being promotion. He co-authored the books *Psicologia dei Videogiochi* (Psychology of Videogames) (Apogeo, 2013) and *Patient Engagement: a consumer-centered model to innovate healthcare* (De Gruyter Open, 2015) and other publications among journal articles and contributions to edited books in the field of cyberpsychology.

Tony Zordich After 20 years of face to the customer business development roles in the medical imaging space with Fortune 500 organizations, Tony's career focus has shifted to advancing emerging technologies in the patient engagement and management services. He launched the Consortium for Patient Engagement www.CoPE.tips in September 2014, a venue for providers, payers, and developers to find, assess, and collaborate on patient engagement opportunities and potential partners.

Index

N

O

P

R

S

www.ingramcontent.com/pod-product-compliance
Lightning Source LLC
LaVergne TN
LVHW080606300926
849162LV00005B/1064